Ultrasonography in Vascular Diseases
A Practical Approach to Clinical Problems

Second Edition

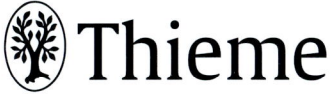

Ultrasonography in Vascular Diseases
A Practical Approach to Clinical Problems

Second Edition

Edward I. Bluth, M.D., F.A.C.R.
Chairman Emeritus
Department of Radiology
Ochsner Health System
New Orleans, Louisiana

Carol B. Benson, M.D.
Professor
Department of Radiology
Harvard Medical School
Director of Ultrasound
Co-Director of High Risk Obstetrical Ultrasound
Brigham and Women's Hospital
Boston, Massachusetts

Philip W. Ralls, M.D.
Professor and Vice Chair
Department of Radiology
Keck School of Medicine
University of Southern California
Los Angeles, California

Marilyn J. Siegel, M.D.
Professor
Departments of Radiology and Pediatrics
Washington University School of Medicine
Division of Diagnostic Radiology
Mallinckrodt Institute of Radiology
Saint Louis, Missouri

Thieme
New York • Stuttgart

Thieme Medical Publishers, Inc.
333 Seventh Ave.
New York, NY 10001

Editor: Timothy Hiscock
Editorial Assistant: David Price
Vice President, Production and Electronic Publishing: Anne T. Vinnicombe
Production Editor: Print Matters, Inc.
Vice President, International Marketing: Cornelia Schulze
Chief Financial Officer: Peter van Woerden
President: Brian D. Scanlan
Compositor: Compset, Inc.
Printer: Everbest Printing Co.

Library of Congress Cataloging-in-Publication Data

Ultrasonography in vascular diseases / [edited by] Edward I. Bluth . . . [et al.]. — 2nd ed.
  p.; cm.
  Includes bibliographical references and index.
  ISBN 978-1-58890-610-6 (alk. paper)

  1. Blood-vessels—Ultrasonic imaging. I. Bluth, Edward I.
  [DNLM: 1. Vascular Diseases—ultrasonography. 2. Diagnosis, Differential. 3. Extremities—
ultrasonography. 4. Ultrasonography—methods. WG 500 U473 2007]
  RC691.6.U47U48 2007
  616.1'307543—dc22 2007015100

Copyright ©2008 by Thieme Medical Publishers, Inc. This book, including all parts thereof, is legally protected by copyright. Any use, exploitation, or commercialization outside the narrow limits set by copyright legislation without the publisher's consent is illegal and liable to prosecution. This applies in particular to photostat reproduction, copying, mimeographing or duplication of any kind, translating, preparation of microfilms, and electronic data processing and storage.

Important note: Medical knowledge is ever-changing. As new research and clinical experience broaden our knowledge, changes in treatment and drug therapy may be required. The authors and editors of the material herein have consulted sources believed to be reliable in their efforts to provide information that is complete and in accord with the standards accepted at the time of publication. However, in view of the possibility of human error by the authors, editors, or publisher of the work herein or changes in medical knowledge, neither the authors, editors, or publisher, nor any other party who has been involved in the preparation of this work, warrants that the information contained herein is in every respect accurate or complete, and they are not responsible for any errors or omissions or for the results obtained from use of such information. Readers are encouraged to confirm the information contained herein with other sources. For example, readers are advised to check the product information sheet included in the package of each drug they plan to administer to be certain that the information contained in this publication is accurate and that changes have not been made in the recommended dose or in the contraindications for administration. This recommendation is of particular importance in connection with new or infrequently used drugs.

Some of the product names, patents, and registered designs referred to in this book are in fact registered trademarks or proprietary names even though specific reference to this fact is not always made in the text. Therefore, the appearance of a name without designation as proprietary is not to be construed as a representation by the publisher that it is in the public domain.

Printed in China

5 4 3 2 1

The Americas   ISBN 978-1-58890-610-6
Rest of the World ISBN 978-3-13-129142-4

We dedicate this book to our families and friends, who supported us in this project:

Ed Bluth to Elissa, Rachel, Jonathan, Marjorie, Irene, and Lawry
with gratitude and love.

Carol Benson to her husband, Peter, and her children, Nicole and Benjamin.

Phil Ralls to Renee, Colin, and Whitney with love.

Marilyn Siegel to her husband, Barry.

Contents

Preface ix

Contributors x

1 Leg Swelling with Pain or Edema 1
   Edward I. Bluth

2 Painful Legs after Walking 17
   William J. Zwiebel

3 Pulsatile Groin Mass in the Postcatheterization Patient 28
   Barbara A. Carroll

4 Carotid Arteries in Patients with Transient Ischemic Accidents, Stroke, or Carotid Bruits 42
   Joseph F. Polak

5 Arm Swelling 53
   Janis G. Letourneau and Thomas R. Beidle

6 Hypertension and Bruit 67
   Laurence Needleman

7 Acute Scrotal Pain: Diagnosing with Color Duplex Sonography 81
   Thomas A. Stavros and Cynthia L. Rapp

8 Acute Pelvic Pain 102
   John S. Pellerito

9 Intraoperative Ultrasound 112
   Robert A. Kane

Index 129

Preface

We have been pleased by the considerable popularity achieved by the first edition of *Ultrasonography in Vascular Diseases: A Practical Approach to Clinical Problems*. The second edition builds on the foundation that was originally laid at the Special Course on Ultrasound at the Meeting of the Radiological Society of North America in 1996, and then was further developed in the first edition of this text published in 2000. This new edition greatly expands and updates that previous work.

The overall aim of this textbook is to help the clinician assess and decide whether sonography or another imaging modality is the most appropriate for evaluating a clinical problem. In contrast to standard textbooks, our chapters are divided according to clinical questions rather than by organ systems. Our aim is to review the most important clinical issues faced by clinicians in their daily practice and to outline approaches for the effective use of sonography and other imaging modalities. Most chapters in the second edition have been extensively revised with new illustrations and images being added. The authors have attempted to incorporate the latest advances in ultrasound as well as to revise earlier recommendations based on advances in MRI, CT, and PET.

All of the authors are recognized authorities in the fields of ultrasound and radiology. The role of the radiologist and sonologist is changing. It is important to develop not only accurate diagnostic skills but also the appropriate consultative skills to help direct the workup of clinical problems. It is hoped that this textbook will assist radiologists, residents, medical students, and midlevel providers in developing their consultative skills regarding the use of ultrasound.

Each chapter includes practical, technical sonographic hints for studying an area or problem, basic sonographic anatomy, and the sonographic findings that can be seen in different clinical entities with the same clinical presentation. Additionally, the authors have included their recommendations regarding the use of alternative imaging modalities for solving clinical problems. The intended outcome is for the clinician to receive guidance in directing the imaging workup and in selecting the best imaging examination for a given clinical problem. New chapters have been added on acute scrotal pain, acute pelvic pain, and intraoperative ultrasound.

Although some of what is included in this book might be considered an opinion, our goal for the second edition of *Ultrasonography in Vascular Diseases: A Practical Approach to Clinical Problems* is to provide a readable and manageable book which will offer guidance for clinicians and diagnosticians on the appropriate use of sonography to solve important clinical problems.

Acknowledgments

The authors would like to thank Drs. Peter Arger, Barbara Hertzberg, William Middleton, and Carol Stelling for their help with the conceptual origins for this project. Additionally, the authors would like to thank Dr. Peter Arger for his role as an editor of the first edition.

Contributors

Edward I. Bluth, M.D., F.A.C.R.
Chairman Emeritus
Department of Radiology
Ochsner Health System
New Orleans, Louisiana

Thomas R. Beidle, M.D.
Reno Radiological Associates
Reno, Nevada

Barbara A. Carroll, M.D., F.A.C.R.
Professor Emeritus of Radiology
Duke University Medical Center
Durham, North Carolina

Robert A. Kane, M.D., F.A.C.R.
Associate Chief
Department of Radiology
Director of Ultrasound
Harvard Medical School
Beth Israel Deaconess Medical Center
Boston, Massachusetts

Janis G. Letourneau, M.D.
Professor of Radiology and Surgery
Louisiana State University Health Sciences Center
School of Medicine
New Orleans, Louisiana

Laurence Needleman, M.D.
Associate Professor
Department of Radiology
Jefferson Medical College
Thomas Jefferson University
Philadelphia, Pennsylvania

John S. Pellerito, M.D.
Chief
Department of Radiology
Division of Ultrasound, CT, and MRI
North Shore Hospital
Manhasset, New York

Joseph F. Polak, M.D., M.P.H.
Professor
Department of Radiology
Tufts University School of Medicine
New England Medical Center
Boston, Massachusetts

Cynthia L. Rapp, B.S., R.D.M.S., R.D.C.S.
Sonographic Practitioner
Radiology Imaging Associates
Swedish Medical Center
Englewood, Colorado

Thomas A. Stavros, M.D.
Assistant Clinical Professor
Medical Director for Clinical Site Sonographer
  Training Program
University of Colorado School of Medicine
Denver, Colorado

William J. Zwiebel, M.D.
Professor of Radiology and Staff Radiologist
University of Utah School of Medicine
University of Utah Medical Center and
VA Medical Center
Salt Lake City, Utah

1 Leg Swelling with Pain or Edema

Edward I. Bluth

Patients who present with leg swelling with pain or edema are of great clinical concern because they are at risk for having acute deep venous thrombosis (DVT). Acute DVT is an important public health problem because it affects over 20 million individuals yearly in the United States. Estimates of the incidence of DVT range from between 100 and 180 per 100,000 persons per year.[1] DVT occurs in both sedimentary outpatients as well as hospital inpatients, although rarely in children. Among the predisposing factors are prolonged congestive heart failure, pelvic and lower extremity surgery, pregnancy, obesity, inactivity, airplane travel, coagulopathy, and paraplegia.[2]

The diagnosis of DVT has other significant implications as well. It has been known for more than a century that DVT may be a presenting feature of an occult neoplasm. Recently, a definite association between DVT and a subsequent clinically occult cancer has been shown, particularly in the first 6 to 12 months of follow-up.[3] However, in the study by Sorensen et al 40% of the patients diagnosed with cancer within 1 year of the diagnosis of DVT had distant metastases. As a result, it is uncertain whether an extensive search for an occult neoplasm would be cost-effective or warranted because early diagnosis may not change outcomes. The types of cancers most strongly associated with DVT in this Swedish study of more than 15,000 patients were cancer of the pancreas, ovary, liver (primary hepatic cancer), and brain.[3]

Presently, it is important to diagnose acute DVT because of its relationship with acute pulmonary embolism. The presence of DVT does not equate with pulmonary embolism, but detecting DVT may prevent pulmonary embolism from developing. It is reported that when significant acute venous thrombosis is diagnosed but not treated, pulmonary embolism is likely to occur in up to 50% of the cases.[4] More importantly, it is believed that in up to 30% of the episodes of pulmonary embolism the outcome is death.[4] Pulmonary embolism is reported to be the cause of death in more than 10,000 hospitalized patients each year in the United States.[5] Mortality can be significantly reduced when acute DVT is treated with anticoagulation. Because an estimated 90% of pulmonary emboli arise from the lower extremities, there is a great clinical need to accurately assess the venous system of the lower extremities when there is clinical suspicion of acute DVT.

Accuracy of Presentation in Diagnosing Deep Venous Thrombosis

Patients who present with the clinical symptomatology of leg swelling with pain or edema certainly are at risk for acute DVT. However, the clinical accuracy of diagnosing this entity is known to be very poor. Every clinical sign

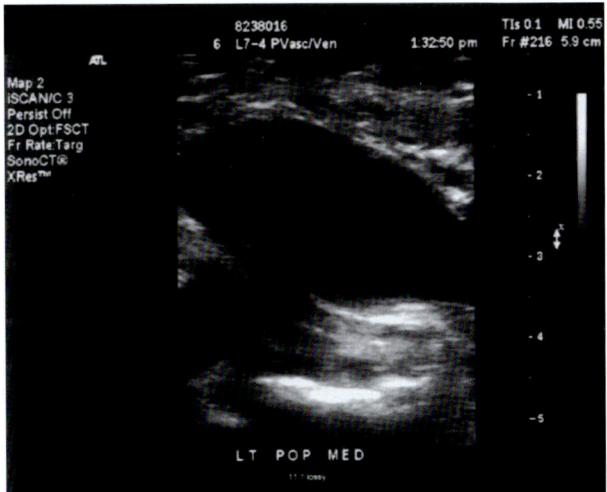
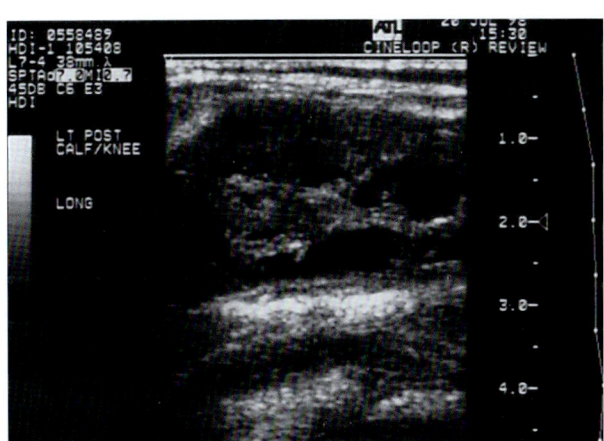

Figure 1–1 (A) Oblique view of a large sonolucent mass located in the popliteal fossa separate and apart from the artery and vein on sagittal color flow Doppler imaging. This is consistent with a Baker's cyst. **(B)** Oblique image of a complex mass in the popliteal space of another patient. This mass is separate and medial to the artery and vein and is characteristic of a ruptured Baker's cyst.

attributed to DVT has been statistically analyzed and found to be of no value in reliably determining the presence or absence of DVT.[6] The location of signs and symptoms of pain or swelling is usually unrelated to the extent or location of clot within the veins. Symptoms localized to the calf may have an etiology in the femoral veins, and thigh pain may be related to occlusion of calf veins.[7] The specificity for clinical diagnosis is low because the symptomatology associated with acute DVT can have, among other causes, a musculoskeletal or lymphatic basis. Furthermore, asymptomatic DVT can commonly occur, and the sequelae can even be severe enough to cause death by pulmonary embolism.

In patients who present with bilateral leg symptoms, in the absence of significant risk factors (such as malignancy, paralysis, bed rest of more than 3 days, major surgery, strong family history of DVT, or leg, thigh, or calf swelling)[8] the first assumption should be that the etiology is cardiac disease or chronic peripheral vascular disease.[9] However, in patients with risk factors, the possibility of bilateral clot must be seriously considered, and a bilateral ultrasound examination is warranted.

Accuracy of D-Dimer Test in Diagnosing Deep Venous Thrombosis

D-dimer has emerged as a clinically useful serological test. D-dimer represents a breakdown of the cross-linked fibrin clot. It is elevated in almost all patients with acute DVT, having a sensitivity of 97%, but it is nonspecific (less than 50%). D-dimer is also elevated in patients who have had recent surgery, trauma, sepsis, and malignancy.[1] However, it is very useful in excluding DVT having a negative predictive value of 97%.[10] In certain patient groups, D-dimer combined with clinical assessment has been shown to safely reduce or eliminate the need for noninvasive testing.[10]

Differential Diagnosis

The differential diagnosis for the symptoms of leg swelling with pain or edema includes acute DVT, Baker's (popliteal) cyst, cellulitis, lymphedema, chronic venous insufficiency, superficial thrombophlebitis, popliteal venous aneurysm, popliteal artery aneurysm, iliac artery aneurysm, femoral artery pseudoaneurysm, enlarged lymph nodes extrinsically compressing the veins, heterotopic ossification, hematoma, muscular tears, and diabetic muscle infarction.[7,11-19] The appropriate use of imaging studies, and, in particular, the appropriate use of ultrasound, enables us to distinguish which of these clinical entities is present.

Baker's cysts appear as sonolucent or complex masses more commonly medial than lateral. When they rupture, the surface margins become irregular (**Fig. 1–1A,B**). They appear separate and distinct from the popliteal artery or vein. The normal popliteal artery measures less than 1 cm. Veins and arteries should taper normally, and an outpouching would suggest aneurysmal dilatation (**Fig. 1–2**). Frequently, thrombus may surround the residual lumen of an arterial aneurysm. Aneurysms or pseudoaneurysms, owing to their expanded size, can compress the venous structures that surround them, resulting in swelling or edema of the distal extremity. The visualization of a concomitant vascular abnormality should, therefore, not preclude further evaluation of the more distal venous structures because the resultant stasis may be a predisposing factor to the development of DVT (**Fig. 1–3**). Patients with superficial thrombophlebitis have an increased risk of progressing to DVT. In one report, 11% of patients who initially had isolated superficial venous thrombus progressed to DVT.[20] In another study, 23% of patients with superficial thrombophlebitis had occult DVT of the lower extremities.[21] As a result, if superficial venous thrombosis is noted, then the deep venous system should be carefully studied. Similarly, enlarged lymph nodes can also extrinsically compress adjacent venous structures, resulting in lower extremity symptoms (**Fig. 1–4**). This has been noted in patients with acquired immunodeficiency syndrome (AIDS). On rare occasions, pain or swelling of the lower extremity may be the presenting symptom of lymphoma. Lymph nodes appear separate from the vascular structures and are easily distinguished using color flow Doppler imaging (CFDI). Hematomas are also separate and distinct from the arteries and veins and, depending on their age, appear as either complex or sonolucent masses.

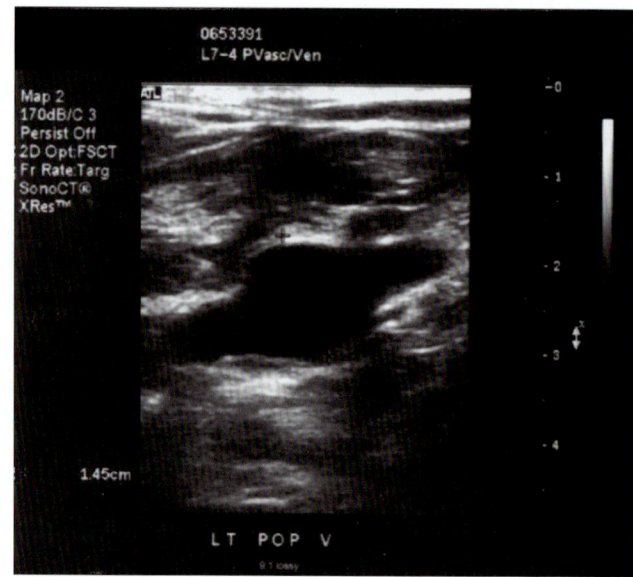

Figure 1–2 Sagittal color flow Doppler imaging of a 1.5 cm popliteal venous aneurysm.

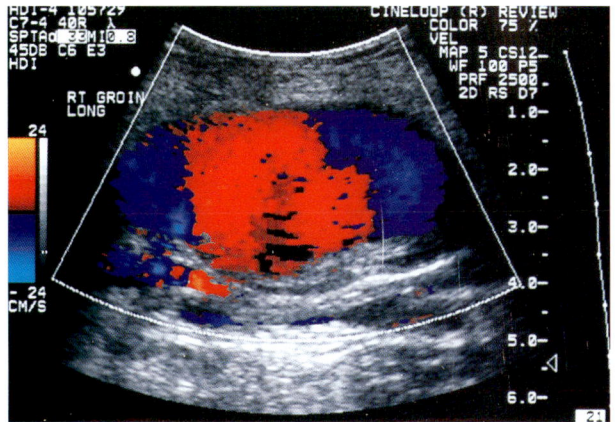

Figure 1–3 (A) Large pseudoaneurysm of the right common femoral artery (CFA) postcardiac catheterization compressing the common femoral vein (CFV). **(B)** Transverse image showing the more expanded hypoechoic noncompressible proximal superficial femoral vein (SFV) consistent with acute thrombus. PFV, profunda femoris vein.

Diagnostic Imaging Evaluation

Tests to evaluate the lower extremities include contrast venography, venous ultrasound including CFDI and Doppler spectral analysis, impedance plethysmography (IPG), various radionuclide approaches, magnetic resonance (MR) venography, computed tomography (CT), nonimaging continuous wave Doppler, and thermography. All evaluation methods were studied by the Cardiovascular Appropriateness Panel of the American College of Radiology (ACR), and each of these methods was rated for appropriateness in 1995 and reassessed in 1999 (**Table 1–1**).[22]

Contrast venography has been the gold standard by which other examination methods have been rated; however, in 5 to 10% of patients it may not give a reliable result, and because it also requires the use of intravenous contrast with the associated risks of renal failure, extravasation, chemical-induced thrombophlebitis, and idiopathic contrast reactions, its appropriateness rating was only intermediate. In contrast, duplex Doppler compression ultrasound received the highest possible rating and, therefore, now should be used as the study of choice to evaluate symptomatic patients.

The panel reported also that thermography and nonimaging continuous wave Doppler analysis were inappropriate and should not be performed. IPG was given an intermediate appropriateness rating as was MR venography. The accuracy of IPG is reported to be close to 90% for DVT above the knees, but it requires meticulous technique. Heijboer et al reported that serial ultrasonography is a more accurate means of detecting DVT than is IPG. An abnormal IPG had a positive predictive value of 83% for DVT compared with a 94% rate for an ultrasound abnormality in patients with DVT.[23]

Radionuclide venography was given a lower intermediate rating. The accuracy of detecting large obstructive thrombi is reported to be close to 90%. Another approach that can be used and appears best to diagnose DVT below the knee or in the lower thigh is the active uptake of radionuclide-labeled fibrinogen, platelets, peptides, fibrin, and plasmin by thrombi. New imaging agents may also be helpful in differentiating acute recurrent from chronic DVT. CT is most useful for imaging thrombosis related to the iliac veins and is not particularly suitable for studying the femoropopliteal veins. It is also valuable in identifying sources of extrinsic compression of the iliac veins. Recently, CT venography has been recommended as a quick and safe means to evaluate the deep venous system after multidetector row CT (MDCT) angiography of the pulmonary arteries (within the same examination), particularly if the patient is clinically unstable and requires immediate diagnosis.[24,25] This methodology has a reported sensitivity ranging between 71 and 100%, specificity between 93 and 97%, positive predictive value between 53 and 92%, and negative predictive value between 92 and 97%.[24,26,27] However, the estimated median cumulative effective radiation dose is 8.26 mSv

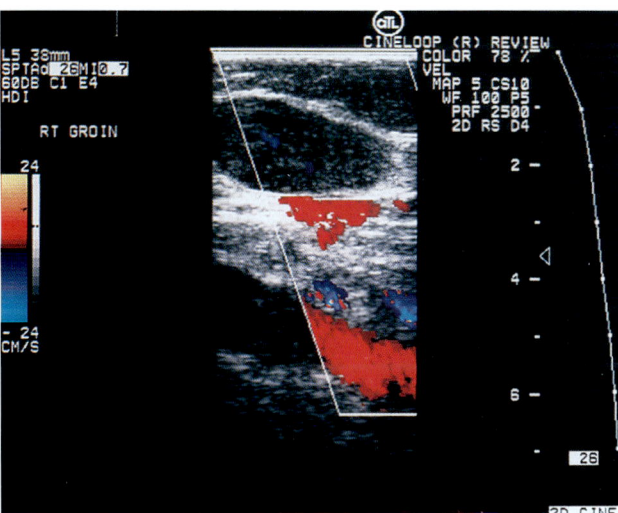

Figure 1–4 Solid mass density in the right inguinal area separate and apart from the common femoral artery and common femoral vein. On biopsy this mass of nodes was diagnosed as non-Hodgkin's lymphoma.

Table 1–1 American College of Radiology ACR Appropriateness Criteria for Clinical Condition: Suspected Lower Extremity Deep Vein Thrombosis

	Clinical Condition	
Radiologic Procedure	Appropriateness Rating	Comments
US, lower extremity, duplex Doppler compression	9	
MRI, venography, lower extremity	6	Demonstrated to be useful, but insufficient supporting data so far.
INV, venography, pelvis	6	When other studies equivocal or an intervention is planned.
CT, pelvis, with contrast	6	As an adjunct to CTPA done for suspected PE.
INV, venography, lower extremity	5	When other studies equivocal or an intervention is planned.
CT, venography, lower extremity (following arm injection)	5	As an adjunct to CTPA done for suspected PE.
NM, venography (MAA), lower extremity	3	
IPG, lower extremity	2	
X-ray, lower extremity	2	
Continuous wave Doppler (nonimaging), lower extremity	1	

Appropriateness Criteria Scale:
1 = Least appropriate, 9 = Most appropriate
INV = interventional venography

[compared with 2.5 mSv for CT angiography (CTA) of pulmonary arteries] for all patients with an effective gonadal dose of 3.87 mSv. This dose is more than 300% of the median effective dose for CTA of the pulmonary arteries (2.5 mSv). This dose must be significantly reduced before it could become a routine clinical method to evaluate for DVT in clinically stable patients, particularly for those who are young.

MR venography has also been suggested as a useful technique to detect DVT in the lower extremities.[28,29] It appears to be particularly useful in detecting femoral and iliac vein thrombi and may be particularly valuable in determining the proximal extent of disease in these vessels. Newer techniques such as venous enhanced subtracted peak arterial (VESPA) MR venography,[30] flow-independent MR venography,[5] and direct thrombus MR imaging,[31,32] may allow MR to play a more significant role in DVT imaging in the future.

One major limitation of both MR and CT is the significant increase in cost relative to ultrasound. Presently, both may be most useful for evaluating the more proximal venous structures when a satisfactory study is not achieved with ultrasound. But when considering the overall sensitivities, specificities, and costs of the various testing options, ultrasound remains the screening test of choice for lower extremity DVT.

Ultrasound Imaging

Evaluating patients with symptoms of leg swelling with pain or edema should involve using all the capabilities of ultrasound when available, including Doppler spectral analysis, CFDI, transducer compression, and high-resolution B-mode imaging. The examination should integrate all these methodologies into the complete study of the venous structures of the lower extremity. Extended field of view sonography, a new option of some machines, may be useful in demonstrating more easily the full extent of disease. The use of contrast agents and harmonic imaging may be helpful, in the future, in cases in which the complete occlusion of vessels is uncertain.

Normal Findings

With Doppler spectral analysis and CFDI, three parameters of normal lower extremity veins can be identified: respiratory phasicity, spontaneous flow, and augmentation (**Fig. 1–5A–E**). During the respiratory cycle, the change in venous flow is termed respiratory phasicity (**Fig. 1–5A**). During inspiration, an increase in intraabdominal pressure causes compression of the inferior vena cava and a decrease in the Doppler signal. In expiration, there is an increase in visualized flow and in the Doppler spectral analysis signal (**Fig. 1–5B**). The Valsalva maneuver leads to stasis and venous dilatation. The normal physiological response of the femoral vein is a 50 to 200% increase in diameter. At the end of the Valsalva maneuver, augmented venous flow normally occurs (**Fig. 1–5C**). In a normal venous system, augmentation also occurs with distal mechanical compression (**Fig. 1–5B,D,E**). Spontaneous venous flow is easily detected in the large leg vessels, but is frequently not seen in some of the smaller calf vessels. Augmentation will frequently be required to prove patency.

A normal vein also demonstrates compressibility, has unidirectional flow, and is free of internal echoes. Compressibility is best demonstrated when the transducer is

1 Leg Swelling with Pain or Edema 5

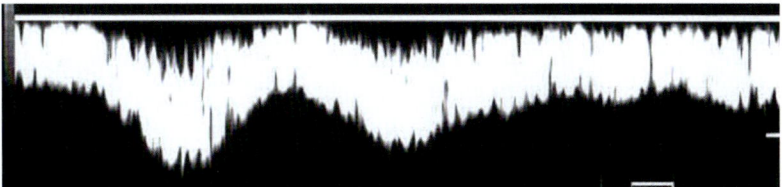

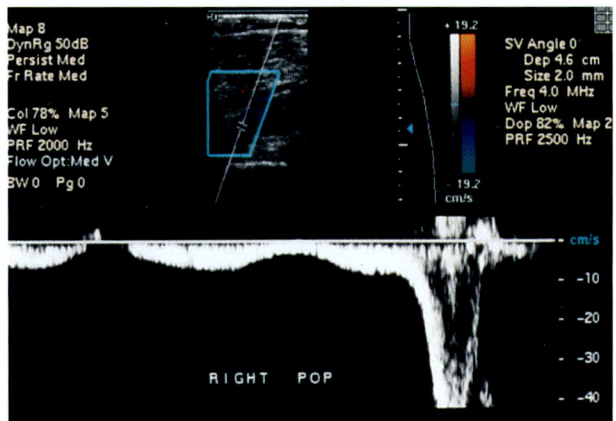

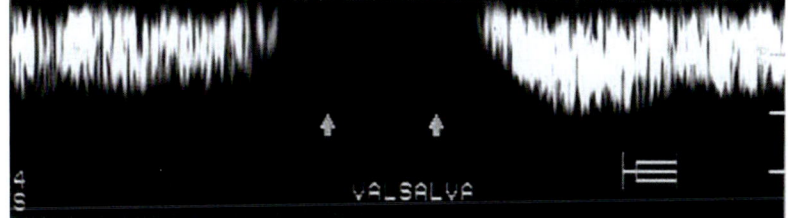

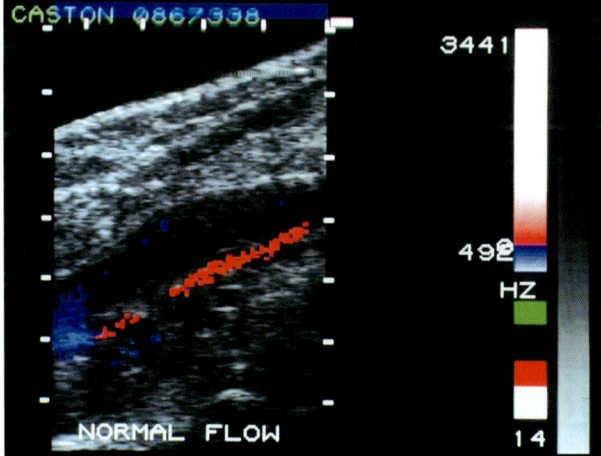
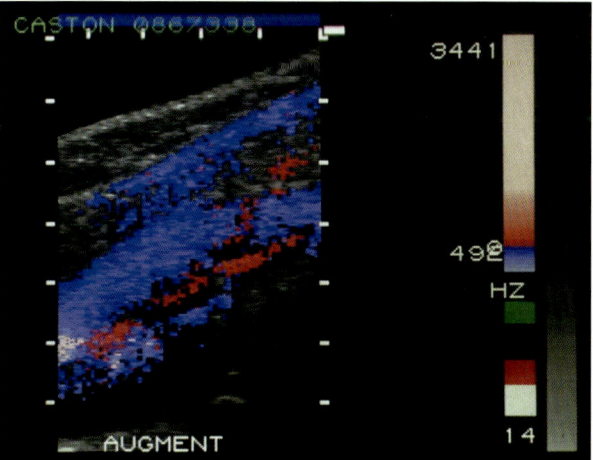

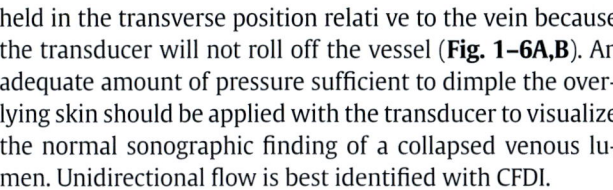

Figure 1–5 **(A)** Normal parameters of lower extremity veins include respiratory phasicity, **(B)** augmentation following distal compression, and **(C)** absence of flow during the Valsalva maneuver and then slight augmentation following the maneuver. These are demonstrated with Doppler spectral analysis. **(D)** Augmentation can also be demonstrated with color flow Doppler imaging following **(E)** distal compression.

held in the transverse position relative to the vein because the transducer will not roll off the vessel (**Fig. 1–6A,B**). An adequate amount of pressure sufficient to dimple the overlying skin should be applied with the transducer to visualize the normal sonographic finding of a collapsed venous lumen. Unidirectional flow is best identified with CFDI.

Technique

The choice of transducers for studying the lower extremities depends on the patient's body habitus and the depth of the vessel being studied. For the average patient, a 5 to 10 MHz linear transducer is most appropriate. Vessels ranging in size

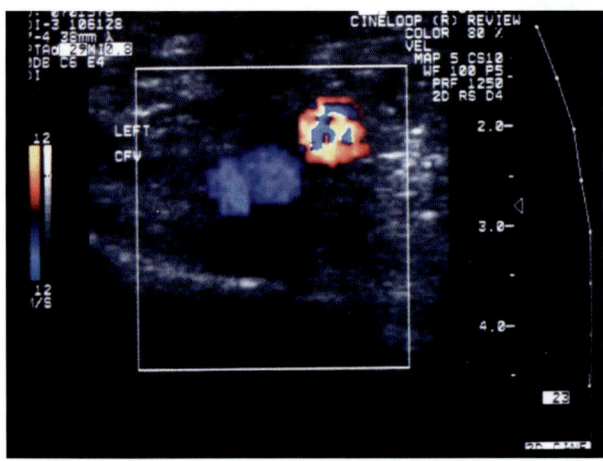 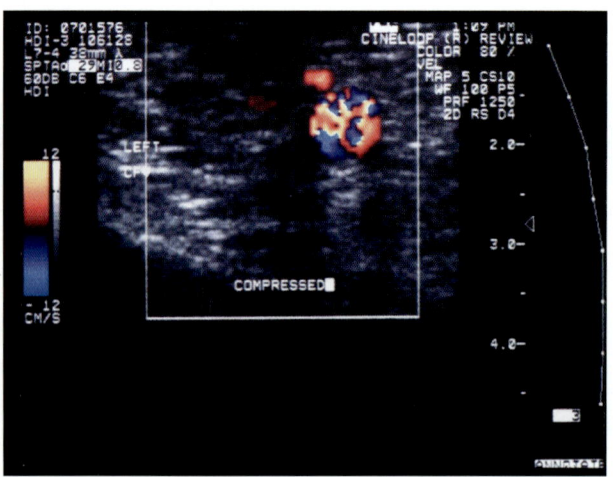

Figure 1–6 **(A)** Transverse color flow Doppler imaging demonstrating the normal common femoral vein (CFV–blue) and the common femoral artery (CFA–red) without and **(B)** with compression. Note the collapse of the normal vein.

from 1 mm to slightly over 1 cm can be clearly visualized over a depth of 6 cm. For large-body-habitus patients, transducers of lower MHz can be used. Linear array transducers permit long segments of vessels to be imaged more rapidly and are therefore preferred. Transducers will frequently need to be switched when the examiner moves from the inguinal region to the thicker thigh or the calf veins.

Vessels that can be studied include the common femoral veins; saphenous veins; superficial femoral veins (SFVs); popliteal veins; calf veins, including the anterior tibial, posterior tibial, and peroneal veins; and if possible, the iliac veins (**Fig. 1–7**). The external iliac, common femoral, saphenous, and superficial femoral veins are best evaluated with the patient supine. The popliteal veins can be studied in any of three different positions: with the patient prone and the leg flexed 20 to 30 degrees, with the patient decubitus and the study side up, and by elevating the foot and leg and scanning from below. At times, a combination of these techniques is necessary. Flow augmentation of the calf veins can be achieved by having the patients plantar flex the foot. This self-augmentation technique helps in better visualization of these vessels. Some have advocated studying the calf veins by having the patient sitting up and dangling the legs over the side of the examining table.

The calf veins can be studied by using either an anterolateral or a posteromedial approach (**Fig. 1–8**). To evaluate the posterior tibial veins, it is recommended to turn the foot outward and place the probe posterior medial to the medial malleolus (**Fig. 1–9**). The color box can also be directed to the left to optimize flow. For the study of the peroneal and anterior tibial veins, the foot should be turned inward and the probe should be placed parallel with the fibula and tilted outward (**Fig. 1–9**). Additionally, the color box can be directed straight to better visualize the veins. Also, if a linear probe is not technically adequate, a curved array transducer can be substituted. Additionally, it has been noted that if the posterior tibial and peroneal veins are patent, it is exceedingly rare to have an isolated thrombus in the anterior tibial vein. Therefore, if the other two venous pairs are patent, examination for the anterior tibial vein is unnecessary.

Figure 1–7 Vessels commonly visualized when evaluating the veins of the lower extremities.

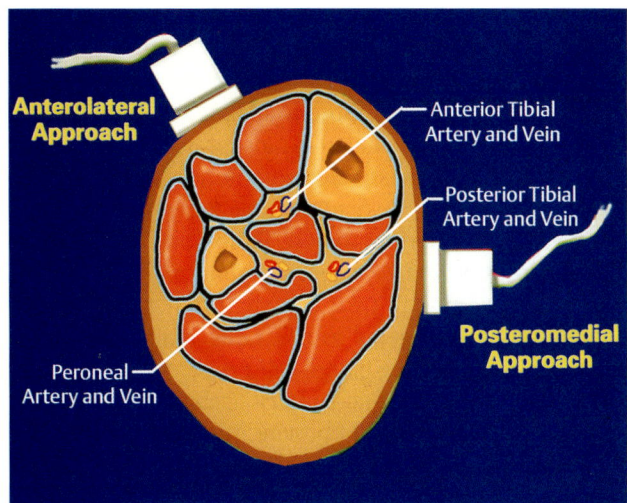

Figure 1-8 Diagram demonstrating practical anatomical approaches used to study the calf veins.

Sonographers and sonologists should carefully scan the femoral veins to look for duplicated vessels. In a recent report, Screaton et al demonstrated that multiple femoral veins were present in 177 (46%) of 381 venograms.[33] This is much more than the generally accepted frequency of duplication of 20 to 25%.[34] However, even with this high frequency of duplication, Screaton et al demonstrated only a 6% false-negative rate for DVT, which was not statistically significant compared with the 1% (4/402 patients) false-negative rate found in patients with single femoral veins. Quinlan et al also demonstrated that variations in lower limb venous anatomy were common, showing that in 31% of 404 bilateral venograms, the SFV was duplicated.[53] For the inexperienced, it is important to realize that the incidence of duplication for femoral veins is significant and, therefore, special attention must be directed to insure that a duplicated thrombosed vessel is not ignored.

Examination Protocol

Recently, there has been considerable debate about what constitutes an adequate and appropriate examination. The traditional protocol described in the American College of Radiology Standard for Performance of the Peripheral Venous Ultrasound Examination adopted in 1993 and reassessed in 1999 and 2005 calls for the careful examination of the full length of the common femoral vein, superficial femoral vein, and popliteal vein.[22] Images with and without compression should be recorded at the common femoral, midsuperficial femoral, and midpopliteal veins. We use CFDI as an adjunct in nearly all our examinations because it helps speed identification of vessels. Power Doppler imaging can sometimes be useful in identifying early recanalization, but because there is no directionality of flow, it is not as useful as CFDI alone. Doppler spectral analysis is useful in assessing phasicity and augmentation responses and is particularly helpful as a secondary means of evaluating the patency of the iliac veins. Some centers also include the study of the greater saphenous vein where it enters the common femoral vein as part of the routine examination because of the risk of superficial thrombophlebitis extending into the deep system. In the future, ultrasound contrast may be included as a means to improve indeterminate or uncertain studies.

Limited Compression Examinations

Pezzullo, Perkins, and Cronan reported in a prospective study of 53 symptomatic patients and a retrospective study of 155 symptomatic patients that a limited compression

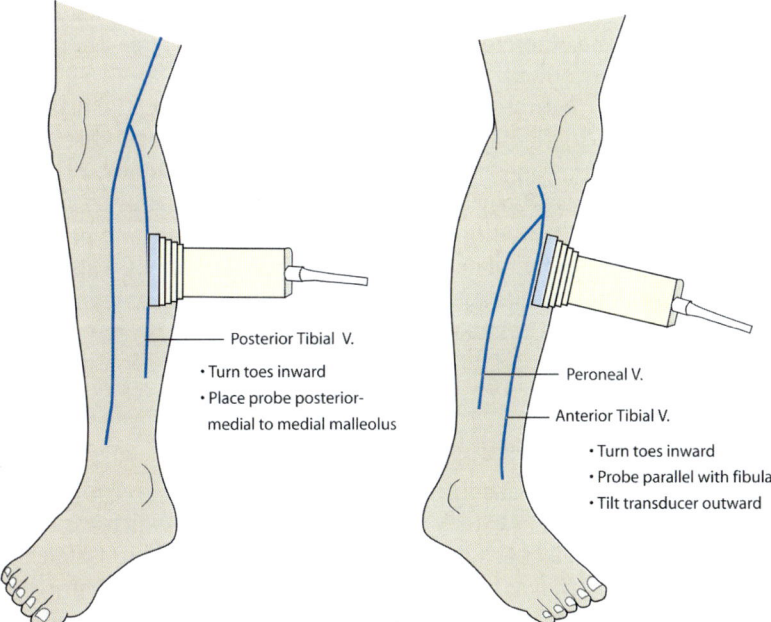

Figure 1-9 How to evaluate calf veins.

examination of the common femoral (from the inguinal ligament to the takeoff of the profunda femoral vein) and of the popliteal vein (above and below the knee) depicted each case of DVT that was detected with the traditional more complete examination.[36] Additionally, they found a 54% reduction in examination time (9.7 min) with the limited study. As a result, they recommended studying just the common femoral and popliteal veins and repeating the study in 2 to 5 days if the patient was still symptomatic. In reaction, Frederick et al prospectively studied 721 symptomatic patients and determined after 755 examinations that DVT limited to a single vein occurs with sufficient frequency that the study could not be abbreviated without loss of diagnostic accuracy.[37] They found that DVT was limited to the common femoral vein in eight studies (6.1%), to the superficial femoral vein in six studies (4.6%), and to the popliteal vein in 14 studies (10.7%). They found no statistically significant difference between the frequency of isolated thrombus in any of these three veins. Maki et al, in a study of 2704 lower extremities, found that acute DVT was isolated to the superficial femoral vein in 22.3% of those patients who had DVT.[38] Considering these two major studies, a limited examination is not recommended.

Scanning Calf Veins

The issue of what to do about studying the calf veins is also controversial. The ACR standard does not require the study of calf veins. Gotlieb et al found no significant adverse outcomes between patients who participated in a study in which the calf veins were only evaluated if physical signs or symptoms were present.[39] However, although most calf vein thromboses resolve spontaneously, ~20% extend to the proximal venous system.[10,36] This suggests that if symptoms persist or worsen, a repeat study should be performed even if an initial study was negative. In 2% of patients who had an initial normal examination, abnormalities were evident on serial testing due to extension of calf vein thrombosis.[8] Even in the most careful and detailed examination of the calf veins, it is difficult to be certain that all of the possibly duplicated vessels are free of thrombus. Reported rates on nondiagnostic studies vary in the literature from 19.3% to 82.7%.[10] Additionally, as a result, some have suggested repeating a negative ultrasound in 7 days to look for propagation of thrombus.[40] It has been suggested, however, that a negative ultrasound combined with a normal plasma D-dimer value or low pretest risk factor probability can exclude DVT without further tests.[8] With the more recent aggressive interventional approaches to thrombolytic therapy for treating DVT, the accurate identification of calf vein thrombosis that might propagate proximally is becoming increasingly important. Additionally, with the advent of low molecular weight heparin/warfarin and the introduction of the safer fixed dose ximelgratan, which does not require coagulation monitoring, some clinicians are now beginning to advocate treating isolated calf vein thrombosis and rescanning in 1 week to determine if there is a need to continue therapy or if the calf thrombosis has resolved.[41,42] Including the calf veins in the assessment of the lower extremity therefore is advisable when possible.

Although not yet included in most protocols, the identification of occluded distended communicating and perforating veins, most particularly the gastrocnemius and soleal veins, is important to note. Perforating veins greater than 3 mm in size are considered abnormal. Some clinicians are beginning to treat acutely thrombosed gastrocnemius and soleal veins in the same manner as acute thrombosis of the three paired calf veins.

Microbubble ultrasound contrast agents are reported to be particularly useful in improving the evaluation of calf veins. Bucek et al reported that the use of Levovist (Schering, Berlin, Germany) reduced the rate of indeterminate examinations from 55 to 20% and improved the specificity for detection of calf vein DVT from 25 to 67% without compromising sensitivity (10 to 86%).[43] Contrast was thought to be particularly helpful in improving the quality of difficult examinations caused by significant leg swelling and patient obesity.

How to Scan Carefully

How carefully the vessels are studied depends on the history and symptomatology. Usually, it is adequate to scan every 1 to 2 cm of the veins. In most symptomatic patients, the clot usually involves multiple or whole venous segments. However, orthopedic patients, particularly those who had hip fractures and joint replacements, have short and focal segments of thrombus above the knee and extensive thrombus in the calf veins. As a result, if the calf veins are not studied, the examiner should study the veins above the knee in shorter intervals than they might otherwise plan to do. Additionally, absent flow augmentation tells the examiner that there should be an obstruction between the site of Doppler sampling and the site of augmentation, and, therefore, a detailed study of this area should be performed.

Several studies have recently reported that in orthopedic patients with joint replacements (hips and knees) and in postoperative foot and ankle surgical patients, although calf DVT may be present, the thrombus disappears spontaneously without developing more significant proximal propagation or embolization when the patient is appropriately anticoagulated.[44-46] Therefore, careful assessment of the calf veins is important in these patients when possible so appropriate therapy can be instituted.

Unilateral or Bilateral Scanning

Another controversial issue regarding technique is whether to study both lower extremities, which has traditionally been done. However, in a recent article, Naidich et al[47] showed that in only 1% of patients was the thrombus found in the asymptomatic leg when evaluation of the

1 Leg Swelling with Pain or Edema

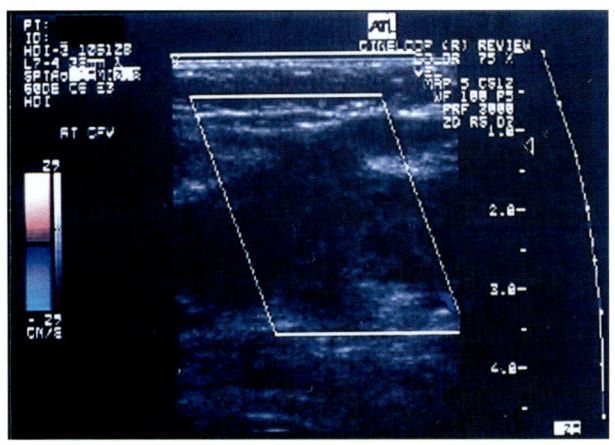
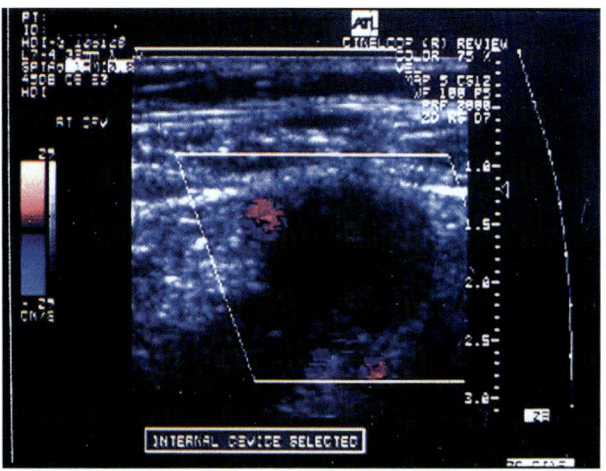

Figure 1–10 **(A)** Sagittal and **(B)** transverse images of the right common femoral vein (CFV) and profunda femoral vein (PFV) demonstrating hyperexpanded vessels filled with hypoechoic thrombus consistent with acute deep venous thrombosis.

symptomatic leg was negative. Cronan[9] described that the likelihood of finding clots solely in the asymptomatic leg was between 0 and 1% and therefore questioned the routine evaluation of the asymptomatic leg. However, the status of the venous structures is important, particularly in differentiating acute recurrent thrombus from chronic venous thrombus. Therefore, routine bilateral studies are probably worthwhile, if for no other reason than as a baseline for future comparison.

Benefits of Ultrasound

Classic Findings of Acute Deep Venous Thrombosis

When classic findings are present, acute venous thrombosis appears to be hypoechoic. On CFDI it can be demonstrated as an intraluminal defect or color void. Acute DVT expands the venous lumen; it is noncompressible, does not

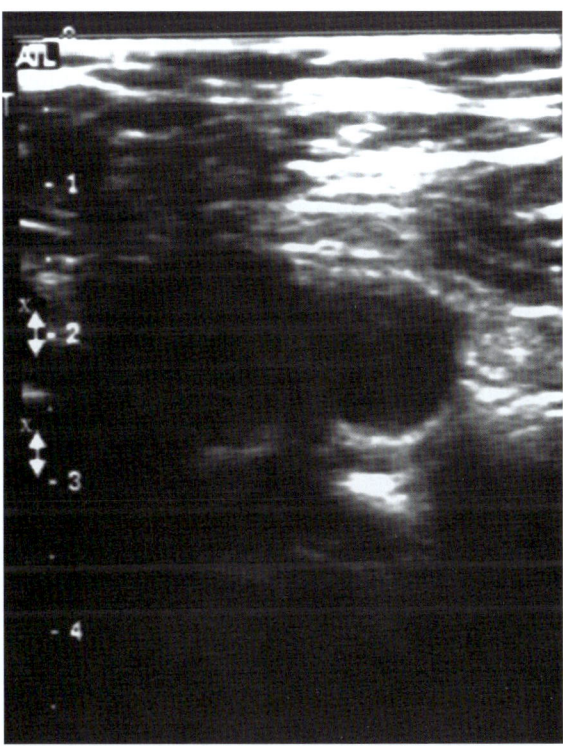
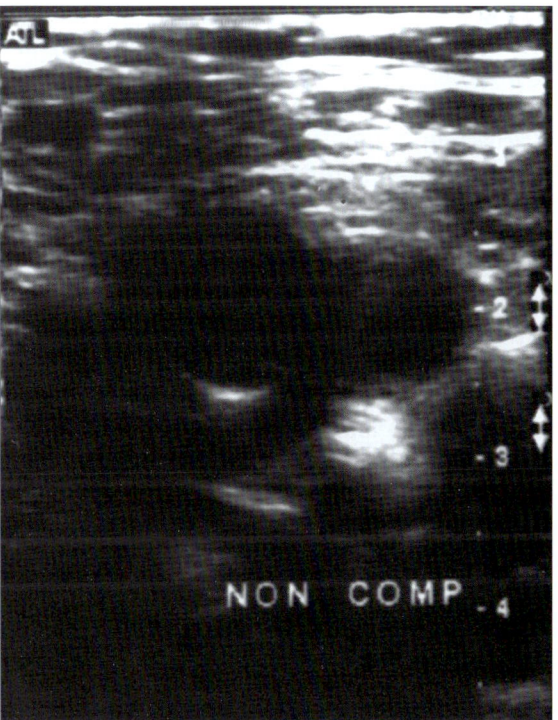

Figure 1–11 **(A)** Transverse images without and **(B)** with compression of a popliteal vein. The vein **(B)** remains hyperexpanded and is filled with hypoechoic plaque. It does not collapse, consistent with acute deep venous thrombosis.

10 Ultrasonography in Vascular Diseases

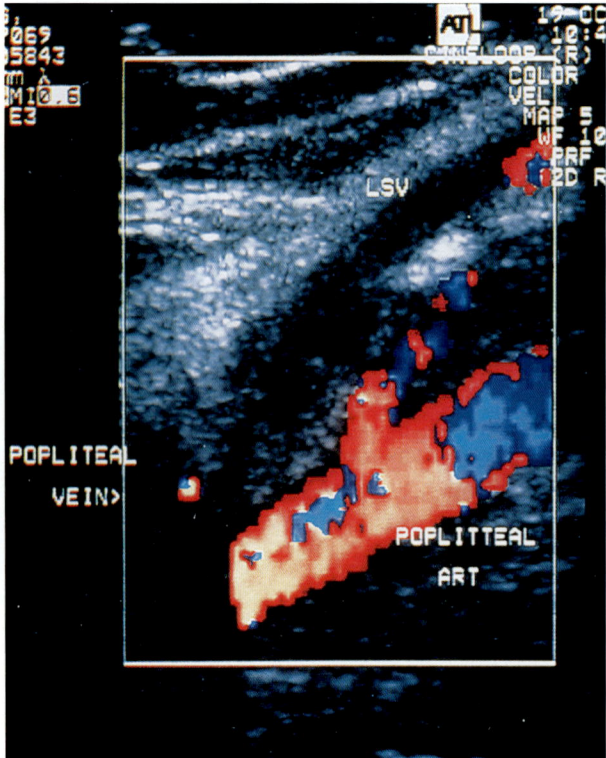

Figure 1–12 Sagittal color flow Doppler imaging of an acutely occluded popliteal vein (PV) and lesser saphenous vein (LSV). Note that the thrombosed veins appear expanded and hypoechoic.

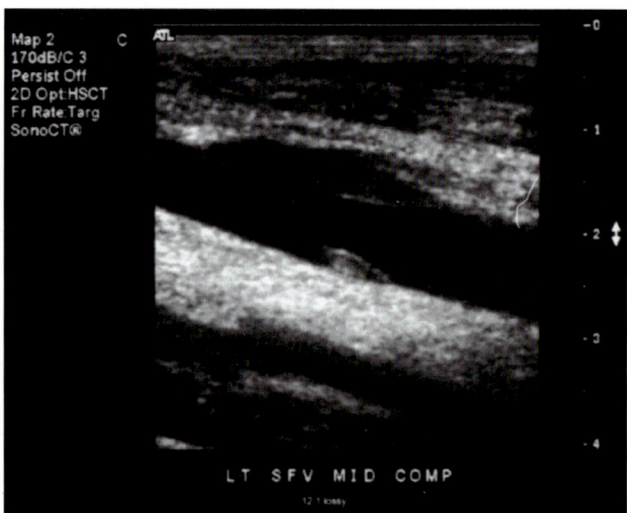

Figure 1–13 Gray-scale sagittal image demonstrating acute thrombus developing along a posterior leaflet of a venous valve. Resolution of thrombus involving valves can result in valve destruction leading to venous incompetence and the venous insufficiency syndrome.

demonstrate augmentation, and, as an indirect sign, the distal vein demonstrates nonvariable venous signals or loss of phasicity (**Fig. 1–10A,B, Fig. 1–11, Fig. 1–12, Fig. 1–13, Fig. 1–14**). The latter finding is particularly important when the iliac veins are not well visualized and they can only be secondarily evaluated by interrogating the common femoral veins (**Fig. 1–15A–D**). As an early manifestation of acute DVT, irregularities corresponding to acute thrombus can be noted on the venous valves (**Fig. 1–13**).

Accuracy

Loss of compressibility of the veins is the most important of the criteria and is the most universally accepted as being highly accurate (**Fig. 1–11A,B**). Cronan pooled the results of several series that totaled 1619 lower extremities and compared compression ultrasonography with ascending venography. This pooling resulted in a 95% sensitivity and a 98% specificity for compression ultrasound.[6] Many studies have similarly shown the high accuracy of compression sonography in diagnosing acute DVT. The sensitivities range from 88 to 100% and the specificities from 92 to 100%.[23,48–60] Additionally, in several outcome studies, patients who had negative compression ultrasounds and therefore were followed but not treated with anticoagulation did not have any evidence of developing pulmonary emboli.[61,62] This adds further credence to the accuracy of this technique. With CFDI, the normal vessels are usually completely filled in with color, indicating patency. Additionally, compression, phasicity, and augmentation responses can be studied. Several studies have reported that CFDI was comparable to compression sonography.[63,64] Lewis et al reported a sensitivity of 95%, a specificity of 99%, an accuracy of 98%, a positive predictive value of 95%, and a negative predictive value of 99%.[65] For isolated calf vein thrombosis, the sensitivity is significantly lower, ranging between 60 and 80%. Lewis et al also reported that the rate for indeterminate results in their patients was 6% with CFDI, which was comparable to the rate of indeterminate examinations reported for compression sonography.

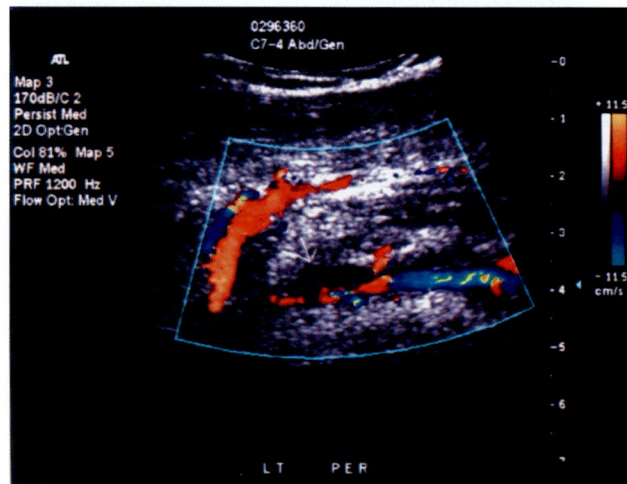

Figure 1–14 Nonoccluding acute thrombus located in the anterior tibial and peroneal veins. Note the calf vessels are hyperexpanded and the acute thrombus is hypoechoic. Color flow does not extend to the outer margin of the vessels.

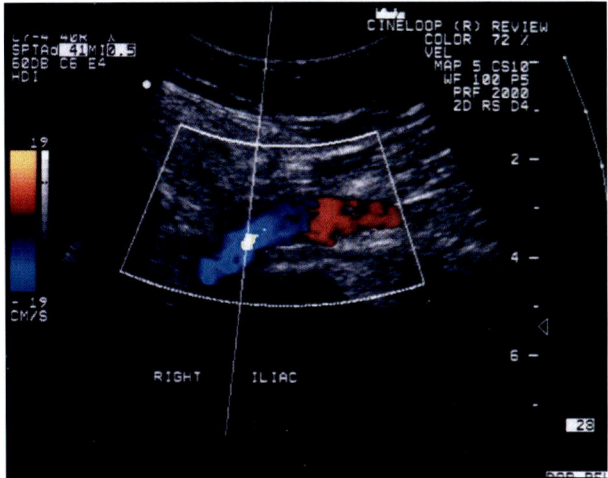
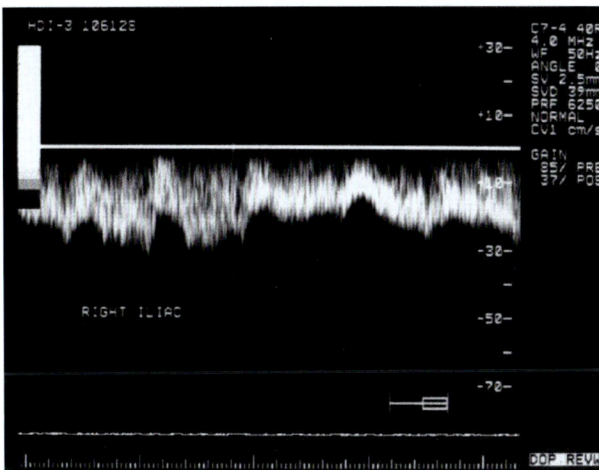
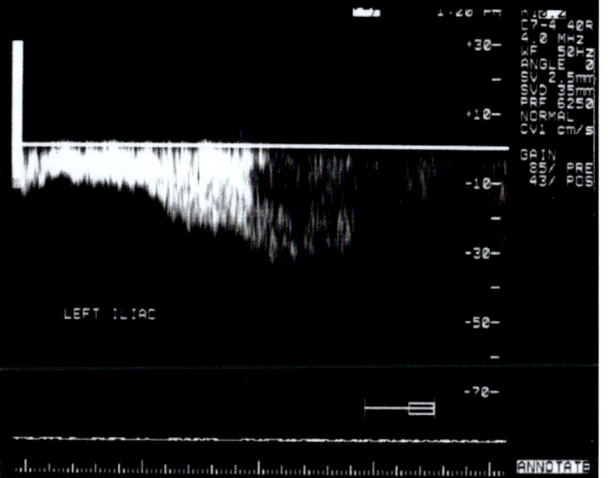

Figure 1–15 **(A)** Sagittal color flow Doppler imaging of the right and **(B)** left iliac veins demonstrating flow. **(C)** There is loss of respiratory phasicity in the right common femoral vein Doppler spectral analysis pattern compared with **(D)** the normal left, indicating a more proximal obstruction on the right.

It is hoped that in the future, accuracy can be improved with the use of ultrasound contrast agents.[43]

Although with the use of careful techniques and state of the art equipment and with the potential use of ultrasound contrast the accuracy of lower extremity venous ultrasound will remain excellent, it is unlikely for it to be 100%. As in all tests, false-negatives can occur. Theodorou et al reported that the pulmonary embolism rate was 1.6% even after a negative ultrasound was performed in a laboratory that had a sensitivity of 93%, specificity of 98%, and accuracy of 97%.[66] Sonography, similar to all tests, is not foolproof.

Complications

There are very few complications attributed to ultrasound. Although no complications are generally assumed to be the result of compression ultrasound, a few case reports have described documented cases of a pulmonary embolism developing as a result of a compression study of a superficial femoral vein.[67] Gentle compression is therefore advised, particularly when acute thrombus is present.

Limitations

The limitations of this technique include proximal obstruction by an extrinsic mass such as adenopathy, hematoma, or tumor, which may, therefore, limit compressibility of the venous structures and suggest a false-positive diagnosis. Additionally, congestive heart failure with secondary venous distension may also lead to an inaccurate assessment and false-positive diagnosis.

Other significant problems relate to differentiating chronic thrombus from an acute exacerbation. This is particularly difficult in patients with chronic DVT who have residual changes of a thickened venous wall and who have decreased compliance. When recurrent thrombus occurs in these patients, the venous wall cannot acutely expand, and diagnostic certainty decreases.

False-negative examinations can occur in obese patients and patients with edematous extremities, which are therefore difficult to examine. Small nonocclusive thrombi less than 3 cm in length in the profunda femoral vein and the distal popliteal vein in particular are prone to being missed.[63,64] The presence of nonocclusive thrombus can be identified by noting subtle changes in respiratory phasicity while maintaining the augmentation response (**Fig. 1–16**). Additionally, careful attention to detail relative to technical optimization can help in visualization, particularly in the calf (**Fig. 1–14**). Nevertheless, nonobstructing thrombus may lead to false-negative examinations if collateral vessels are present, and as a result there are no changes in blood flow patterns. The adductor canal is a particularly difficult site to produce a technically adequate examination, but, luckily, isolated thrombus in this location is rare.[50] Another pitfall is to mistake a patent lesser saphenous vein at the saphenopopliteal junction for a distal popliteal vein that is thrombosed (**Fig. 1–12**). Usually, the saphenous vein is more superficial and is smaller than the 3 to 4 mm popliteal vein.

Frequently, iliac veins are difficult to visualize, but if careful attention is paid to the spectral analysis patterns of the visualized portions of the distal iliac and femoral veins and loss of phasicity is noted, a secondary sign of proximal thrombosis will not be missed and the correct diagnosis will be suggested (**Fig. 1–15**). Collateral vessels can also be mistaken for occluded vessels. Collaterals can be differentiated by appreciating the fact that the true venous structure is adjacent to the artery, whereas collateral veins have a more random relationship

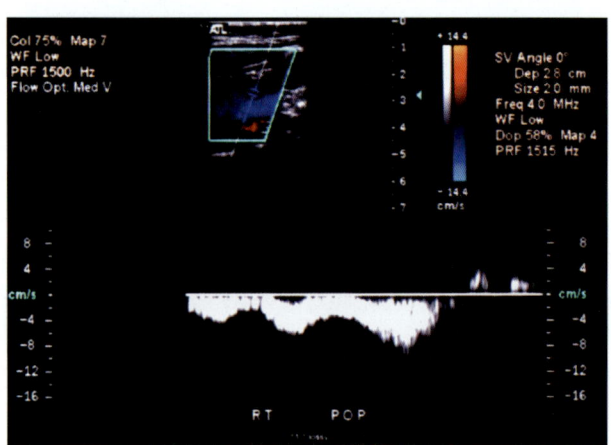
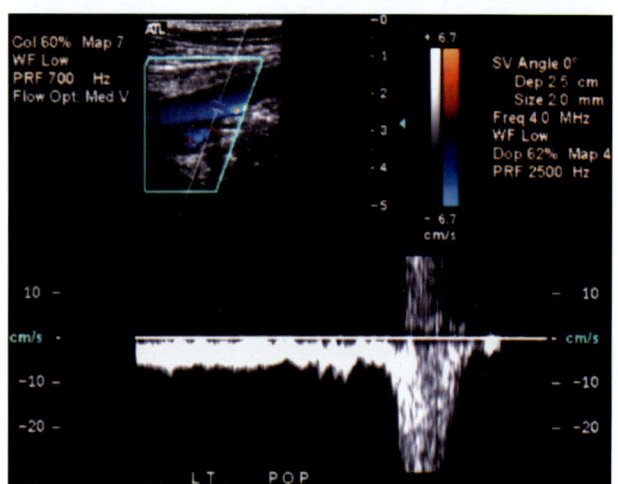
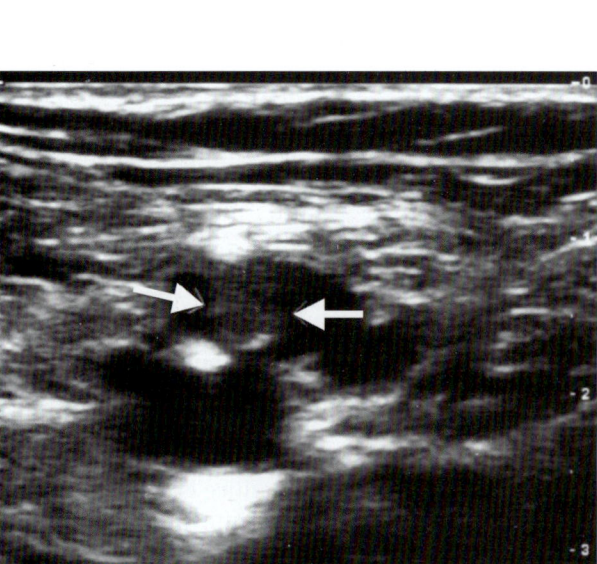
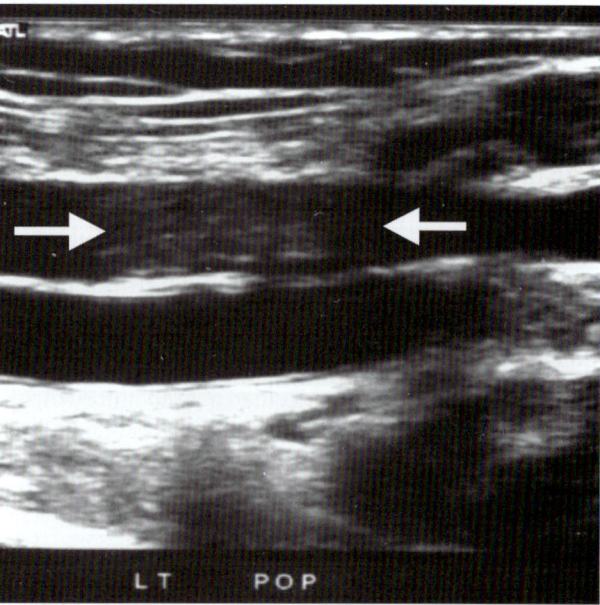

Figure 1–16 (**A**) Sagittal color flow Doppler imaging and Doppler spectral analysis of the right and (**B**) left popliteal veins. Note normal respiratory phasicity on the right and subtle decrease in phasicity on the left. This suggests proximal thrombus. However, there is good augmentation response on the left (**B**), indicating that the thrombus is nonoccluding. (**C**) Corresponding transverse and (**D**) sagittal gray-scale images demonstrate nonoccluding thrombus in the more proximal left popliteal vein.

1 Leg Swelling with Pain or Edema

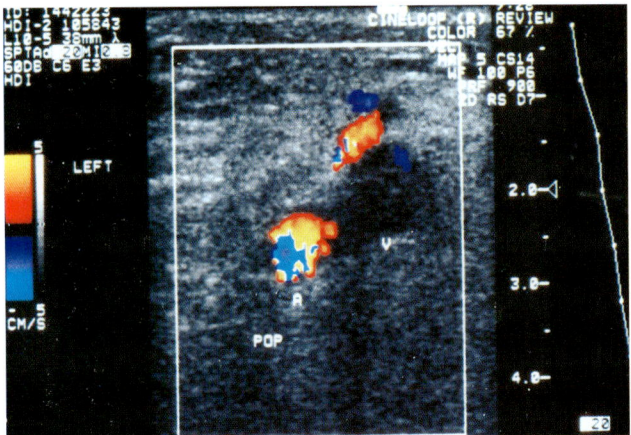

Figure 1–17 Large collateral vessel adjacent to an occluded popliteal vein. Note that the collateral vein is not immediately adjacent to the artery.

(**Fig. 1–17**). Lastly, the venous structures are frequently duplicated, and this duplication cannot always be visualized, even with CFDI. Thrombosis in one of these duplicated vessels may go undetected. In the future, it is hoped that the use of ultrasound contrast agents may reduce these limitations.

Diagnosing Chronic Venous Thrombosis

Cronan has reported that after 6 months of acute DVT, 48% of veins will still have demonstrable abnormalities on ultrasound examination. In this study, 14% of the abnormal veins remained completely occluded.[6] A larger number of veins recanalized to some extent, but remained with residual clot as organized thrombus material along the vein wall. This organized fibrous intimal venous thickening results from an ingrowth of inflammatory cells, which begins to occur soon after acute thrombus adheres to the venous endothelium. This thickened vein will now resist compression, causing confusion with nonocclusive thrombosis, and can lead to the incorrect diagnosis of acute recurrent thrombosis.

Some findings that can help distinguish chronic from acute thrombosis include the fact that chronic thrombus does not expand the venous lumen, that chronic thrombus is generally more echogenic than acute thrombus, that collateral vessels when seen particularly with CFDI suggest a chronic etiology, and that flow is seen within the central venous lumen with CFDI and the wall changes may be better appreciated (**Fig. 1–18, Fig. 1–19**). Linkins et al reported success in diagnosing DVT by comparing the change in thrombus length over two ultrasound examinations.[68] A change in length of 9 cm or greater is supportive of a diagnosis of recurrent DVT. Less than 9 cm was reported to be measurement error. However, in many cases, distinguishing recurrent acute venous thrombosis from chronic thrombosis is a very difficult diagnostic dilemma. Perhaps there may be a role for radionuclide imaging or MR in some of these indeterminate cases. In a small study, Fraser et al showed that VESPA MR venography demonstrated contrast enhancement of the vessel wall in cases of acute thrombosis, but not in cases of chronic thrombosis. If confirmed, this may mean that this technique could be used to resolve nondiagnostic ultrasound cases.[30]

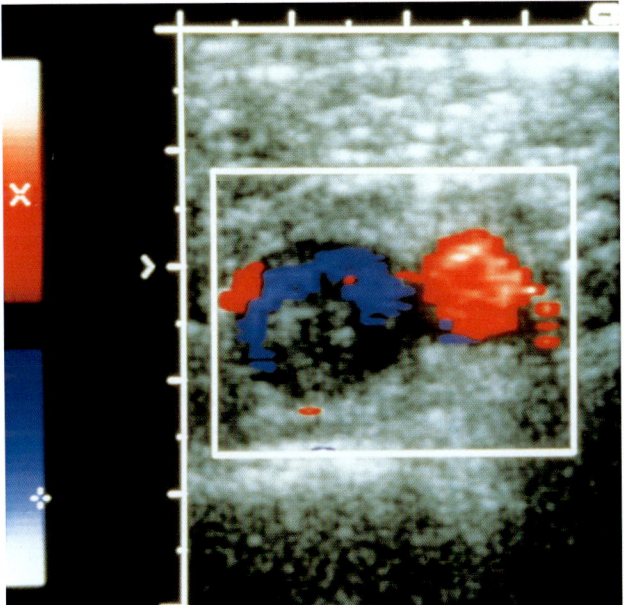
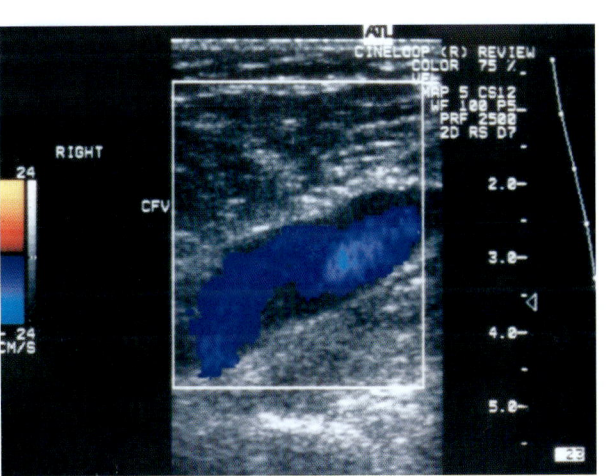

Figure 1–18 Transverse **(A)** and sagittal **(B)** images demonstrating recanalized flow around chronic thrombus in two different patients. The vein is not expanded and the thrombus is echogenic.

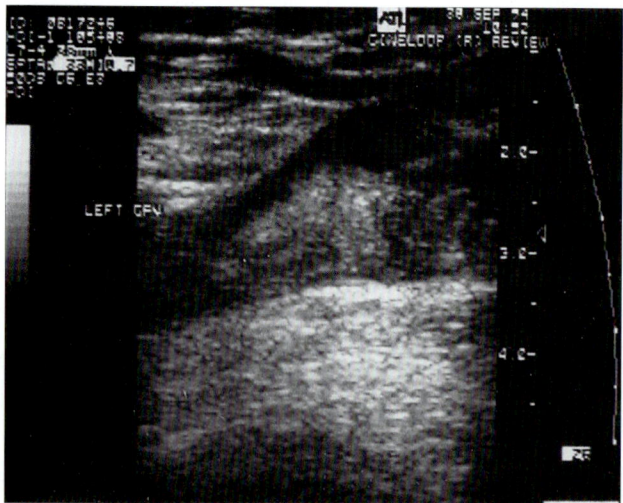

Figure 1–19 Sagittal image of a left CFV which contains chronic residual thrombus from a previous episode of DVT but now has superimposed acute recurrent thrombosis as evidenced by the expanded noncompressible CFV.

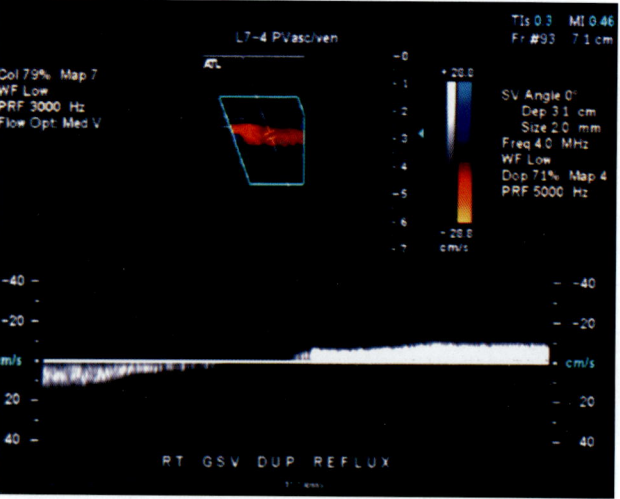

Figure 1–20 Sagittal image of the superficial femoral vein demonstrating reversal of flow after a Valsalva maneuver lasting several seconds. This is characteristic of venous reflux.

Diagnosing Chronic Venous Insufficiency Syndrome and Ultrasound-Guided Treatment

The chronic venous insufficiency syndrome occurs as a result of destruction of venous valves secondary to acute DVT, allowing blood to flow from the deep to the superficial venous system (**Fig. 1–13**). The resulting volume overload and distension or obstruction of these veins produces a clinical picture of pain, swelling, skin changes, necrosis, and superficial ulcerations. This syndrome can be identified by seeing reverse flow with CFDI for more than 1 second when the patient performs the Valsalva maneuver (**Fig. 1–20**). Other methods to test for reflux include applying compression to the limb above the area being evaluated and producing augmentation by squeezing the calf with the patient standing and then observing the venous response.[69] Johnson et al reported that after an episode of DVT, 41% of patients developed features of the chronic venous insufficiency syndrome, although only 13% of patients developed skin complications.[70] The magnitude of the reflux detected by ultrasound appears to be related to the likelihood of developing ulcerations.[69]

Radiofrequency ablation and laser ablation of the refluxing greater saphenous vein (GSV) have been introduced as a new option for treatment of complications of venous reflux, particularly varicosities. Ultrasound is used for mapping the GSV, for guidance in cannulating the GSV, and for positioning the tip of the interventional catheter within 1 cm of the origin of the inferior epigastric vein (the first GSV tributary) to perform the procedure. Hingorani et al have reported that DVT was noted in 16% of 66 patients treated (12 of 73 limbs). Eleven had extension of the occlusive clot into the proximal GSV and one had one calf DVT. None of these patients developed pulmonary embolism, however.[71] Early postoperative venous ultrasound of the lower extremities is therefore essential and should be performed in all patients undergoing noninvasive closure of the GSV.

Summary

Ultrasound continues to be recognized as the first and most appropriate study to perform when a patient presents with symptomatic lower extremities suggesting acute venous thrombosis. There are numerous advantages to performing a sonographic study of the lower extremities. These evaluations can be performed portably, generally cause no complications, and generally do not involve the use of contrast media or radiation. In ~10% of patients, other abnormalities such as Baker's cysts, arterial aneurysms, or hematomas can be detected and can explain the symptoms (**Fig. 1–2, Fig. 1–4**). The limitations of ultrasound are that it requires experienced operators, it is frequently hard to define the iliac and calf veins, it is difficult to distinguish chronic from acute recurrent thrombosis, and the presence of duplicated vessels can be a significant challenge to achieving an accurate study. In the future, with the introduction of contrast agents, some of these limitations should be resolved or eliminated. Nonetheless, at the present time, because it is the study of choice, it is important for all those involved in diagnostic ultrasound to be comfortable in performing and interpreting these examinations.

References

1. Jacobson AF. Diagnosis of deep venous thrombosis: a review of radiologic, radionuclide, and non-imaging methods. Q J Nucl Med 2001;45:324–333
2. Foley WD. Extremity venous disease. In: Foley WD, ed. Color Doppler Flow Imaging. Reading, MA: Andover Press; 1991:129–151
3. Sorensen HT, Mellemkjaer L, Steffensen FH, Olsen JH, Nielsen GL. The risk of a diagnosis of cancer after primary deep venous thrombosis or pulmonary embolism. N Engl J Med 1998;338:1169–1173
4. Needleman L, Polak J. Suspected lower extremity deep vein thrombosis. In: American College of Radiology Appropriateness Criteria for Imaging and Treatment Decisions. Reston VA: ACR; 1995: CV-8.1–8.6
5. Gallix B, Achard-Lichere C, Dauzat M, Bruel JM, Lopez FM. Flow-independent magnetic resonance venography of the calf. J Magn Reson Imaging 2003;17:421–426
6. Cronan JJ. Venous thromboembolic disease: the role of US. Radiology 1993;186:619–630
7. Hirsh J, Hull RD. Venous thromboembolism: natural history, diagnosis and management. In: Hirshi J, Hull RD, eds. Diagnosis of Venous Thrombosis. Boca Raton, FL: CRC Press; 1987:23–28
8. Ginsberg JS. Management of venous thromboembolism. N Engl J Med 1996;335:1816–1828
9. Cronan JJ. Controversies in venous ultrasound. Semin Ultrasound CT MR 1997;18:33–38
10. Fraser JD, Anderson DR. Venous protocols, techniques, and interpretations of the upper and lower extremities. Radiol Clin North Am 2004;42:279–296
11. Melikian N, Bingham J, Goldsmith DJ. Diabetic infarction: an unusual cause of acute limb swelling in patients on hemodialysis. Am J Kidney Dis 2003;42:1102–1103
12. Bluth EI, Merritt CR, Sullivan MA. Gray-scale evaluation of the lower extremities. JAMA 1982;247:3127–3129
13. Borgstede JP, Clagett GE. Types, frequency, and significance of alternative diagnoses found during duplex Doppler venous examinations of the lower extremities. J Ultrasound Med 1992;11:85–89
14. Sandler DA, Mitchell JR. How do we know who has had deep venous thrombosis? Postgrad Med J 1989;65:16–19
15. Grice GD III, Smith RB III, Robinson PH, Rheudasil JM. Primary popliteal venous aneurysm with recurrent pulmonary emboli. J Vasc Surg 1990;12:316–318
16. Ross GJ, Violi L, Barber LW, Vujic I. Popliteal venous aneurysm. Radiology 1988;168:721–722
17. Lutter KS, Kerr TM, Roedersheimer LR, Lohr JM, Sampson MG, Cranley JJ. Superficial thrombophlebitis diagnosed by duplex scanning. Surgery 1991;110:42–46
18. Ikeda M, Fujimori Y, Tankawa H, Iwata H. Compression syndrome of the popliteal vein and artery caused by popliteal cyst. Angiology 1984;35:245–251
19. Swett HA, Jaffe RB, McIff EB. Popliteal cysts: presentation as thrombophlebitis. Radiology 1975;115:613–615
20. Chengelis DL, Bendick PJ, Glover JL, Brown OW, Ranval TJ. Progression of superficial venous thrombosis to deep vein thrombosis. J Vasc Surg 1996;24:745–749
21. Jorgensen JO, Hanel KC, Morgan AM, Hunt JM. The incidence of deep venous thrombosis in patients with superficial thrombophlebitis of the lower limbs. J Vasc Surg 1993;18:70–73
22. American College of Radiology. ACR Standards for Performance of the Peripheral Venous Ultrasound Examination. Reston, VA: ACR; 1993
23. Heijboer H, Buller HR, Lensing AW, Turpie AG, Colly LP, ten Cate JW. A comparison of real-time compression ultrasonography with impedance plethysmography for the diagnosis of deep venous thrombosis in symptomatic outpatients. N Engl J Med 1993;329:1365–1369
24. Begemann PG, Bonacker M, Kemper J, et al. Evaluation of the deep venous system in patients with suspected pulmonary embolism with multi-detector CT: a prospective study in comparison to Doppler sonography. J Comput Assist Tomogr 2003;27:399–409
25. Loud P, Katz D, Bruce D, Klippenstein D, Grossman Z. Deep venous thrombosis with suspected pulmonary embolism: detection with combined CT venography and pulmonary angiography. Radiology 2001;219:498–502
26. Duwe KM, Shiau M, Budorick NE, Austin JH, Berkmen YM. Evaluation of the lower extremity veins in patients with suspected pulmonary embolism: a retrospective comparison of helical CT venography and sonography. 2000 ARRS Executive Council Award I. American Roentgen Ray Society. AJR Am J Roentgenol 2000;175:1525–1531
27. Peterson DA, Kazerooni EA, Wakefield TW, et al. Computed tomographic venography is specific but not sensitive for diagnosis of acute lower-extremity deep venous thrombosis in patients with suspected pulmonary embolus. J Vasc Surg 2001;34:798–804
28. Evans AJ, Sostman HD, Knelson MH, et al. Detection of deep venous thrombosis: prospective comparison of MR imaging with contrast venography. AJR Am J Roentgenol 1993;161:131–139
29. Spritzer CE, Norconk JJ Jr, Sostman HD, Coleman RE. Detection of deep venous thrombosis by magnetic resonance imaging. Chest 1993;104:54–60
30. Fraser DG, Moody AR, Davidson IR, Martel AL, Morgan PS. Deep venous thrombosis: diagnosis by using venous enhanced subtracted peak arterial MR venography versus conventional venography. Radiology 2003;226:812–820
31. Fraser DGW. Using magnetic resonance direct thrombus imaging to diagnose deep-vein thrombosis in the lower legs. Ann Intern Med 2002;136:I26
32. Fraser DGW, Moody AR, Morgan PS, Martel AL, Davidson I. Diagnosis of lower-limb deep venous thrombosis: a prospective blinded study of magnetic resonance direct thrombus imaging. Ann Intern Med 2002;136:89–98
33. Screaton NJ, Gillard JH, Berman LH, Kemp PM. Duplicated superficial femoral veins: a source of error in the sonographic investigation of deep vein thrombosis. Radiology 1998;206:397–401
34. Cronan JJ. Venous duplex US of the lower extremities: effect of duplicated femoral veins [editorial]. Radiology 1998;206:308–309
35. Quinlan DJ, Alikhan R, Gishen P, Sidhu PS. Variations in lower limb venous anatomy: implications for US diagnosis of deep vein thrombosis. Radiology 2003;228:443–448
36. Pezzullo JA, Perkins AB, Cronan JJ. Symptomatic deep venous thrombosis: diagnosis with limited compression US. Radiology 1996;198:67–70
37. Frederick MG, Hertzberg BS, Kliewer MA, et al. Can the US examination for lower extremity deep venous thrombosis be abbreviated? A prospective study of 755 examinations. Radiology 1996;199:45–47
38. Maki DD, Kumar N, Nguyen B, Langer JE, Miller WT Jr, Gefter WB. Distribution of thrombi in acute lower extremity deep venous thrombosis: implications for sonography and CT and MR venography. AJR Am J Roentgenol 2000;175:1299–1301
39. Gottlieb RH, Voci SL, Syed L, et al. Randomized prospective study comparing routine versus selective use of sonography of the complete calf in patients with suspected deep venous thrombosis. AJR Am J Roentgenol 2003;180:241–245

40. Kraaijenhagen RA, Piovella F, Bernardi E, et al. Simplification of the diagnostic management of suspected deep vein thrombosis. Arch Intern Med 2002;162:907–911
41. Fiessinger JN, Huisman MV, Davidson BL, et al. Ximelagatran vs low-molecular-weight heparin and warfarin for the treatment of deep vein thrombosis. JAMA 2005;293:681–689
42. Gurewich V. Ximelagatran: promises and concerns. JAMA 2005; 293:736–739
43. Bucek RA, Kos T, Schober E, et al. Ultrasound with Levovist in the diagnosis of suspected calf vein thrombosis. Ultrasound Med Biol 2001;27:455–460
44. Elias A, Cadene A, Elias M, et al. Extended lower limb venous ultrasound for the diagnosis of proximal and distal vein thrombosis in asymptomatic patients after total hip replacement. Eur J Vasc Endovasc Surg 2004;27:438–444
45. Wang CJ, Wang JW, Weng LH, Hsu CC, Lo CF. Outcome of calf deep-vein thrombosis after total knee arthroplasty. J Bone Joint Surg Br 2003;85:841–844
46. Solis G, Saxby T. Incidence of DVT following surgery of the foot and ankle. Foot Ankle Int 2002;23:411–447
47. Naidich JB, Torre JR, Pellerito JS, Smalberg IS, Kase DJ, Crystal KS. Suspected deep venous thrombosis: is US of both legs necessary? Radiology 1996;200:429–431
48. Rosner NH, Doris PE. Diagnosis of femoropopliteal venous thrombosis: comparison of duplex sonography and plethysmography. AJR Am J Roentgenol 1988;150:623–627
49. White RH, McGahan JP, Daschbach MM, Hartling RP. Diagnosis of deep-vein thrombosis using duplex ultrasound. Ann Intern Med 1989;111:297–304
50. Vogel P, Laing FC, Jeffrey RB Jr, Wing VW. Deep venous thrombosis of the lower extremity: US evaluation. Radiology 1987;163:747–751
51. Cronan JJ, Dorfman GS, Scola FH, Schepps B, Alexander J. Deep venous thrombosis: US assessment using vein compression. Radiology 1987;162(1 Pt 1):191–194
52. Cronan JJ, Dorfman GS, Grusmark J. Lower-extremity deep venous thrombosis: further experience with and refinements of US assessment. Radiology 1988;168:101–107
53. George JE, Smith MO, Berry RE. Duplex scanning for the detection of deep venous thrombosis of lower extremities in a community hospital. Curr Surg 1987;44:202–204
54. Appelman PT, De Jong TE, Lampmann LE. Deep venous thrombosis of the leg: US findings. Radiology 1987;163:743–746
55. Lensing AWA, Prandoni P, Brandjes D, et al. Detection of deep venous thrombosis by real-time B-mode ultrasonography. N Engl J Med 1989;320:342–345
56. Froehlich JA, Dorfman GS, Cronan JJ, Urbanek PJ, Herndon JH, Aaron RK. Compression ultrasonography for the detection of deep venous thrombosis in patients who have a fracture of the hip: a prospective study. J Bone Joint Surg Am 1989;71:249–256
57. O'Leary DH, Kane RA, Chase BM. A prospective study of the efficacy of B-scan sonography in the detection of deep venous thrombosis in the lower extremities. J Clin Ultrasound 1988;16:1–8
58. Aitken AGF, Godden DJ. Real-time ultrasound diagnosis of deep vein thrombosis: a comparison with venography. Clin Radiol 1987;38:309–313
59. Killewich LA, Bedford GR, Beach KW, Strandness DE Jr. Diagnosis of deep venous thrombosis: a prospective study comparing duplex scanning to contrast venography. Circulation 1989;79:810–814
60. Becker DM, Philbrick JT, Abbitt PL. Real-time ultrasonography for the diagnosis of lower extremity deep venous thrombosis: the wave of the future? Arch Intern Med 1989;149:1731–1734
61. Vaccaro JP, Cronan JJ, Dorfman GS. Outcome analysis of patients with normal compression US examinations. Radiology 1990;175: 645–649
62. Sarpa MS, Messina LM, Smith M, et al. Significance of a negative duplex scan in patients suspected of having acute deep venous thrombosis of the lower extremity. J Vasc Tech 1989;13:222–226
63. Rose SC, Zweibel WJ, Nelson BD, et al. Symptomatic lower extremity deep venous thrombosis: accuracy, limitations, and role of color duplex flow imaging in diagnosis. Radiology 1990;175:639–644
64. Foley WD, Middleton WD, Lawson TL, Erickson S, Quiroz FA, Macrander S. Color Doppler ultrasound imaging of lower extremity venous disease. AJR Am J Roentgenol 1989;152:371–376
65. Lewis BD, James EM, Welch TJ, Joyce JW, Hallet JW, Weaver AL. Diagnosis of acute deep venous thrombosis of the lower extremities: prospective evaluation of color flow Doppler imaging versus venography. Radiology 1994;192:651–655
66. Theodorou SJ, Theodorou DJ, Kakitsubata Y. Sonography and venography of the lower extremities for diagnosing deep vein thrombosis in symptomatic patients. Clin Imaging 2003;27:180–183
67. Perlin SJ. Pulmonary embolism during compression US of the lower extremity. Radiology 1992;184:165–166
68. Linkins LA, Pasquale P, Paterson S, Kearon C. Change in thrombus length on venous ultrasound and recurrent deep vein thrombosis. Arch Intern Med 2004;164:1793–1796
69. Polak JA. Peripheral artery and veins: contributions of CFDI. In: Bluth EI, Divon MY, Laurel MD, eds. Update in Duplex, Power and Color Flow Imaging. American Institute of Ultrasound in Medicine; 1996:51–62
70. Johnson BF, Manzo RA, Bergelin RO, Strandness DE Jr. Relationship between changes in the deep venous system and the development of the postthrombotic syndrome after an acute episode of lower limb deep venous thrombosis: a one- to six-year follow-up. J Vasc Surg 1995;21:307–313
71. Hingorani AP, Ascher E, Markevich N, et al. Deep venous thrombosis after radiofrequency ablation of greater saphenous vein: a word of caution. J Vasc Surg 2004;40:500–504

2 Painful Legs after Walking
William J. Zwiebel

Leg pain after walking immediately brings to mind intermittent claudication resulting from arterial insufficiency, but it is important to recognize that other disorders also may cause leg pain after walking, including neuropathy, sciatica, acute venous thrombosis, chronic venous insufficiency, rupture of a popliteal cyst, and muscular hematoma.[1-4] The starting point for differentiating among the possible causes of walking-related leg pain is the history and physical examination (H&P). For certain diagnoses, including arterial insufficiency, the H&P is generally quite specific and useful. For other causes of leg pain, however, the H&P findings are nonspecific and do not permit definitive diagnosis. Furthermore, the H&P may be nondiagnostic when two conditions coexist, both of which might cause leg pain (e.g., arterial insufficiency and peripheral neuropathy). In such circumstances, it may be difficult to determine which condition is causing the symptoms.

This chapter reviews the clinical diagnosis of arterial insufficiency, with emphasis on the role played by duplex ultrasound (imaging combined with Doppler) and other diagnostic methods. First the capabilities and limitations of the major diagnostic methods, including ultrasound, are described, followed in some detail by the ultrasound methods and diagnostic parameters used for evaluating the lower extremity arterial tree, and then postprocedure ultrasound surveillance after surgical bypass grafting and angioplasty.

Diagnostic Evaluation for Arterial Insufficiency

History and Physical Examination

As already noted, the patient's history is often quite helpful in cases of arterial insufficiency because the patient describes a fairly specific symptom complex called intermittent claudication. The term *claudication* is derived from a Latin word for limping or lameness.[5] *Intermittent claudication* refers to leg pain, weakness, or other discomfort that is absent at rest, commences after a period of ambulation, and subsides promptly when the patient stops walking.[1-4] In most instances, intermittent claudication is a sign of arterial insufficiency. At rest, the circulation is sufficient to meet the metabolic demands of the leg muscles and other tissues, but blood flow is insufficient to keep up with the metabolic demands of exercise.

Lactic acid and other metabolites accumulate in the ischemic muscles, causing cramping pain. Because intermittent claudication occurs specifically in areas of muscle ischemia, the location of pain is a fairly good indication of the location of arterial obstruction. The most common site of intermittent claudication is in the calf, implying femoropopliteal arterial occlusive disease, or arterial obstruction in the tibial and peroneal arterial trunks of the calf. Claudication may also occur in the thigh, implying external iliac or common femoral artery obstruction, or in the buttock, implying aortic or common iliac artery blockage.[1-4] The severity of arterial insufficiency is implied by the amount of exercise that results in claudication, and it is routine, therefore, to grade intermittent claudication according to the distance the patient can walk before symptoms develop or limit ambulation (e.g., one- or two-block claudication).

Most patients with lower extremity arterial insufficiency present with typical intermittent claudication symptoms; however, atypical claudication symptoms also occur, including foot pain or burning. These atypical symptoms are particularly confusing from a diagnostic perspective because they could be due to conditions other than arterial insufficiency, such as diabetic neuropathy or spinal nerve root compression resulting from degenerative disease of the lower lumbar spine. The clinical diagnosis of arterial insufficiency is also based on physical examination of the extremities.[1-4] Arterial pulses in the foot are diminished or absent, depending on the degree of arterial obstruction. Other findings include absence of leg hair and coolness of the skin. With severe arterial insufficiency, rubor (redness of the skin) may be evident in the leg and foot with the limb dependent, accompanied by pallor of the skin when the leg is elevated.

Moderate or severe arterial insufficiency is generally easy to diagnose clinically, but mild arterial insufficiency often cannot be confirmed clinically, especially when the only physical finding is diminished pulses—a subjective determination. Clinical assessment is further hampered when symptoms produced by other conditions mimic those of arterial insufficiency, as mentioned previously. Finally, clinical evaluation is inherently qualitative (subjective). A stoic patient may describe mild symptoms that another patient would describe as moderate or severe, and one clinician's assessment of disease severity may vary from another. Such problems make it difficult to compare one patient's condition with another and also complicate the assessment of disease progression over time.

18 Ultrasonography in Vascular Diseases

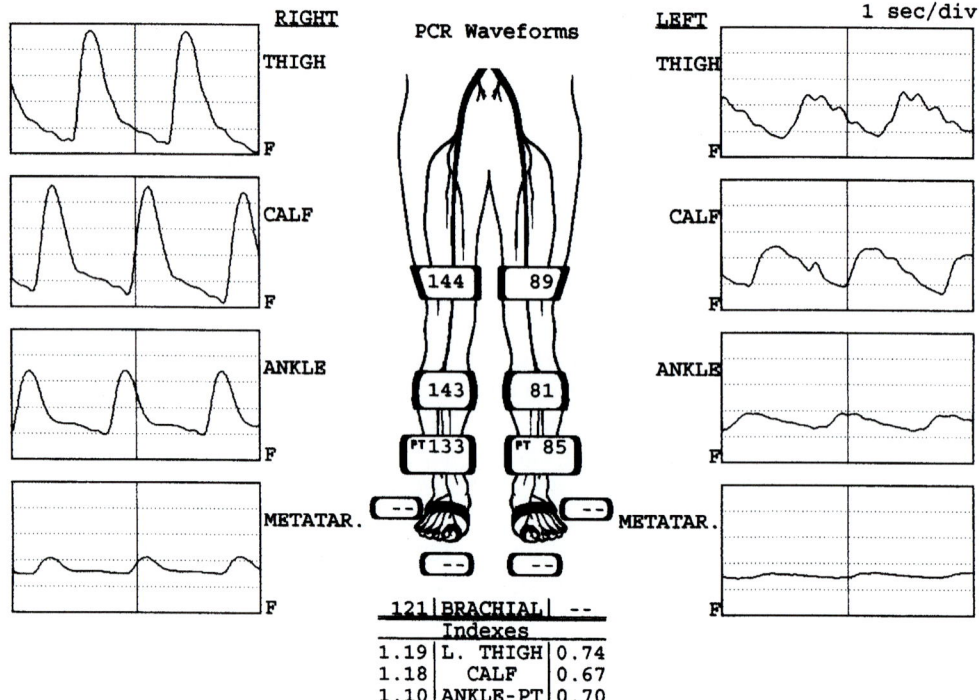

Figure 2-1 Physiological study. Segmental pressure and plethysmographic examination reveals left lower extremity arterial insufficiency resulting from inflow (iliac) obstruction. At all levels on the left, the systolic blood pressure is significantly reduced and pulse volume waveforms are damped. The left ankle/brachial index is 0.70, consistent with mild claudication. There is no evidence of arterial insufficiency on the right.

Tests Other than Imaging Tests

The deficiencies of clinical evaluation (H&P) led to the development of physiological tests for the assessment of lower-extremity arterial insufficiency,[1–4,6,7] including the ankle/brachial index (ABI), segmental pressure measurements (thigh, calf, ankle, foot), plethysmography (which measures changes in limb volume with each arterial pulse), and Doppler waveform analysis (**Fig. 2-1, Fig. 2-2**). Treadmill ambulation may be incorporated with these examinations to evaluate the capacity of the arterial system to respond to increased metabolic demand. The physiological tests serve well to answer several important questions, as listed below, that are not adequately addressed by clinical evaluation.

1. Are the patient's symptoms truly due to arterial insufficiency or should another cause be sought? A normal resting ABI, coupled with a normal postexercise ABI response, effectively excludes arterial insufficiency as a cause of ambulation-related symptoms.
2. How severe is arterial insufficiency? Pressure measurements provide a reliable way of quantifying arterial insufficiency and a fairly precise way for comparing one patient's condition with another's. For example, an ABI of 0.7 or 0.8 generally corresponds to mild arterial

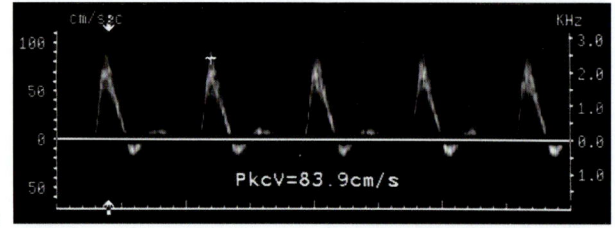
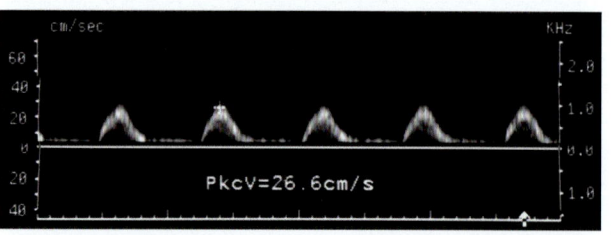

Figure 2-2 Doppler extremity arterial evaluation. **(A)** The normal, triphasic arterial signal in this common femoral artery suggests an absence of arterial insufficiency. Peak systolic velocity (PkcV) is within the normal range (**Table 46-1**). **(B)** The damped resting arterial waveform in this popliteal artery indicates arterial obstruction proximal to the examination site. Note the broad systolic peaks, slow upstroke in systole, low PkcV, and forward flow in diastole.

insufficiency and relatively mild claudication, whereas an ABI of 0.4 or less corresponds to severe arterial insufficiency, possibly with rest pain.

3. Is arterial insufficiency stable or progressing? Physiological studies provide quantitative data that are more reliable than changes in symptomatology. In some cases the patient may describe lessening of symptoms, yet physiological tests show worsening of arterial insufficiency, and vice versa.
4. Has the patient responded to therapy? The effects of medical or surgical therapy can be gauged quantitatively with physiological tests.

The principal disadvantage of physiological studies is the limited information these methods provide about the extent and location of arterial obstruction. These methods also do not differentiate effectively between arterial stenosis and occlusion. Historically, catheter angiography was required to accurately determine the location and severity of arterial obstruction for purposes of surgical planning. More recently, however, noninvasive angiography and duplex ultrasound have emerged as the predominant methods for definitive evaluation of arterial insufficiency.

Imaging Tests Other than Ultrasound

Magnetic Resonance Angiography and Computed Tomographic Angiography

Initially, magnetic resonance angiography (MRA)[8] appeared to have greater potential than computed tomographic angiography (CTA)[9] for lower-extremity arterial diagnosis, but the recent introduction of multidetector-row computed tomography (CT) has given the edge to CTA. Diagnostic-quality images of the entire lower extremity arterial tree can be obtained with CT within the time taken for a bolus of iodinated contrast to flow from the aorta to the feet. Similar diagnostic quality can be obtained with MRA, which offers the advantage of a less nephrotoxic contrast agent; however, the time frame for MRA examination is longer than that for CT. Owing to advancements in MRA and CTA, catheter-based angiography will soon virtually disappear from the *diagnostic* armamentarium for extremity arterial disease in Western nations, and arterial catheterization will be used only for therapeutic measures.

Duplex Ultrasound Imaging

The clinical utility of duplex ultrasound for lower-extremity arterial diagnosis[10-42] was advanced significantly by the development of color Doppler and power Doppler flow imaging; nevertheless, duplex examination of extremity arteries can be arduous and time consuming. Iliac artery imaging may be significantly limited by interference from bowel contents, as well as vessel tortuosity. The femoral and popliteal arteries are relatively easy to examine, but even here difficulties may arise if there are multiple areas of obstruction or if the vessels are heavily calcified. Duplex examination of calf arteries (anterior tibial, posterior tibial, and peroneal arteries) is limited by the small size of the vessels, acoustic shadows from calcification, and difficulty in identifying/following diseased arteries.[13] Even the use of ultrasound contrast agents does not substantially improve duplex results for calf vessel evaluation.[14]

These technical limitations have, in general, restricted the use of duplex sonography to relatively focused objectives, rather than comprehensive assessment of lower-extremity arterial disease. However, some centers do use duplex ultrasound routinely for comprehensive surgical planning and report excellent results, in terms of both examination success and surgical outcome. Advocates of comprehensive duplex arterial evaluation point out that ultrasound is cost-effective and noninvasive, and can be done in a clinical outpatient setting without the need for specialized facilities.[15-19] These advantages notwithstanding, most medical facilities continue to use ultrasound in a more tailored way, to answer specific questions raised by the H&P, physiological studies, or arteriography. The following are examples of clinical questions that can be addressed with this approach.

1. Where are significant arterial obstructions located? As noted previously, the H&P and physiological tests provide some information about the location of arterial occlusive disease, but this information may be quite sketchy. In addition, it may not be clear whether the disease is localized or diffuse, or whether the problem is stenosis or occlusion. An example is the patient with reduced upper thigh pressure on a segmental pressure examination. It may be unclear if obstruction is in the iliac system, the common femoral artery, the superficial femoral artery, or in more than one area. This information can be conveniently obtained with duplex examination of the common femoral artery and the origin of the superficial femoral artery, possibly supplemented with direct evaluation of the iliac arteries.
2. Is an arterial segment stenotic or occluded? Duplex sonography can reliably differentiate between arterial stenosis and occlusion, which is something that physiological tests and physical examination cannot do accurately.
3. Is there an iliac artery obstruction that is amenable to angioplasty? Iliac lesions are generally considered amenable to angioplasty when they are localized (not multisegment), less than 5 cm in length, and reduce the lumen diameter by at least 50%.[16] Eighty percent of iliac artery stenoses can be adequately evaluated with ultrasound, and the concordance between sonography and angiography is 92% for determining if the stenosis

can be treated with angioplasty or is better treated surgically.[15–19]

4. Is an arteriographically identified stenosis hemodynamically significant? Even when carefully performed, CTA, MRA, or catheter arteriography may produce indeterminate results regarding the hemodynamic significance of stenotic lesions. Duplex examination of the arteriographically equivocal stenosis may be very useful for assessing the hemodynamic significance of such lesions, facilitating interventional or surgical planning.

5. What is the status of potential run-off vessels in the calf? Arteriography, regardless of the method used, sometimes fails to adequately define the presence, condition, and length of potential arterial bypass run-off vessels in the calf. Although duplex sonography, as noted previously, is far from perfect for evaluating infrapopliteal arteries,[13,20] it *can* visualize some infrapopliteal arteries with great clarity when the vessels are relatively disease free and not heavily calcified. Thus, ultrasound is sometimes very useful as a means for determining which of the three main arterial trunks in the calf (anterior tibial, posterior tibial, or peroneal arteries) are patent, and which is sufficiently disease-free for use as a bypass target.

6. Is a pseudoaneurysm or arteriovenous fistula present? Pseudoaneurysms (false aneurysms or pulsating hematomas) and arteriovenous fistulas may be caused by violent or iatrogenic trauma (usually in the context of cardiac catheterization or angiographic procedures). These conditions cannot be accurately diagnosed clinically, but are readily detected with ultrasound.

7. Guidance for angioplasty. In recent years, it has become apparent that ultrasound is an excellent means for directing angioplasty in both the iliac and femoral arteries. Eighty percent of angioplasties can be completed successfully with ultrasound guidance alone, assuming that preprocedure case selection (see earlier discussion) is thorough.[21] Ultrasound performs as well as angiography for determining balloon size, monitoring guidewire passage, directing dilatation, and judging procedure success.

8. What is the status of the circulation following arterial bypass grafting or angioplasty? Perhaps the most widespread use of duplex arterial ultrasound is for sequential postprocedure evaluation of arterial bypass grafts and femoropopliteal stents. Ultrasound effectively detects graft or postangioplasty stenosis before signs or symptoms of ischemia occur and before change is apparent in the physiological tests, such as the ABI. There is substantial evidence that timely detection of stenoses with ultrasound improves primary graft patency and is beneficial postangioplasty, as compared with surveillance by physical examination or pressure measurements.[22–25]

Duplex Ultrasound for Arterial Examination of Extremity

Ultrasound examination of extremity arteries should be conducted in a warm room to avoid vasoconstriction. The patient should be comfortable because the examination may take some time. The diagnostic criteria that are widely used for grading stenoses have been described for resting patients. Additional postexercise assessment may be conducted, as discussed later. Because duplex examinations are usually focused on specific areas of concern, the sonographer should clearly understand the diagnostic objective before beginning the study. This may entail discussion with the referring practitioner, chart review, or review of other imaging studies, such as MRA or CTA.

Begin the duplex examination with color Doppler imaging of the artery of interest, and get oriented. Trace the course of the artery to get an overview of the entire arterial segment (e.g., the entire common and external iliac segment) rather than initially focusing on a specific obstructive lesion. During this survey, look for areas of high velocity or disturbed flow, as well as arterial occlusion (absence of flow). If obstructive lesions are present, first determine where they are located anatomically, and systematically record color and spectral Doppler information related to individual lesions. Important color Doppler findings include the approximate length of the stenosis, the size of the residual lumen (if adequately visualized), the presence or absence of high-velocity flow, and the presence or absence of poststenotic flow disturbances.

Doppler stenosis assessment entails the recording of Doppler spectral waveforms, including measurements of peak-systolic and end-diastolic velocities, proximal to the stenosis, within the stenotic segment, immediately distal to the stenosis (for poststenotic turbulence), and farther distal (to detect waveform damping). This information should be obtained for each discrete region of narrowing within the arterial segment of interest.

Duplex Doppler Criteria for Grading Stenoses

The normal values for arterial diameter and peak systolic velocity (PSV) have been determined for lower extremity arteries in adults (**Table 2–1**).[26,27] Lower-extremity arterial stenoses generally reach hemodynamic significance, meaning that a pressure gradient can be measured across the stenosis, when the lumen diameter is reduced by 50%.[28] Doppler diagnostic criteria have been established for this degree of stenosis, as well as severe stenosis that reduces the lumen diameter by 70% or more. The principal Doppler criterion is the systolic velocity ratio, which is the PSV in the stenosis divided by the PSV *proximal* to the stenosis. A ratio of 2 or greater (i.e., a doubling of the PSV) generally indicates ≥ 50% stenosis, and a ratio of 3.3 generally indicates ≥ 70% stenosis.[10–12,26,29–32] Other criteria for grading stenoses are the shape of the Doppler waveform in and distal to the

Table 2-1 Normal Diameters and Peak Systolic Velocities for Lower Extremity Arteries*

Artery	Diameter (mm)	Peak Systolic Velocity (cm/s)
Common iliac	7.9–12.1	
Common femoral	6.6–9.6	89–141
Superficial femoral	4.3–7.2	77–108
Popliteal	4.1–6.3	55–82

*Common iliac diameter measurements from Pedersen OM, Aslaksen A, Vik-Mo H. Ultrasound measurement of the luminal diameter of the abdominal aorta and iliac arteries in patients without vascular disease. J Vasc Surg 1993;17:596–601. Remainder of data from Jager KA, Ricketts HI, Strandness DE. Duplex scanning for the evaluation of lower limb arterial disease. In: Bernstein EF, ed. Noninvasive Diagnostic Techniques in Vascular Disease. St. Louis: Mosby; 1985:876–892. Note: Pedersen OM et al report that the common iliac arteries in older adults are commonly ectatic and should not be considered abnormal unless they exceed 14 mm diameter in men or 12 mm in women, or are focally dilated.

stenosis, and the degree of poststenotic flow disturbance. The entire Doppler system for grading lower extremity arterial stenoses is summarized in **Table 2–2**. After reviewing the diagnostic criteria in this table, the reader should examine the examples of minor, moderate, and severe stenosis illustrated in **Fig. 2–3, Fig. 2–4, Fig. 2–5**. These examples convey a sense of how different levels of stenosis are differentiated with Doppler sonography.

Duplex Doppler Accuracy in Grading Stenoses

Table 2–3[10–12,26,29–32] lists the results of validation studies of lower extremity duplex sonography, using the Doppler criteria summarized in **Table 2–2**. On review of these data, it is apparent that false-positive diagnosis of stenosis (≥ 50% diameter) is uncommon because specificity is high in all reported series. False-negative examinations are more of a problem, as **Table 2–3** shows. This problem has also been emphasized by Coffi et al,[33] who report that a systolic ratio of 2.0 is only ~74% sensitive for pressure-reducing iliac artery lesions when Doppler findings are compared with intraarterial pressure measurements (which more accurately define hemodynamic significance than angiography). This means that up to one fourth of iliac artery stenoses of proven hemodynamic significance may go untreated when evaluated solely with duplex sonography. Although Coffi et al only studied the iliac arteries, it is possible that the same problem applies to femoral and popliteal stenoses.

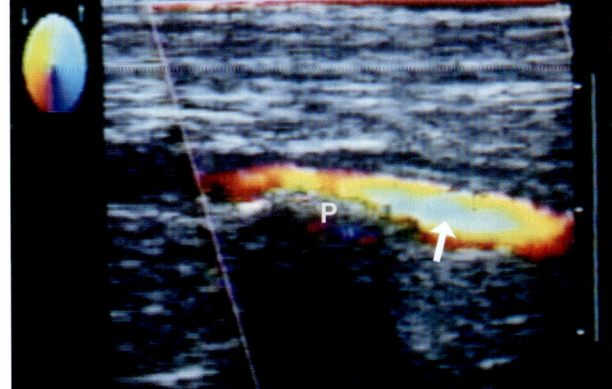

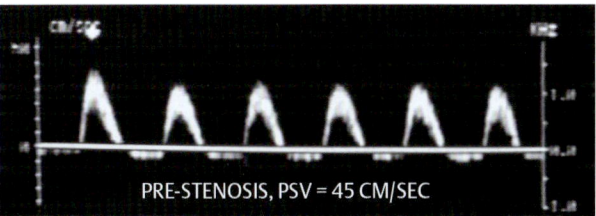

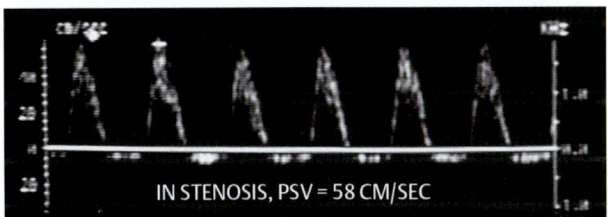

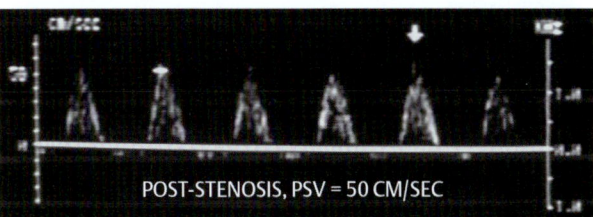

Figure 2–3 Mild arterial stenosis that is not hemodynamically significant. **(A)** Color Doppler image shows plaque (P) in the superficial femoral artery that generates a region of increased velocity (arrow), but no appreciable poststenotic flow disturbance. **(B)** Prestenotic peak systolic velocity is 45 cm/s. **(C)** In the stenotic region, the Doppler waveform is biphasic and the peak systolic velocity is 58 cm/s. Systolic velocity ratio is 1.3. **(D)** Poststenotic Doppler waveforms are biphasic and not damped, with peak systolic velocity similar to the prestenotic velocity. This constellation of findings indicates that lumenal diameter reduction is less than 50%, and the stenosis is not hemodynamically significant.

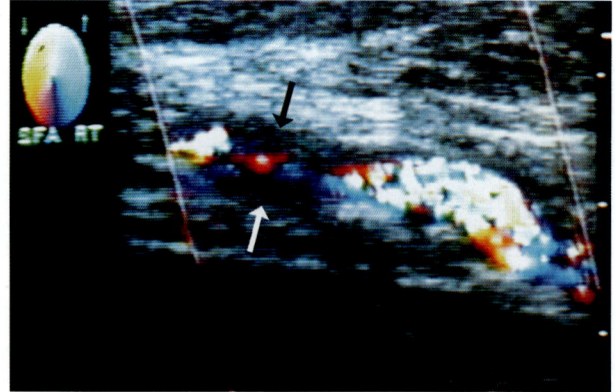
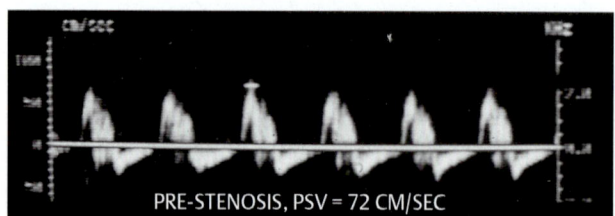
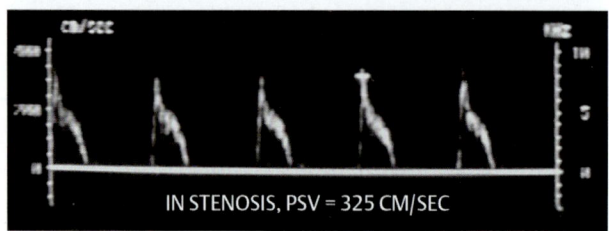
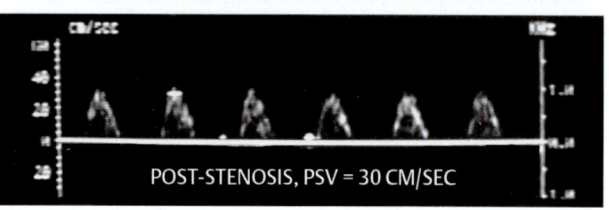

Figure 2–4 Moderate arterial stenosis. **(A)** Color Doppler image shows substantial narrowing of the superficial femoral artery accompanied by moderate poststenotic flow disturbance. **(B)** In the prestenotic region, the peak systolic velocity is 72 cm/s, and the Doppler waveforms are biphasic. **(C)** In the stenosis, the peak systolic velocity is 325 cm/s, and the systolic velocity ratio is 4.5. The Doppler waveforms are monophasic, but without diastolic flow. **(D)** In the poststenotic region, Doppler waveforms are monophasic and slightly damped, and peak systolic velocity is low.

Table 2–2 Doppler Criteria for Lower Extremity Arterial Stenosis

Minor stenosis (<50% diameter reduction)

Within stenosis
1. PSV < double prestenosis PSV
2. Biphasic or triphasic waveform
3. Reverse flow waveform component present

Pre-/poststenosis
1. Waveforms and flow velocity normal prestenosis
2. Disturbed flow immediately beyond stenosis. Normal waveforms farther distal to stenosis

Severe stenosis (50–75% diameter reduction)

Within stenosis
1. PSV ≥ 2 times prestenotic PSV
2. Reverse component absent
3. End diastolic velocity < prestenotic PSV

Pre-/poststenosis
1. Possible reduced velocity pre- and poststenosis (due to flow reduction)
2. Disturbed flow immediately poststenosis
3. Possible damped waveforms farther distal to stenosis

Very severe stenosis (> 75% diameter reduction)
1. Same as 50–75% stenosis, but–
2. End diastolic velocity in stenosis > PSV prestenosis

Dual-phase Doppler stenosis evaluation has been proposed as a method for boosting duplex ultrasound sensitivity for hemodynamically significant stenoses. With this method, Doppler evaluation is conducted first with the patient at rest and then either following exercise or following administration of papaverine (vasodilator). A postexercise/papaverine PSV increase of 140 to 160 cm/s (or greater) *within the stenosis* proves hemodynamic significance with sensitivity of 93% or greater and no substantial loss of resting measurement specificity (~88%).[34–36] Postexercise or papaverine testing is not needed for stenoses with a systolic ratio of 3.5 or greater because the hemodynamic significance of such lesions is unquestioned.

Localized stenoses are most easily and accurately evaluated with duplex ultrasound. Diffuse disease is a diagnostic problem because it is difficult to get a visual sense of stenosis location and severity. This problem is compounded by plaque calcification and tortuosity, which make it difficult to visualize and follow the arterial lumen. As a result, patients with diffuse, severe arterial disease are better evaluated angiographically. Diffuse or multisegment occlusive disease also reduces the accuracy of Doppler measurements because each area of stenosis imposes physiological effects on more distal stenoses.[37] Finally, stenoses at vessel origins are also problems because no prestenotic velocity is available for measuring the systolic velocity ratio.

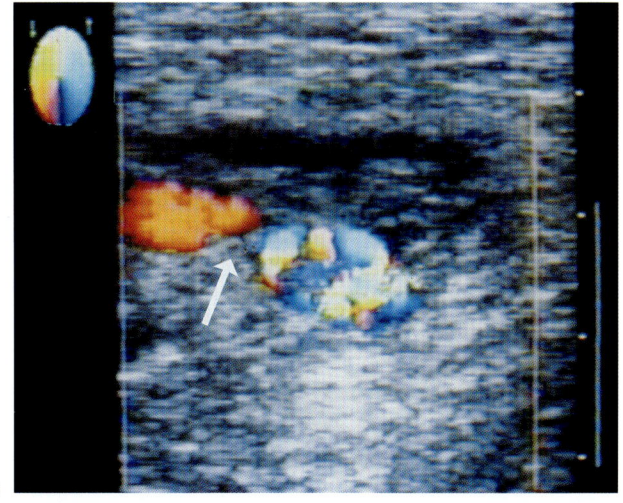
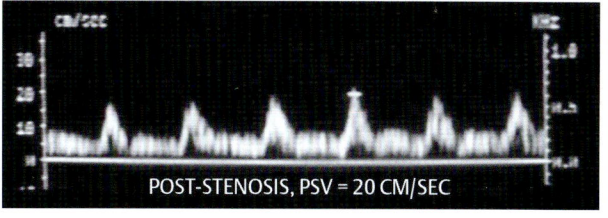
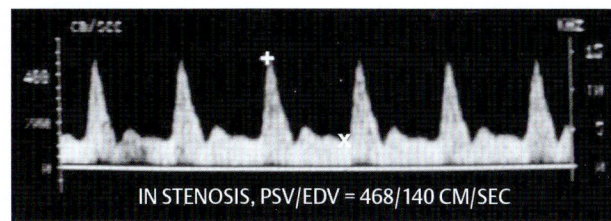
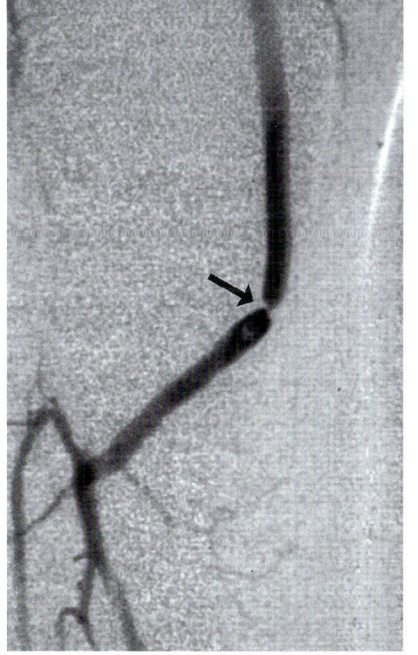

Figure 2–5 Severe arterial stenosis. **(A)** Color Doppler examination of this reversed vein graft shows an eccentric, focal area of narrowing (*arrow*) accompanied by severe poststenotic flow disturbance. **(B)** The prestenotic peak systolic velocity is 42 cm/s. **(C)** Within the stenosis, peak systolic velocity is 468 cm/s, there is a large amount of diastolic flow, and end diastolic velocity is 140 cm/s. The systolic velocity ratio is 11.2, and the end diastolic velocity exceeds the prestenotic peak systolic velocity. **(D)** Poststenotic Doppler waveforms are damped, peak systolic velocity is very low, and there is a large amount of flow throughout diastole. **(E)** Digital subtraction arteriogram confirming the ultrasound findings.

Duplex Doppler Diagnosis of Occlusion

Arterial occlusion is diagnosed on the basis of absent blood flow and damped arterial Doppler waveforms distal to the occluded segment. The diagnosis of occlusion is generally straightforward, but a few words of caution are in order. First, be sure that your instrument is set to detect low-velocity flow. Otherwise, you may miss a "trickle" of flow in a highly stenosed vessel and make a false-positive diagnosis of occlusion. Second, double check with spectral Doppler to confirm the color Doppler impression of arterial occlusion. Spectral Doppler may be more sensitive to low-flow states than color Doppler.

Duplex Doppler Bypass Graft Examination

The great majority of infrainguinal lower extremity bypass grafts are created with autologous vein (usually

Table 2-3 Accuracy, Lower Extremity Arterial Duplex

	% Stenosis*	Sensitivity	Specificity
Jager et al 1985[26]	≥ 50	77	98
Kohler et al 1987[29]	≥ 50	82	92
Moneta et al 1993[31]	≥ 50	67–89	97–99
Visser and Hunink 2000[32]**	≥ 50	88	95

*Diameter reduction.
**Pooled data from 21 published series.

greater saphenous). Much less commonly, synthetic graft material is used in the femoropopliteal area. Vein graft stenosis or occlusion usually occurs during the first 2 postoperative years, and surveillance (clinical, ABI, and duplex ultrasound) is most frequent during this period—generally at 3, 6, 12, 18, and 24 months. After 2 years, the graft failure (occlusion) rate is only ~2 to 4% per year[38]; therefore, the surveillance interval is reduced to yearly. Duplex graft surveillance substantially improves graft patency rates and has become a standard of care in Western nations.[22–24,39,40] Additional details about graft procedures and follow-up not covered here can be found elsewhere.[24]

It is generally much easier to examine grafts with duplex sonography than native arteries; nonetheless, you can still save a lot of time and aggravation (and avoid errors) if you know the surgical anatomy before setting out on a duplex graft examination. If a preceding graft study is available, the findings should always be reviewed prior to starting the current examination.

We begin the duplex examination at the proximal anastomosis because this is usually more easily found than the distal anastomosis. Using color Doppler, the sonographer examines the inflow (supply) artery and then follows the course of the graft to the distal anastomosis, noting the location of any visibly narrowed segment or flow abnormality (elevated flow velocity or turbulence). If the graft appears normal, the sonographer pauses during the survey examination to obtain Doppler waveform and PSV measurements at three or four locations within the graft, as well as in the inflow artery proximal to the graft, the proximal and distal anastomoses, and the run-off artery distal to the graft. It is extremely important to identify the proximal and distal anastomoses of arterial bypass grafts because stenoses commonly occur at these locations. That being said, however, it should be noted that slight velocity elevation and flow disturbances are commonly encountered at the anastomoses in normally functioning grafts, and these findings should not be overdiagnosed as functionally significant. It is also important to visualize several centimeters of the run-off vessel distal to the graft to detect stenoses that may put the graft at risk of failure.

There is no "normal" definition for graft Doppler findings because every graft is, in a sense, a rule unto itself. Nevertheless, Doppler waveforms within the graft and runoff vessel should have a sharp upstroke in systole and high resistance features (with the patient at rest), including a sharp, narrow systolic peak and absence of late diastolic flow. Graft waveform shape is frequently biphasic but ranges from monophasic to triphasic in normally functioning grafts. The most important normal feature of graft waveforms is stability over time, both in shape and in PSV. Femoral–distal grafts generally have PSVs under 100 cm/s, but graft diameter varies from place to place, and higher PSVs may be encountered in relatively narrow portions of normally functioning grafts. A midgraft PSV of less than 40 cm/s (possibly indicating a low level of flow) is worrisome with respect to potential graft failure, but this finding is not an absolute predictor of doom because low flow velocity has not proven to be an accurate predictor of graft failure.[24,39,40] This is particularly true for grafts that feed into small, distal tibial arteries that have limited flow capacity. Damped Doppler waveforms, with a pulsus parvus tardus configuration, are never normal in a graft or run-off vessel and should prompt a search for arterial obstruction in the graft or inflow artery.

Despite the earlier statement, forward flow late in diastole is commonly seen in grafts for several months following surgery. Ordinarily, forward flow throughout diastole is a sign of tissue ischemia distal to the graft and is worrisome, but in the postoperative period this represents an unexplained physiological phenomenon that is self-limiting. In patients with far-distal tibial anastomoses, forward diastolic flow may be present permanently, probably due to persistent low resistance in the large volume of tissues supplied by a relatively small artery.

When focal flow disturbance and high velocity are detected during graft examination (**Fig. 2–5**), the diagnostic criteria described in **Table 2–2** should be used to evaluate stenosis severity. A PSV of 125 cm/s is the threshold value for concern about graft stenosis; however, velocities up to 180 cm/s, or even higher, can occasionally be seen in normally functioning grafts.

Furthermore, it is well documented that stenoses in the first few months after surgery commonly regress spontaneously.[24,39] Progression of stenosis severity over time, therefore, is often the most important indication of functional significance. Graft stenoses with PSVs exceeding 300 cm/s and systolic velocity ratios exceeding 3.5 generally benefit from surgical repair or angioplasty, whereas those with lower values can generally be followed.[24,39,40] In clear-cut, uncomplicated cases, surgical repair can be performed on the basis of ultrasound findings, and arteriography is not needed. The location of the stenosis is simply marked on the skin before the patient is taken to the operating room.

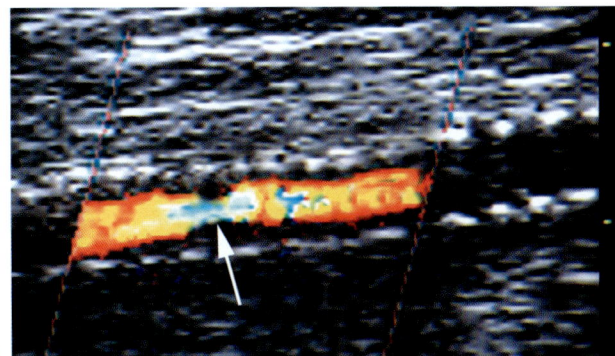
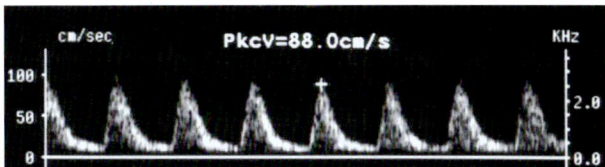
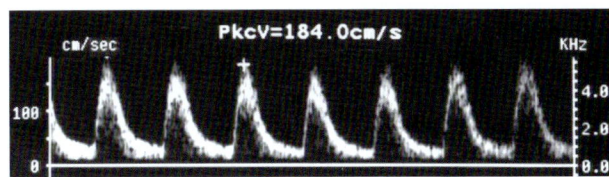
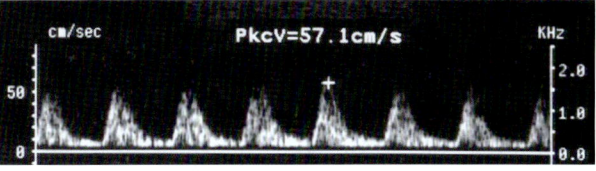

Figure 2–6 Arterial stent stenosis. **(A)** Strong reflections from the metallic stent are easily seen on this color Doppler image. Note the flow void between the stent and the lumen due to fibrointimal hyperplasia. A stenosis results that is moderately severe by visual assessment. **(B)** The prestenotic Doppler waveforms are monophasic due to diffuse arterial disease with stenosis proximal to the stent. Peak systolic velocity (PckV) is 88 cm/s. **(C)** Within the stent stenosis, PckV is slightly more than doubled, at 184 cm/s, indicating hemodynamic significance, but not critical narrowing. **(D)** Doppler waveforms distal to the stenosis are slightly more damped and lower in velocity (PckV 57 cm/s) than those recorded proximal to the stenosis, suggesting that this stenosis is affecting blood flow.

Duplex Doppler Postangioplasty Examination

Balloon angioplasty, with or without stenting, is the principal means for treating isolated iliac artery stenoses. Postprocedure surveillance after iliac angioplasty is with clinical evaluation, ABI measurement, and femoral Doppler waveform assessment. Duplex Doppler is not routinely used. It has been shown that femoral artery Doppler waveforms are highly accurate for detection of hemodynamically significant iliac artery stenosis. For monophasic or biphasic common femoral Doppler waveforms (rather than normal triphasic waveforms) are 95% sensitive and 85% specific for ≥ 50% iliac artery stenosis. A monophasic femoral artery waveform with PSV ≤ 45 cm/s is 97% specific for iliac artery occlusion.[24,25,41,42] Postangioplasty Duplex sonography of the iliac arteries is reserved for cases with clinical, ABI, and Doppler findings, suggesting recurrent iliac stenosis.

Superficial femoral and popliteal artery angioplasty is routinely followed with duplex surveillance, owing to a high incidence of restenosis from fibrointimal hyperplasia. Wall stents are commonly deployed in conjunction with femoral angioplasty to suppress restenosis. Follow-up duplex surveillance is typically conducted within the first 24 hours after the procedure and then at 3 months, 6 months, and every sixth months thereafter.

On ultrasound examination, it is easy to find the treated portion of stented arteries because the metallic framework of the stent is readily visible (**Fig. 2–6**). Color flow Doppler images of the stented area are important to show that flow extends all the way to the stent surface. Fibrointimal hyperplasia causes a flow void between the stent and the lumen that may extend the full length of the stent and may not be evident on casual ultrasound examination. Postangioplasty stenoses are evaluated with color and spectral Doppler in the same fashion as stenoses in untreated native arteries and grafts. The diagnostic criteria are the same as those listed in **Table 2–2**. Repeat angioplasty or other therapy is considered for stenoses with a PSV of 300 cm/s or more and a systolic velocity ratio of 2 or higher.[24,25]

Summary

Walking-associated leg pain, in the form of intermittent claudication, is classically caused by arterial insufficiency; however, other conditions may cause walking-associated leg pain, including peripheral neuropathy, acute venous thrombosis, chronic venous thrombosis, muscular hematoma, and rupture of a popliteal cyst.

Diagnostic measures commonly used for assessing walking-related leg pain include the H&P, systolic blood pressure measurement (ABI and segmental pressures), plethysmography, Doppler and duplex ultrasound, and angiography. The H&P is accurate for diagnosis of arterial insufficiency that is moderate or severe, but physical examination is qualitative and subjective. Furthermore, mild arterial insufficiency cannot always be detected with physical examination. The ABI and plethysmography are highly sensitive for arterial insufficiency, especially when conducted following exercise, and serve well to differentiate between arterial insufficiency and other causes of leg pain. In addition, the ABI and segmental pressure measurements are quantitative and moderately accurate for localizing and following the progression of arterial obstruction. Duplex sonography is accurate for localizing and grading arterial occlusive lesions, both in native arteries and in arterial grafts (**Table 2–3**). Duplex sonography can be used for comprehensive presurgical planning, but is usually used for more focused diagnostic goals. Normal duplex arterial parameters and criteria for stenosis grading have been established (**Table 2–2**). Duplex ultrasound is well established as an effective method for follow-up surveillance following arterial bypass grafting and angioplasty.

References

1. Carter SA. Clinical problems in peripheral arterial disease: is the clinical diagnosis adequate? In: Bernstein EF, ed. Noninvasive Diagnostic Techniques in Vascular Disease. 4th ed. St. Louis: Mosby; 1993:471–480
2. Carter SA. Role of pressure measurements. In: Bernstein EF, ed. Noninvasive Diagnostic Techniques in Vascular Disease. 4th ed. St. Louis: Mosby; 1993:486–512
3. Nicolaides AN. Basic and practical aspects of peripheral arterial testing. In: Bernstein EF, ed. Noninvasive Diagnostic Techniques in Vascular Disease. 4th ed. St. Louis: Mosby; 1993:481–485
4. Zierler RE. Nonimaging physiological tests for assessment of lower extremity arterial occlusive disease. In: Zwiebel W, ed. Introduction to Vascular Sonography. 5th ed. Philadelphia: Elsevier/Saunders; 2005:275–296
5. Dorland's Medical Dictionary. 27th ed. Philadelphia: WB Saunders; 1988:343
6. DeMasi RJ, Gregory RT, Wheeler JR, et al. Exercise testing: diagnosis and follow-up. J Vasc Tech 1994;18:257–261
7. Macdonald NR. Pulse volume plethysmography. J Vasc Tech 1994;18:241–248
8. Hentsch A, Aschauer MA, Balzer JO, et al. Gadobutrol-enhanced moving-table magnetic resonance angiography in patients with peripheral vascular disease: a prospective, multi-centre blinded comparison with digital subtraction angiography. Eur Radiol 2003;13:2103–2114
9. Jakobs TF, Wintersperger BJ, Becker CR. MDCT-imaging of peripheral arterial disease. Semin Ultrasound CT MR 2004;25:145–155
10. Zierler RE. Ultrasound assessment of lower extremity arteries. In: Zwiebel W, ed. Introduction to Vascular Sonography. 5th ed. Philadelphia: Elsevier/Saunders; 2005:341–356
11. Kohler TR. Duplex scanning for the evaluation of lower limb arterial disease. In: Bernstein EF, ed. Noninvasive Diagnostic Techniques in Vascular Disease. St. Louis: Mosby; 1993:520–526
12. Polak JF. Arterial sonography: efficacy for the diagnosis of arterial disease of the lower extremity. AJR Am J Roentgenol 1993;161:235–243
13. Larch E, Minar E, Ahmadi R, et al. Value of color duplex sonography for evaluation of tibioperoneal arteries in patients with femoropopliteal obstruction: a prospective comparison with anterograde intraarterial digital subtraction angiography. J Vasc Surg 1997;25:629–636
14. Eiberg JP, Hansen MA, Jensen F, Rasmussen JB, Schroeder TV. Ultrasound contrast-agent improves imaging of lower limb occlusive disease. Eur J Vasc Endovasc Surg 2003;25:23–28
15. Kerr TM, Bandyk DF. Color duplex imaging of peripheral arterial disease before angioplasty or surgical intervention. In: Bernstein EF, ed. Noninvasive Diagnostic Techniques in Vascular Disease. 4th ed. St. Louis: Mosby; 1993:527–533
16. Back MR, Bowser AN, Schmacht DC, et al. Duplex selection facilitates single point-of-service endovascular and surgical management of aortoiliac occlusive disease. Ann Vasc Surg 2002;16:566–574
17. Bostrom Ardin A, Karacagil S, Hellberg A, et al. Surgical reconstruction without preoperative angiography in patients with aortoiliac occlusive disease. Ann Vasc Surg 2002;16:273–278
18. Schneider PA, Ogawa DY, Rush MP. Lower extremity revascularization without contrast arteriography: a prospective study of operation based upon duplex mapping. Cardiovasc Surg 1999;7:699–703
19. Ramaswami G, Al-Kutoubi A, Nicolaides AN, et al. The role of duplex scanning in the diagnosis of lower limb arterial disease. Ann Vasc Surg 1999;13:494–500
20. Hofmann WJ, Walter J, Ugurluoglu A, et al. Preoperative high-frequency duplex scanning of potential pedal target vessels. J Vasc Surg 2004;39:169–175
21. Ramaswami G, Al-Kutoubi A, Nicolaides AN, et al. Angioplasty of lower limb arterial stenoses under ultrasound guidance: single-center experience. J Endovasc Surg 1999;6:52–58
22. Beidle TR, Brom-Ferral R, Letourneau JG. Surveillance of infrainguinal vein grafts with duplex sonography. AJR Am J Roentgenol 1994;162:443–448
23. Kundell A, Linblad B, Bergqvist D, Hansen F. Femoropopliteal-crural graft patency is improved by an intensive surveillance program: a prospective randomized study. J Vasc Surg 1995;21:26–34
24. Bandyk DF. Ultrasound assessment during and after peripheral interventions. In: Zwiebel W, ed. Introduction to Vascular Sonography. 5th ed. Philadelphia: Elsevier/Saunders; 2005:257–280
25. Back MR, Novotney M, Roth SM, et al. Utility of duplex surveillance following iliac artery angioplasty and primary stenting. J Endovasc Ther 2001;8:629–637
26. Jager KA, Ricketts HI, Strandness DE. Duplex scanning for the evaluation of lower limb arterial disease. In: Bernstein EF, ed. Noninvasive Diagnostic Techniques in Vascular Disease. St. Louis: Mosby; 1985:876–892
27. Pedersen OM, Aslaksen A, Vik-Mo H. Ultrasound measurement of the luminal diameter of the abdominal aorta and iliac arteries in patients without vascular disease. J Vasc Surg 1993;17:596–601
28. Carter SA. Hemodynamic considerations in peripheral vascular disease. In: Zwiebel W, ed. Introduction to Vascular Sonography. 5th ed. Philadelphia: Elsevier/Saunders; 2005:3–18
29. Kohler TR, Nance DR, Cramer MM, et al. Duplex scanning for diagnosis of aortoiliac and femoro-popliteal disease. Circulation 1987;5:1074–1080
30. Moneta GL, Yeager RA, Antonovic R, et al. Accuracy of lower extremity arterial duplex mapping. J Vasc Surg 1992;15:275–284
31. Moneta GL, Yeager RA, Lee RW, et al. Noninvasive localization of arterial occlusive disease: a comparison of segmental Doppler pressures and arterial duplex mapping. J Vasc Surg 1993;17:578–582
32. Visser K, Hunink MG. Peripheral arterial disease: gadolinium-enhanced MR angiography versus color-guided duplex US: a meta-analysis. Radiology 2000;216:67–77
33. Coffi SB, Ubbink DT, Zwiers I, et al. The value of the peak systolic velocity ratio in the assessment of the haemodynamic significance of subcritical iliac artery stenoses. Eur J Vasc Endovasc Surg 2001;22:424–428
34. Coffi SB, Ubbink DT, Zwiers I, et al. Improved assessment of the hemodynamic significance of borderline iliac stenoses with use of hyperemic duplex scanning. J Vasc Surg 2002;36:575–580
35. Legemate DA, Teeuwen C, Hoeneveld H, Eikelboom BC. How can the assessment of the hemodynamic significance of aortoiliac arterial stenosis by duplex scanning be improved? A comparative

study with intraarterial pressure measurement. J Vasc Surg 1993; 17:676–684
36. Elsman BH, Legemate DA, de Vos HJ, et al. Hyperaemic colour duplex scanning for the detection of aortoiliac stenoses: a comparative study with intra-arterial pressure measurement. Eur J Vasc Endovasc Surg 1997;14:462–467
37. Allard L, Cloutier G, Durand LG, et al. Limitations of ultrasonic duplex scanning for diagnosing lower limb arterial stenoses in the presence of adjacent segment disease. J Vasc Surg 1994;19:650–657
38. Ihnat DM, Mills JL, Dawson DL, et al. The correlation of early flow disturbances with the development of infrainguinal graft stenosis: a 10-year study of 341 autogenous vein grafts. J Vasc Surg 1999; 30:8–15
39. Gahtan V, Payne LP, Roper LD, et al. Duplex criteria for predicting progression of vein graft lesions: which stenoses can be followed? J Vasc Tech 1995;19:211–215
40. Dalsing MC, Cikrit DF, Lalka SG, Sawchuk AP, Schulz C. Femorodistal vein grafts: the utility of graft surveillance criteria. J Vasc Surg 1995;21:127–134
41. Shaalan WE, French-Sherry E, Castilla M, et al. Reliability of common femoral artery hemodynamics in assessing the severity of aortoiliac inflow disease. J Vasc Surg 2003;37:960–969
42. Sensier Y, Bell PR, London NJ. The ability of qualitative assessment of the common femoral Doppler waveform to screen for significant aortoiliac disease. Eur J Vasc Endovasc Surg 1998;15: 357–364

3 Pulsatile Groin Mass in the Postcatheterization Patient

Barbara A. Carroll

Percutaneous catheterization of femoral vessels is a rapidly increasing method for performing diagnostic and therapeutic procedures as an alternative to more invasive surgical interventions. As the number of procedures and their complexity, utilizing larger vascular sheaths, lytic agents, and anticoagulants, increases, the number of postcatheterization groin complications has also grown. Although the majority of groin interventional procedures are followed by little more than a relatively small bruise, significant complications including large hematomas, pseudoaneurysms (PSAs), and arteriovenous fistulas (AVFs) can occur. The frequency of postcatheterization complications varies depending upon the nature of the intervention, whether diagnostic or therapeutic, and relative meticulousness of postsheath removal techniques utilized. Complication frequencies reportedly range from less than 1% for diagnostic catheterizations, up to 9% for coronary angioplasty, and as high as 16% following placement of an intracoronary stent.[1] Color Doppler ultrasound is now the preferred technique for evaluating potential groin complications related to femoral artery catheterization.[2-5] The color Doppler findings characteristic of these complications will be presented, including unusual complications, potential diagnostic pitfalls, and an approach to ultrasound-guided compression pseudoaneurysm repair.

Diagnostic Evaluation

Ultrasound Imaging

The majority of patients referred for a groin ultrasound examination after femoral artery catheterization have a palpable mass. These masses may be pulsatile and/or associated with a new bruit or palpable thrill. Color Doppler ultrasound provides a rapid, relatively pain free, portable imaging technique that can readily discern the cause of these auscultatory and palpable abnormalities. The examination is usually performed using a 5 MHz linear array transducer; however, a 7.5 MHz may be used for thin patients or for superficial lesions, whereas for obese patients or those with large hematomas overlying the vascular structures, a 3.5 MHz transducer may be required.

The examination consists of color and pulsed Doppler evaluation of the groin vessels beginning at the region of the inguinal ligament above the puncture site, then at and below the puncture site. Color Doppler should be used to confirm the patency of the femoral artery and vein and search the extravascular soft tissues for evidence of large hematomas, PSAs, or AVFs. The color Doppler gain threshold and flow detection parameters should be adjusted so that color fills the artery and vein, but does not "bleed over" into the adjacent soft tissues. It may be necessary to decrease the gain or increase the pulse repetition frequency (PRF) to visualize the artery and vein if a significant color Doppler bruit secondary to an AVF is present. Similarly, gain and threshold adjustments may be necessary to eliminate color noise artificially written into soft tissues, such as hematomas, which may be confused with PSAs (**Fig. 3–1A,B**). A complete ultrasound evaluation of the postcatheterization groin rarely takes more than 15 to 20 minutes. Alternative imaging tests are rarely needed; however, occasionally computed tomography (CT) will be obtained to evaluate the extent of a retroperitoneal hematoma related to postcatheterization complications, and arteriography may occasionally be needed before surgical or percutaneous interventions.

Hematomas

Virtually all patients who have undergone a groin catheterization have a small, localized hematoma or bruise. However, when the ecchymosis is extensive or there is a palpable mass, which may be pulsatile, patients are usually referred for color Doppler sonography. Localized hematomas present as discrete hypo- to anechoic masses that do not contain blood flow. Color Doppler noise may appear in a hematoma if gain settings are not optimized; pulsed Doppler interrogation will show the absence of a characteristic signal (**Fig. 3–2**). Large hematomas may compress and displace femoral vessels posteriorly such that they are beyond the penetration range of higher-frequency range transducers (**Fig. 3–3**). A localized hematoma and a thrombosed PSA are indistinguishable in appearance. Occasionally a hypoechoic tract leading from the vessel to the thrombosed PSA will be seen. Although hematomas and thrombosed PSAs are both avascular, inflammatory hypervascularity may be seen surrounding

3 Pulsatile Groin Mass in the Postcatheterization Patient

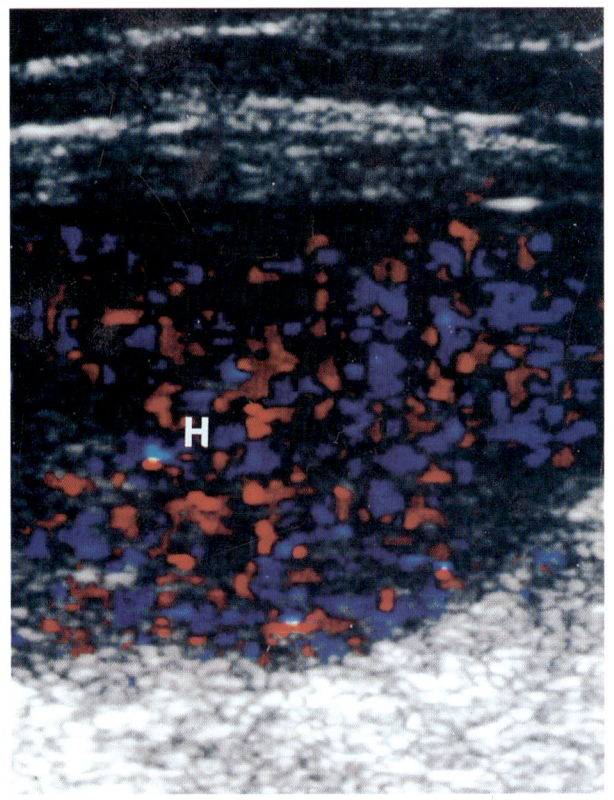
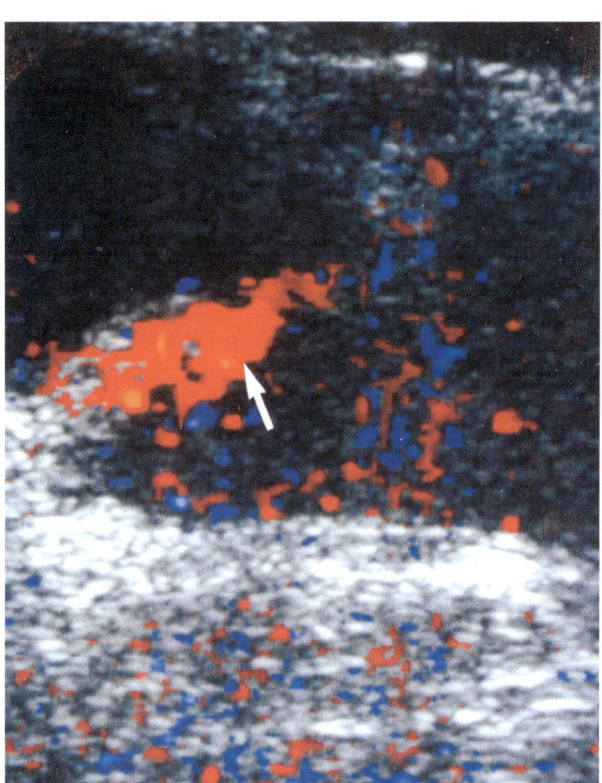

Figure 3–1 (A) A large right thigh hematoma (H) is filled with red and blue color Doppler "noise" related to transmitted motion created by intermittent venous leakage into the large mass. **(B)** The area of the intermittent vascular leak (arrow) is seen. The area of the low-velocity venous leak vanished by the end of the examination.

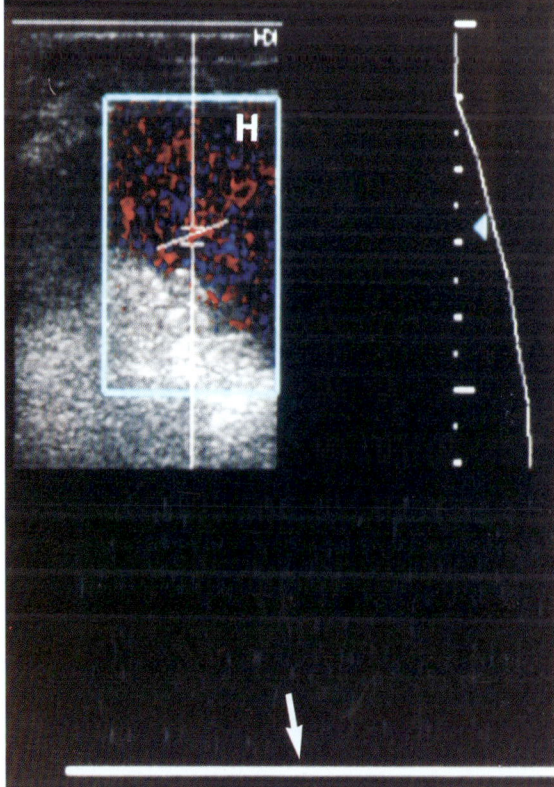

Figure 3–2 Pulsed Doppler analysis of color Doppler noise transmitted into a soft tissue hematoma (H) shows absence of flow (arrow).

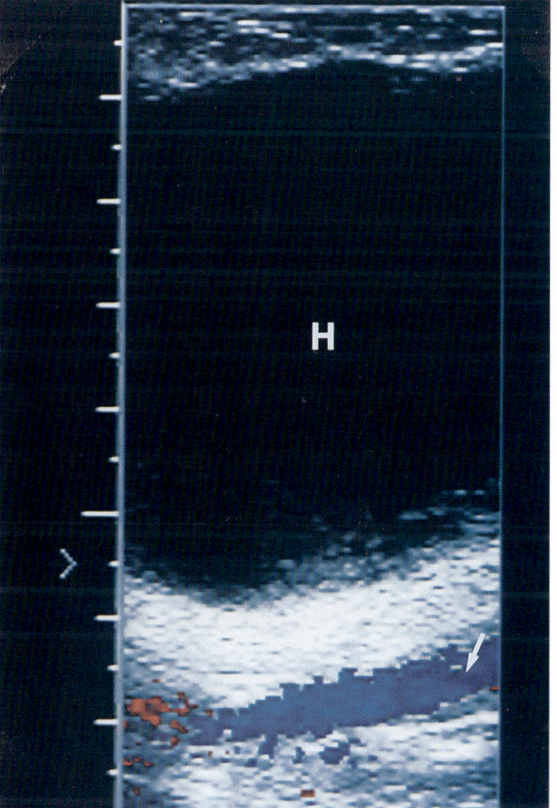

Figure 3–3 Large-groin hematoma (H) displaces the common femoral vein (arrow) posteriorly and compresses it.

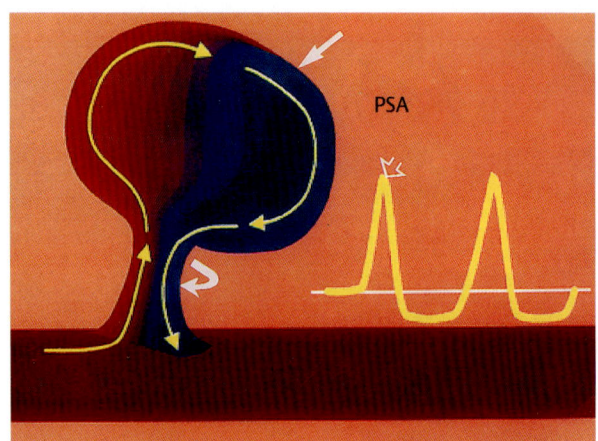

Figure 3–4 **(A)** Diagrammatic representation of a pseudoaneurysm demonstrates the characteristic "yin-yang" color Doppler pattern within the pseudoaneurysm (arrow) and the characteristic to-and-fro waveform (open arrow) obtained from the region of the pseudoaneurysm neck (curved arrow). **(B)** Duplex color Doppler image of a pseudoaneurysm (P). Note the characteristic red and blue flow pattern within the pseudoaneurysm. The pulsed Doppler waveform obtained from the neck (arrow) demonstrates the characteristic to-and-fro (open arrows) waveform.

hematomas. Additionally, actively bleeding jets may be seen into a rapidly expanding hematoma (**Fig. 3–1B**). Many clinically obvious hematomas are difficult to recognize on ultrasound because the hemorrhage has infiltrated diffusely into the soft tissues of the thigh or retroperitoneum, resulting in diffuse distortion of architecture and often suboptimal ultrasound penetration, but no discrete mass. Sonography is relatively insensitive for the evaluation of pelvic side wall or retroperitoneal hematomas. If a patient experiences a significant hematocrit drop or severe back pain following catheterization, CT is usually indicated as a means of evaluating the presence and extent of a retroperitoneal hematoma.

Pseudoaneurysms

Following femoral arterial sheath removal, the artery is manually compressed to assure hemostasis at the puncture site. Typically, 15 minutes of manual compression are required following diagnostic procedures; however, therapeutic procedures may require longer periods of compression, particularly if anticoagulation is continued. A recent study showed that the incidence of PSA development following arterial catheterization was related to the type of intervention, with therapeutic procedures having a higher incidence of PSAs.[5] However, the greatest risk factor for developing a PSA, regardless of the type of intervention, was too brief a period of manual compression following sheath removal. If the arterial wall defect fails to seal, then pulsatile blood jets from the artery into the adjacent perivascular soft tissues. This hematoma connects with the artery via a neck or tract and is largely contained within the soft tissues. Although these contained hematomas are referred to as PSAs, they do not have the characteristic fibrous wall of a true PSA; thus some feel it is more accurate to refer to these masses as pulsatile hematomas.[2]

Color Doppler examination readily distinguishes PSAs from other pulsatile masses in the postcatheterization groin. Sonographic features of a PSA include the detection of a vascular mass connected to the artery by a neck or tract. During systole there is antegrade flow into the PSA through the neck (**Fig. 3–4A,B**). During diastole, the increased pressure in the PSA, vis-à-vis the underlying artery results in a retrograde flow out of the PSA through the neck and back into the artery. This results in a characteristic "to-and-fro" pulsed Doppler waveform in the PSA neck and produces a characteristic "yin-yang" swirling

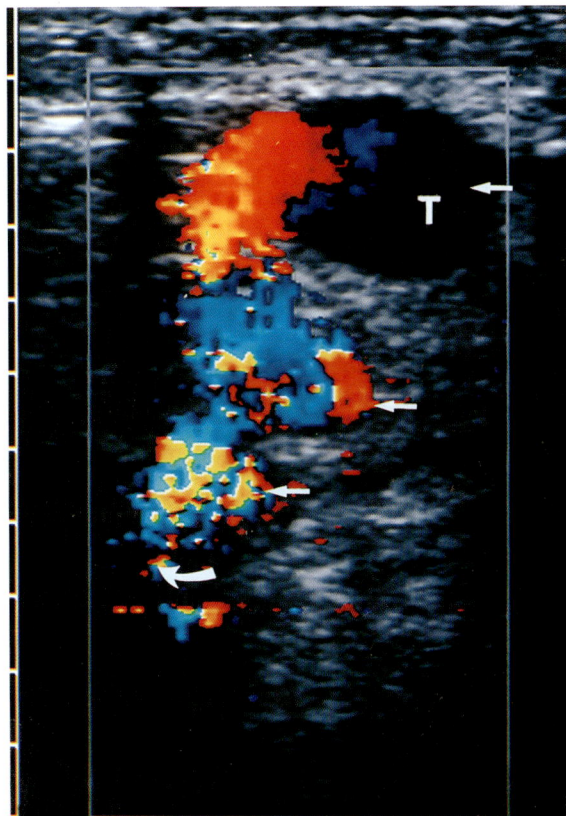

Figure 3-5 Trilobed pseudoaneurysm. The three lobes of the pseudoaneurysm (arrows) are seen arising from a single neck (curved arrow). Thrombus (T) is seen obliterating part of the lumen of the most superficial lobe.

color flow pattern within the body of the PSA. Some PSAs may be multilobed, producing a "string-of-beads" appearance (**Fig. 3-5**). These probably result from more extensive dissection of blood along fascial planes. Although two separate PSAs can occur following multiple punctures, multilobulated PSAs usually arise from a single puncture and interconnect between the artery and the multiple lobes. PSAs may also coexist with AVFs. In such cases, the Doppler features of either or both of the complications may be seen (**Fig. 3-6A-C**). These patients may present with a bruit and a pulsatile mass. Some patients may demonstrate a linear track of blood flow that follows the expected track of the needle or sheath from the artery toward the actual puncture site.[6] These tracks may represent an abortive form of a PSA. However, these are very narrow, with varying waveforms not characteristic for a PSA. These tracks do not seem to be clinically important, nor do they appear to require further imaging or treatment if they are observed as isolated findings.

Complications of PSAs including pain, infection, and compressive neuropathy, and most critically, rupture, can occur. Fortunately, this dire consequence is rare, but because this complication has such a potentially disastrous outcome, PSAs have been considered surgical emergencies. Recent studies have shown that PSAs are more benign and self-limited complications than previously thought.[7-9] Indeed, the majority of PSAs reported in many series have spontaneously thrombosed, suggesting that close monitoring and no further treatment may be sufficient. The majority of PSAs thrombose spontaneously within a week, and if imaged serially will demonstrate progressive thrombus of the PSA. PSAs with relatively small volumes of pulsatile flow and those with long necks are more likely to thrombose than will those with larger-flow volumes and short or wide necks.

Ultrasound-Guided Compression

Ultrasound-guided compression therapy has been enthusiastically welcomed as an alternative to surgery.[10-12] This time-consuming, relatively noninvasive procedure obviates the need for surgical groin incisions, which tend to heal poorly in these patients. Another attractive aspect of this procedure is that there is no need for the expense of operating room time. Although this procedure is less invasive, it is potentially painful, and intravenous sedation is frequently needed.

The procedure consists of obtaining informed consent and administering pain medications and sedation as needed. The ultrasound transducer is then used to locate the PSA neck. Vigorous manual compression is applied directly to the PSA neck to determine if blood flow into the PSA can be completely obliterated (**Fig. 3-7A-C**). Distal arterial pulses are checked to determine that arterial blood flow is maintained during this compression. If the PSA flow is obliterated and the arterial flow distally is maintained, then compression is continued for cycles of 20 minutes followed by a brief check of the status of the PSA. Arterial blood flow can be monitored either with color Doppler or by checking the dorsalis pedis or posterior tibial pulses manually or with a handheld Doppler during the procedure. We have found it helpful to approach this procedure as a tandem, with operators switching after each 20 minute period. We continue compressing the PSA for 20 minute intervals, stopping for as brief a period as possible between intervals until the PSA completely thromboses. Usually PSAs are completely obliterated within 1 hour. However, in some cases compression fails. If after 60 minutes of compression there is no evidence of thrombus formation and no change, or even a slight increase, in size of the PSA, the procedure is terminated. If, however, the PSA has demonstrated significant thrombus but remains patent at 1 hour, we will continue compressing at 20 minute intervals until such time as the PSA is completely obliterated or further observations demonstrate no further progress.

For the past 8 to 9 years, most pseudoaneurysms have been treated with direct injection of thrombin into the PSA under ultrasound guidance.[13,14] The presence of a PSA is

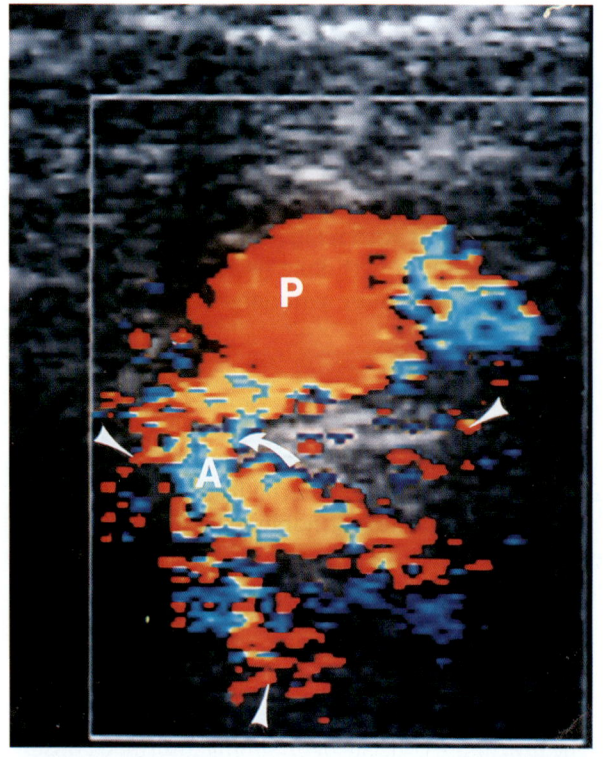
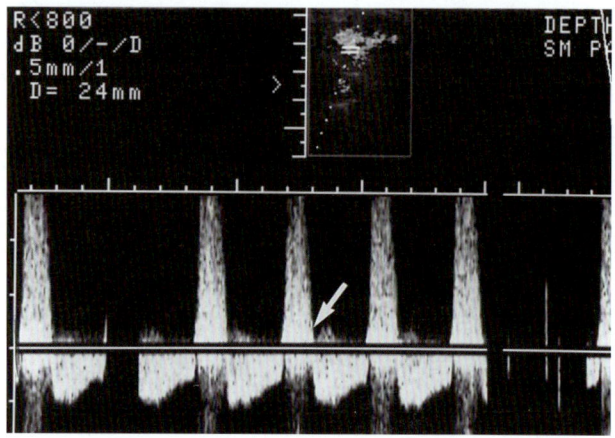
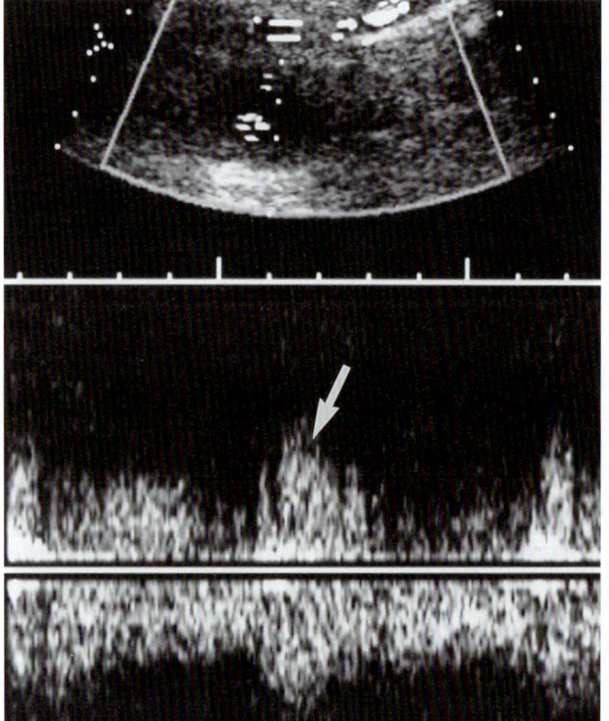

Figure 3–6 (A) A color Doppler image of a pseudoaneurysm–arteriovenous fistula combination demonstrates the pseudoaneurysm (P) with its neck (curved arrow) and a large amount of soft tissue speckling (arrowheads). Common femoral artery (A). **(B)** The neck of the pseudoaneurysm demonstrates characteristic to-and-fro waveforms (arrow). **(C)** Pulsed Doppler waveforms obtained from a small fistulous track arising from the pseudoaneurysm and connecting with the greater saphenous vein demonstrates low-resistance "turbulent" arterial waveforms (arrow).

confirmed by a real-time ultrasound examination. The location of the neck of the PSA is defined and the relationship to the underlying artery is defined. Informed consent is obtained after discussion of the procedure and alternative therapies. The groin is scanned using a 5 to 8 MHz transducer, using a linear or curvilinear array to confirm the anatomy of the PSA and surrounding vessels. A biopsy guide is attached to the transducer and a 22-gauge needle is advanced into the PSA, taking care to avoid the PSA neck. A 1-mL needle is filled with 600 U/mL of bovine thrombin.

The color Doppler is turned off to facilitate localization of the needle during placement. (**Fig. 3–8A-C**). Once

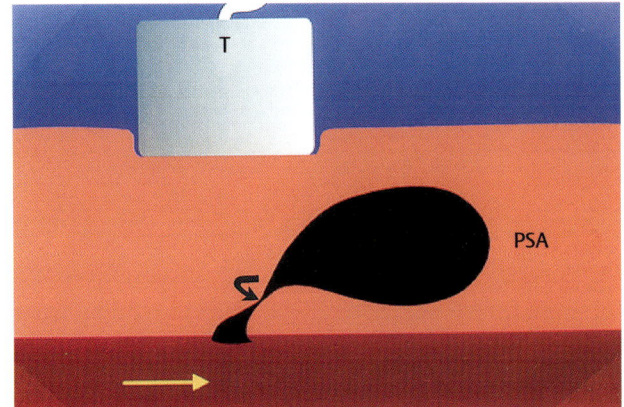

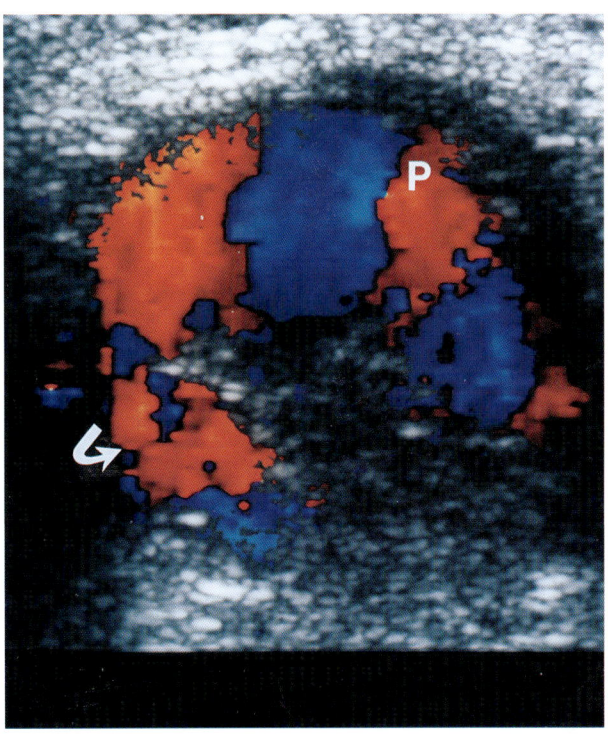

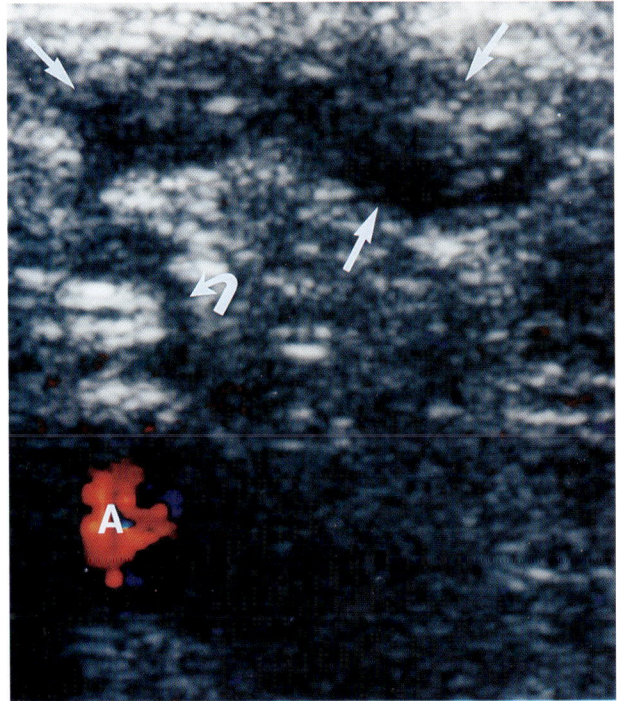

Figure 3–7 (A) A diagrammatic representation of pseudoaneurysm compression demonstrates how the transducer (T) is used to apply pressure over the neck of the pseudoaneurysm (curved arrow) to obliterate flow within the pseudoaneurysm. **(B)** Pseudoaneurysm (P) with a long neck (curved arrow) prior to compression. **(C)** Image obtained following a successful thrombosis of the pseudoaneurysm demonstrates the patent common femoral artery (A) and the thrombosed hypoechoic neck (curved arrow) and body (arrows) of the pseudoaneurysm.

optimal positioning is obtained, the color Doppler is turned on again to monitor flow in the PSA. In ~3 to 5 seconds 100 to 300 units of thrombin are injected and flow within the PSA is monitored. If flow persists after the initial injection, an additional 100 to 300 units of thrombin are injected, often without repositioning the needle. After thrombosis of the PSA, the needle is removed. The presence of pulsation in the dorsalis peditis and posterior tibialis artery is confirmed before, during, and after the procedure.

Routine 24 to 48 hour follow-up to document persistent thrombosis of PSAs is advocated by some; however, we do not do this routinely unless the patient has recurrence of symptoms or an enlarging hematoma in the region of the thrombosed PSA. Successful ultrasound-guided compression repair is reported to range from 66 to 100%. The incidence of success is related to many factors, including the size, multiplicity, and neck length of the PSA, the presence or absence of significant hematoma, the presence of an associated AVF, and most importantly, the presence of concurrent anticoagulation. If PSA compression is desired, we request that the referring physicians discontinue anticoagulation at least 4 hours before the procedure. If the referring physicians believe that the risk of discontinuing anticoagulation outweighs the risk of either PSA rupture or failure to thrombose the PSA, we will attempt compression repair even though the patient is anticoagulated. In such cases, prolonged compression is frequently required and it is possible that mechanical clamp devices may be useful. Multilobed PSAs can be effectively compressed. Although the success rate is slightly less than that for unilobular PSAs, for multilobed PSAs it exceeds 81%. The most important factor enabling success in these multilobulated PSAs is to clarify the

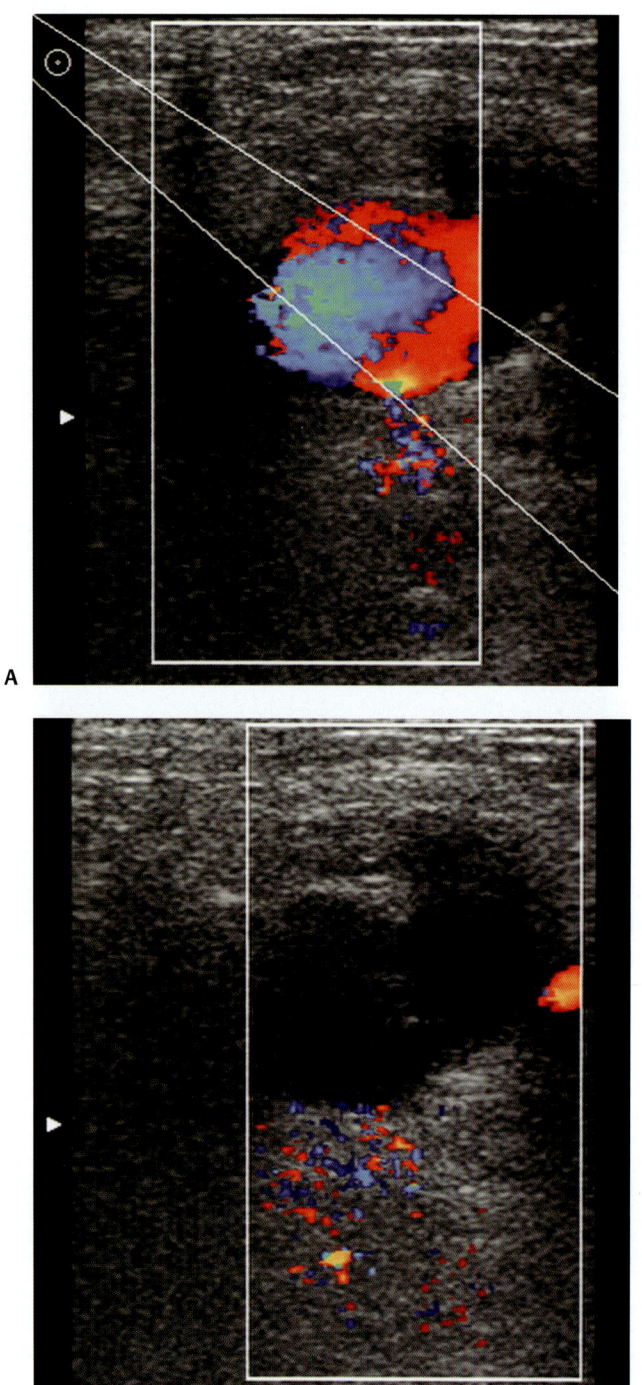
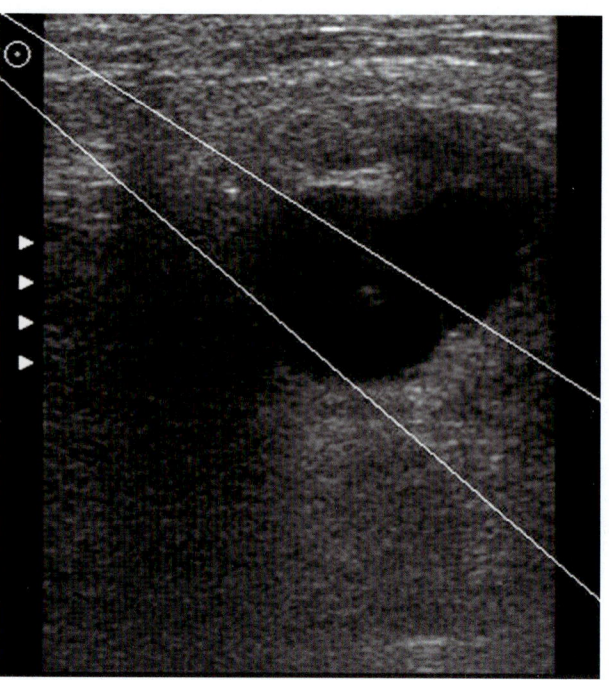

Figure 3–8 (A) A pseudoaneurysm with "yin-yang" flow is seen flanked by a biopsy grid (arrow). **(B)** Color flow is off. **(C)** Biopsy needle (arrow) immediately after injection shows occlusion of the pseudoaneurysm (arrowhead).

course of the blood flow from the native artery. Applying compression to the most proximal neck nearest the artery usually results in obliteration of blood flow to all of the string of PSAs.

Ultrasound-guided compression repair complications are unusual. Reported complications include femoral artery thrombosis, embolization of plaque from compression, deep venous thrombosis, and PSA rupture. Although ultrasound-guided compression therapy has become a very desirable and widely utilized procedure, there are contraindi-

cations. Lower-limb ischemia, the possibility of groin infection (**Fig. 3–9**), skin ischemia overlying the PSA, and active pulsatile bleeding into the groin are contraindications. Although some have suggested that chronic PSAs are difficult to thrombose, success occurs in many cases, and this is not considered an absolute contraindication. Similarly, compression of PSAs associated with AVFs are less likely to be effective. AVFs are not effectively obliterated using this technique; however, the associated PSA may be thrombosed. Percutaneous transcatheter embolization of PSA or

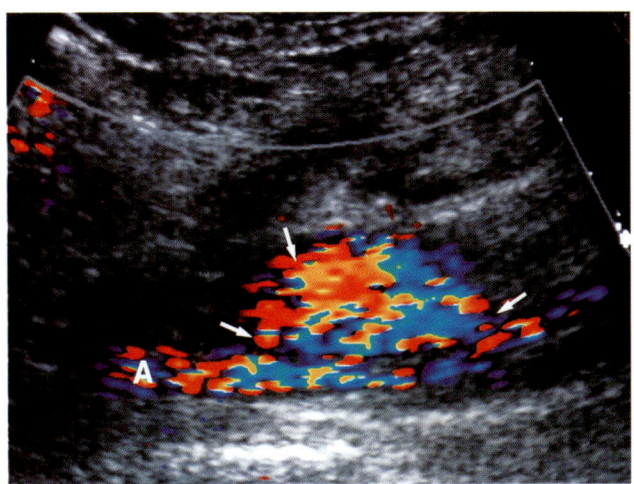

Figure 3–9 A patient several days postcardiac catheterization presents with increasing erythema and pain in the groin as well as a purulent discharge along the puncture site. There is a focal aneurysmal mass (arrows) arising from the common femoral artery (A). The mass has no discernible neck and the distinction cannot be made between a mycotic aneurysm and a pseudoaneurysm. This mass required surgical intervention.

AVF with coils has been done when compression has failed, as a less invasive alternative to surgery.[13] Recent work supports the use of bovine thrombin or human thrombin injections to obliterate pseudoaneurysm.

Duplex sonography has promise for the evaluation of arterial trauma in patients with occult vascular injuries. For many years arterial injury has been perceived as a life- or limb-threatening event requiring immediate angiographic evaluation. Traumatic PSAs caused by knife, bullet, or other penetrating wounds (**Fig. 3–10A,B**) do not seem to have the same propensity to spontaneous thrombosis as does iatrogenic injury. However, ultrasound could provide noninvasive useful information that would allow at least temporary nonoperative observation in a significant number of patients.[14,15] These PSAs are probably best handled by surgical repair, particularly because there is greater vascular injury, significant soft tissue disruption surrounding the PSA, and a greater propensity for infection.

Arteriovenous Fistulas

Simultaneous puncture of the femoral artery and vein can produce an AVF. AVFs most commonly result from the si-

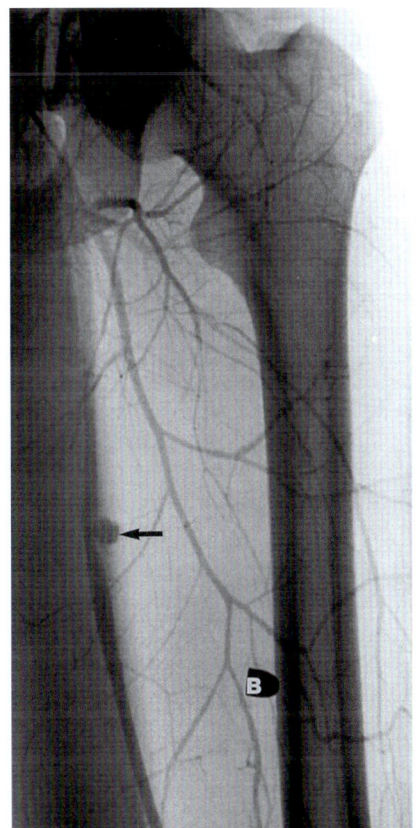

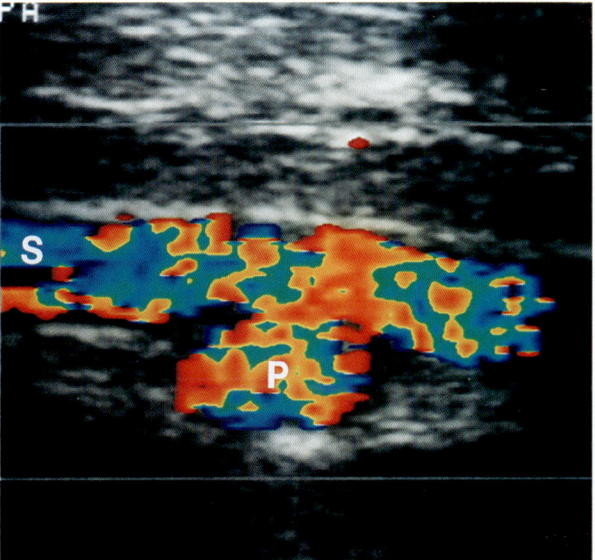

Figure 3–10 (A) A lower-extremity arteriogram demonstrates a traumatic pseudoaneurysm (arrow) and associated vascular spasm involving the superficial femoral artery. The offending projectile (B) lies adjacent to the femur. **(B)** Longitudinal image of the superficial femoral artery (S) demonstrates a broad-based pseudoaneurysm (P) arising from the vessel's posterior aspect. Because of its deep location, as well as significant soft tissue injury, it was decided to observe this patient and perform a follow-up ultrasound.

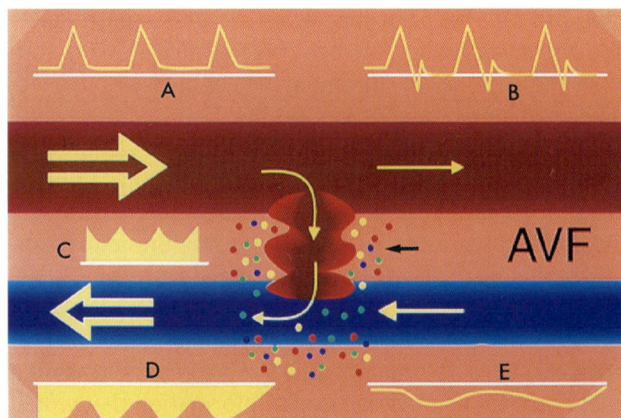

Figure 3–11 A diagram demonstrating the characteristic flow waveform changes seen with arteriovenous fistulas (AVFs). The low-resistance waveform **(A)** seen proximal to the AVF, the more normal triphasic waveform seen distal to the AVF **(B)**, the disturbed low-resistance arterial flow seen within the AVF **(C)**, the high-velocity pulsatile venous flow seen in the vein proximal to the AVF **(D)**, and the more normal undulating low-velocity venous flow seen in the vein distal to the AVF **(E)**, are diagrammed. Note also the soft tissue color Doppler speckling in the region of the AV communication (arrow).

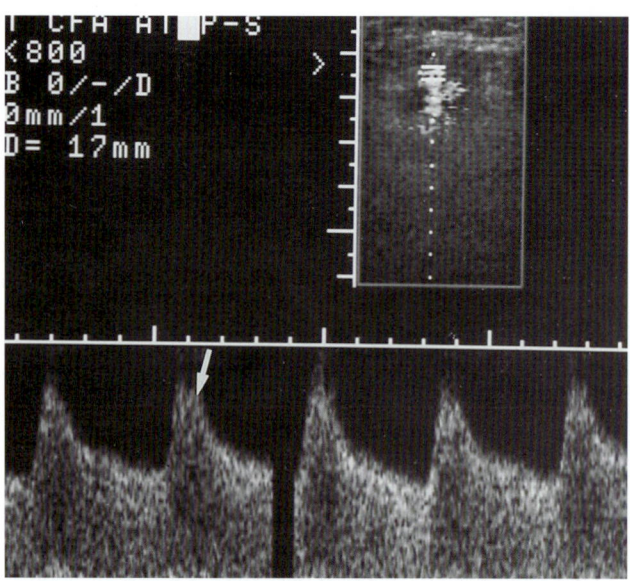

Figure 3–12 Characteristic low-resistance arterial waveforms (arrow) in the artery just proximal to the arteriovenous (AV) communication. Typically, resistive indices are 0.50 or less in the region of the AV communication.

multaneous catheterization of the left and right heart; however, inadvertent venous puncture associated with an arterial study can also result in an AVF. These are less frequently encountered than PSA following groin catheterization. Most AVFs are small and not hemodynamically significant. The majority resolve spontaneously and surgical repair is rarely required except in cases of high-output congestive heart failure, threatened limb ischemia, or severe varicosity. Physical findings of an AVF are most commonly the discovery of a new thrill or bruit at the puncture site. Although a "new" AVF may be discovered, many bruits at the puncture site may be due to preexisting atheroscle-

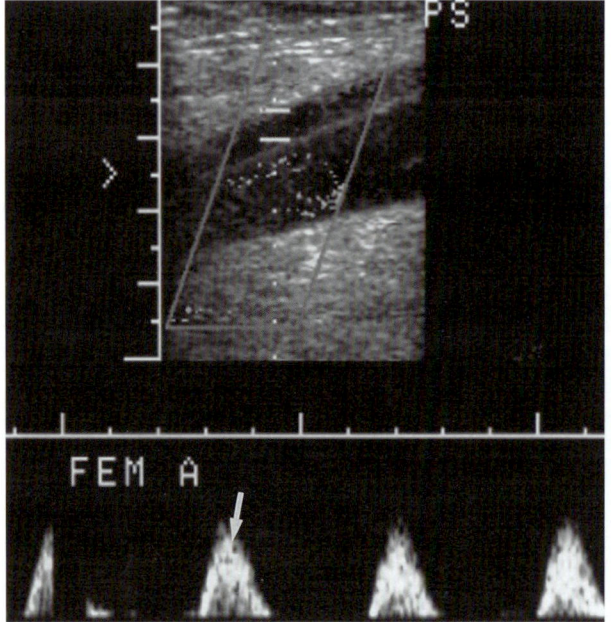

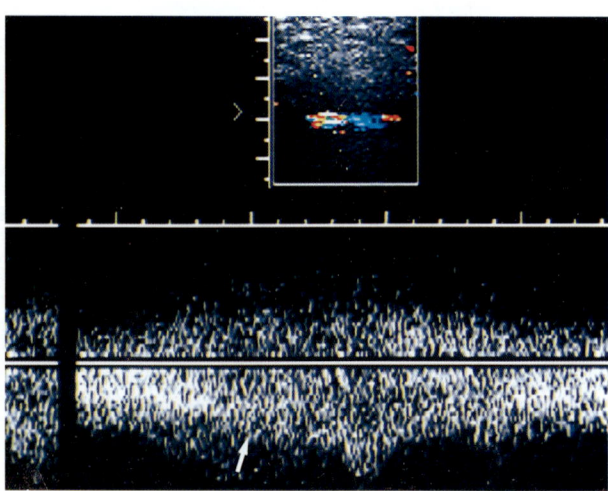

Figure 3–13 (A) Demonstration of arterial waveforms distal to a significant arteriovenous fistula (AVF) in a patient with unilateral decreased dorsalis pedis pulsus. The superficial artery waveform (arrow) demonstrates decreased velocities with loss of the normal triphasic waveform. **(B)** Interrogation of the superficial femoral vein proximal to a more distal AVF demonstrates high-velocity disturbed venous flow (arrow). Pulsed Doppler flow waveform inverted.

rotic disease and/or the inadvertent production of an arterial dissection in the region of the puncture site.

The sonographic features of an AVF mirror the hemodynamic effects of an abnormal communication between a very high-resistance artery and a low-resistance vein without an intervening capillary bed[16,17] (**Fig. 3–11**). Blood flow direction is always toward the region of lower pressures such that arterial blood flow preferentially shunts into the vein. Because the venous pressure is lower, this results in the loss of the high-resistance triphasic waveform in the artery proximal to the fistulous communication (**Fig. 3–12**). If a large enough component of the blood flow is diverted into the fistula, there may be decreased blood flow in the distal artery, as well as increased pulsatile blood flow in the vein proximal to the communication (**Fig. 3–13A,B**). The blood flow disturbance across the fistulous communication can be transmitted into the adjacent soft tissues, resulting in a striking color Doppler soft tissue bruit manifested by extensive heterogeneous color speckling surrounding the AVF (**Fig. 3–14**). This soft tissue color collection contains high-velocity pulsatile flow with extensive spectral broadening and may be so extensive that it actually obscures the site of the AV communication. Appropriate alteration of gain, PRF, wall filter, and persistance settings can decrease or eliminate the soft tissue speckling, allowing one to visualize the AV communication.

AVFs that involve small branch vessels or have a long circuitous communication between the artery and vein may not produce the proximal and distal changes characteristic of an AVF. In such cases, the color Doppler bruit may be localized to the area of the communication with characteristic pulsatile low-resistance disturbed flow localized to the area of the tract (**Fig. 3–15A–E**). The proximal artery and vein may demonstrate relatively normal waveforms.

Because patients with peripheral atherosclerotic disease may have bruits and loss of the normal triphasic waveform associated with significant stenosis or postcatheterization dissection, isolated findings of disturbed, low-resistance arterial flow waveforms and soft tissue speckling should not be considered diagnostic of an AVF (**Fig. 3–16A,B**). The absence of corresponding venous changes and the presence of visible plaque or thrombus within the artery distinguish such arterial disease from an AVF. High-velocity venous flow can also be seen in cases of venous stenosis. Venous compression by hematoma and transmitted pulsations from the adjacent artery can also mimic the venous flow changes seen in AVFs. However, the characteristic AVF communication and corresponding arterial waveform changes are not seen in these situations. Pulsatile venous flow is a frequent manifestation of increased right heart pressure; however, these waveforms manifest significant flow reversal and do not resemble the arterialized pulsatile flow associated with AVFs. Femoral artery dissections may be created by catheterization; however, they may be difficult to distinguish from plaque or thrombus unless arterial flow is seen within the false lumen. Rarely, these dissections may result in arterial occlusions. In the case of an acute arterial occlusion, the ischemic cold leg is usually a surgical emergency such that these patients are not referred for ultrasound examinations. However, color Doppler can diagnose arterial occlusion by showing absence of flow as well as identifying collateral reconstitution. Occasionally, deep venous thromboses may be detected postgroin catheterization (**Fig. 3–17**). Hemorrhage and bleeding into the site of catheterization can result in large hematomas that produce extrinsic compression on the vein. In addition, the groin holding that takes place following the puncture as well as bed rest place the patient at high risk for development of venous thrombosis.

Potential Pitfalls of Ultrasound

Color Doppler accurately diagnoses postcatheterization vascular complications in the groin; however, pitfalls do exist. Hyperemic lymph nodes can produce a pulsatile tender mass that may simulate a PSA on palpation.[18] These hyperemic lymph nodes may be extremely hypoechoic on gray scale and contain extensive internal vascularity with striking increased flow on color or power Doppler (**Fig. 3–18A,B**). Although these inflamed lymph nodes might be mistaken for a partially thrombosed PSA, they do not demonstrate characteristic to-and-fro waveforms. The internal arterial waveforms are characteristically those of a

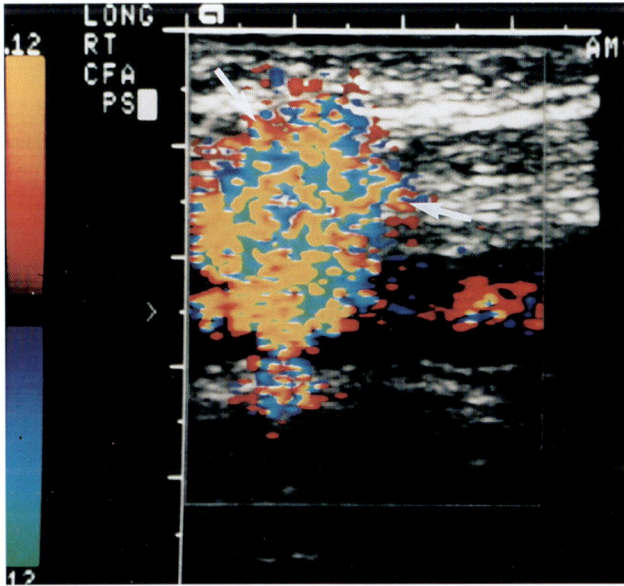

Figure 3–14 A longitudinal color Doppler of the right groin demonstrates a striking heterogeneous ball of color (arrows) produced by the transmitted soft tissue vibrations in the region of the arteriovenous fistula.

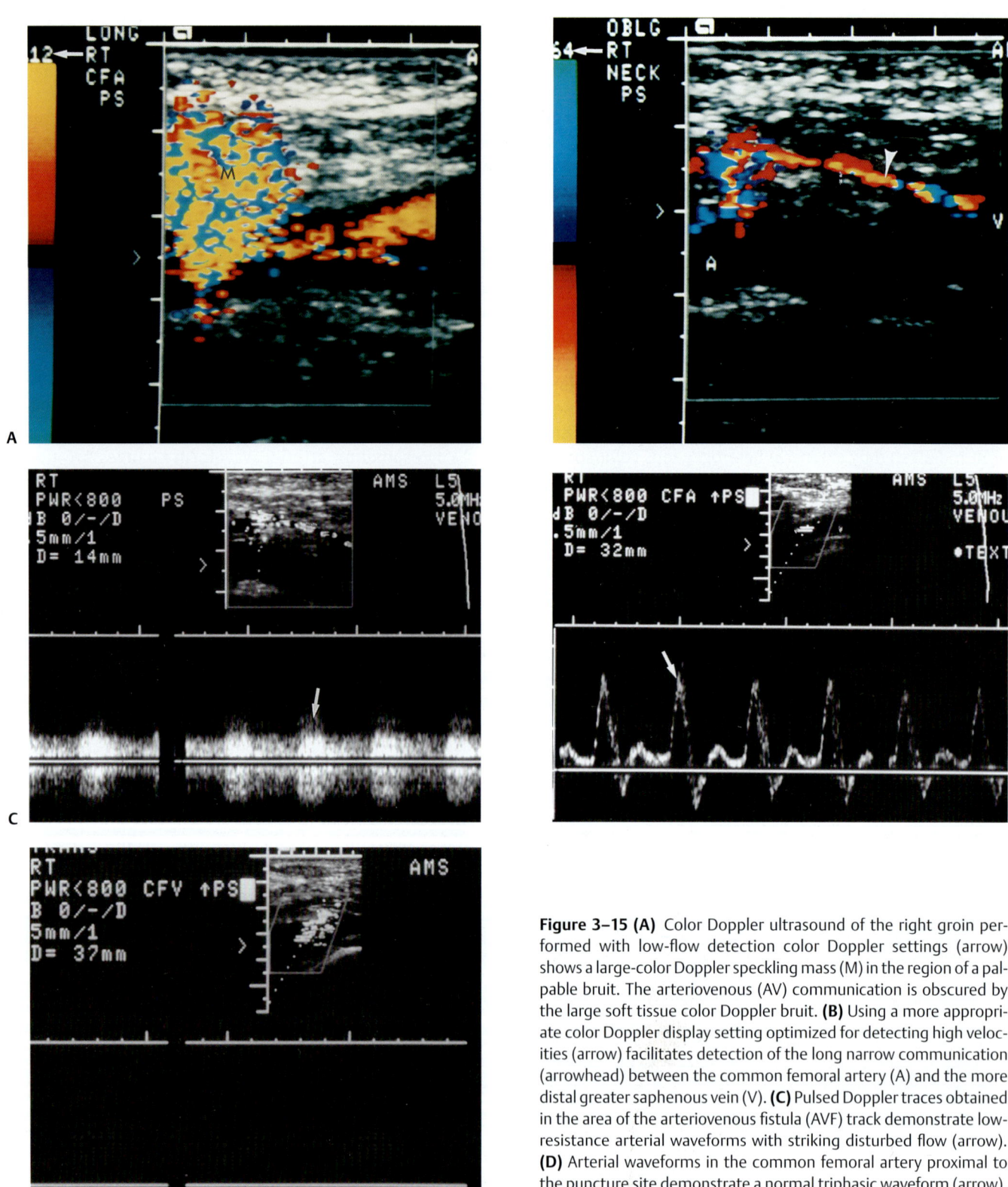

Figure 3–15 (A) Color Doppler ultrasound of the right groin performed with low-flow detection color Doppler settings (arrow) shows a large-color Doppler speckling mass (M) in the region of a palpable bruit. The arteriovenous (AV) communication is obscured by the large soft tissue color Doppler bruit. **(B)** Using a more appropriate color Doppler display setting optimized for detecting high velocities (arrow) facilitates detection of the long narrow communication (arrowhead) between the common femoral artery (A) and the more distal greater saphenous vein (V). **(C)** Pulsed Doppler traces obtained in the area of the arteriovenous fistula (AVF) track demonstrate low-resistance arterial waveforms with striking disturbed flow (arrow). **(D)** Arterial waveforms in the common femoral artery proximal to the puncture site demonstrate a normal triphasic waveform (arrow). **(E)** The common femoral vein above the level of the AVF demonstrates normal respiratory phase change (arrow) without evidence of high-velocity pulsatile flow.

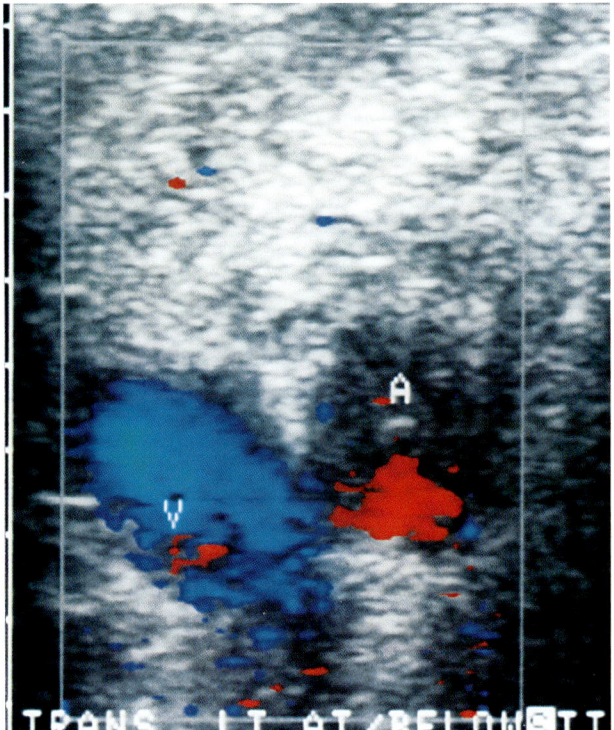

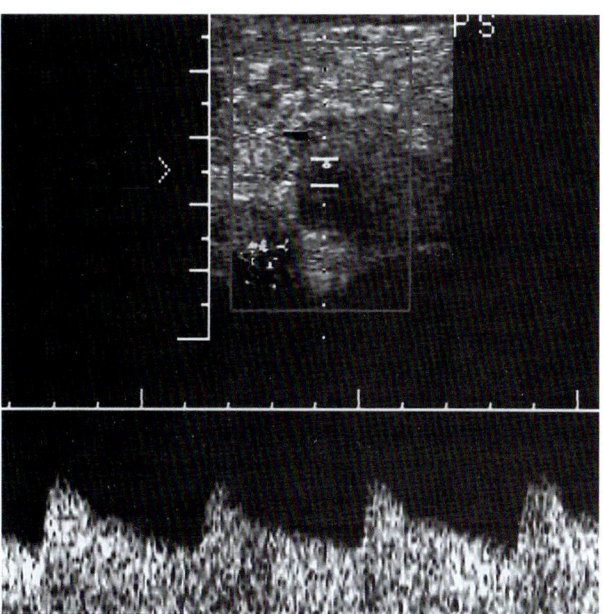

Figure 3–16 (A) Transverse color Doppler ultrasound of the left groin in a patient with a new bruit status postcatheterization demonstrates a hypoechoic mass in the common femoral artery (A), which obliterates roughly two thirds of the vascular lumen. Common femoral vein (V). **(B)** Flow waveforms obtained from the region of this iatrogenic aortic dissection with thrombus demonstrate low-resistance disturbed flow waveforms similar to those that can be seen in the region proximal to an arteriovenous fistula.

normal arterial waveform (**Fig. 3–19A,B**). Furthermore, the gray-scale appearance of these lymph nodes usually shows the characteristic echogenic central hilum of the node with the radial distribution of blood vessels out into the parenchyma. Although many hyperemic lymph nodes have relatively low-resistance waveforms, others may have high-resistance arterial waveforms. There is at least one case report of an inguinal hernia filled with fluid simulating a PSA.[19] In this case the swirling fluid within the hernia sac was shown to have flow that was in synchrony with respiratory motion rather than with the cardiac cycle. We have also seen venous aneurysms (giant varices) of the greater saphenous vein that contained the so-called yin-yang internal blood flow appearance. However, flow on pulsed Doppler was clearly venous in nature and showed a clear-cut response to a Valsalva maneuver.

True aneurysms may also present as a pulsatile groin mass. Furthermore, the flow within these aneurysms may have a swirling pattern reminiscent of a PSA. However, it is usually easy to determine that the aneurysm lies within the arterial lumen rather than outside of the wall of the vessel. If there is any question that a traumatic PSA exists, then further evaluation with angiography may be necessary.

The inferior epigastric artery arises from the distal external iliac artery in the region of the inguinal ligament and ascends to provide arterial blood supply to the anterior abdominal wall musculature. Occasionally, this branch will be visualized in the upper thigh and should not be confused with a PSA neck, a patent needle track, or the arterial limb of an AVF. This vessel does have a relatively low-resistance waveform somewhat atypical of the

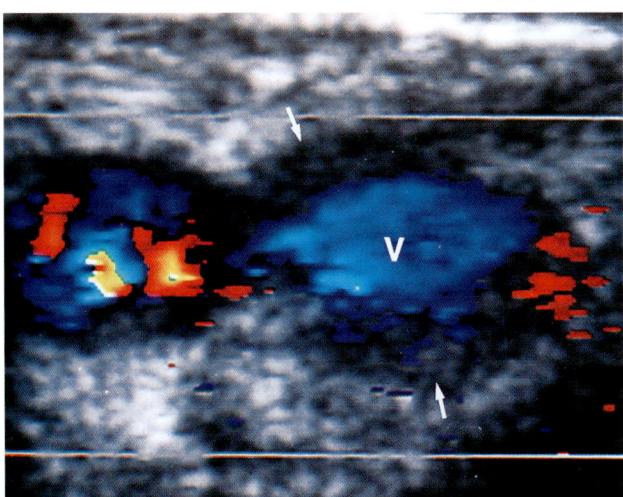

Figure 3–17 A transverse scan of the right groin in a postcatheterization patient demonstrates partial thrombosis (arrows) of the right common femoral vein (V).

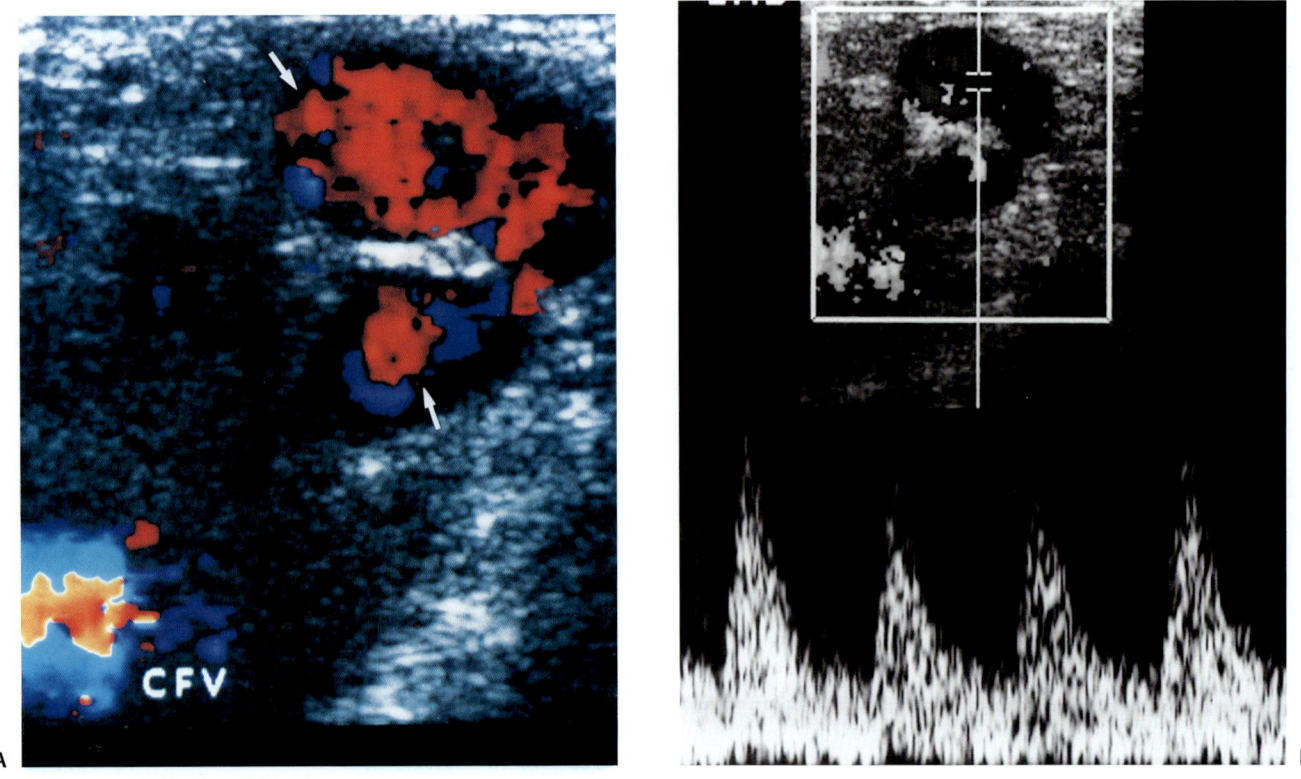

Figure 3–18 **(A)** Hyperemic lymph nodes simulating a pseudoaneurysm (arrows). **(B)** Pulsed Doppler waveforms obtained within these masses demonstrate relatively low-resistance waveforms such as those commonly seen in hyperemic lymph nodes.

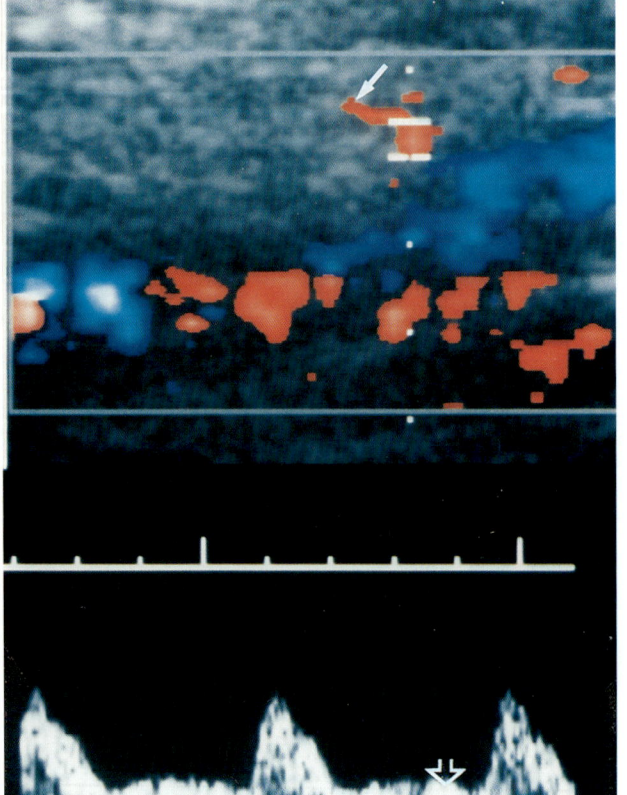

Figure 3–19 A longitudinal color Doppler ultrasound of the groin shows a branch vessel running cranially in the anticipated location of the inferior epigastric artery (arrow). Pulsed Doppler waveforms (open arrow) demonstrate an uncharacteristic waveform with more end-diastolic blood flow than typical for a peripheral artery. The course of this vessel and its waveforms help distinguish it from a pseudoaneurysm neck or an arteriovenous fistula.

femoral arterial system (**Fig. 3–19**). However, its course is different from that anticipated for a needle track or PSA neck, and corresponding venous changes are not present to suggest an AVF. Furthermore, no characteristic PSA to-and-fro flow will be observed along the course of this branch vessel.

Color Doppler imaging has made a significant contribution to the management of the postcatheterization groin. It has become the primary imaging modality for assessing complications and offers an elegant noninvasive method of treatment for PSAs.

References

1. Lumsden AB, Miller JM, Kosinski AS, et al. A prospective evaluation of surgically treated groin complications following percutaneous cardiac procedures. Am Surg 1994;60:132–137
2. Paulson EK, Kliewer MA, Hertzberg BS, et al. Color Doppler sonography of groin complications following femoral artery catheterization. AJR Am J Roentgenol 1995;165:439–444
3. Abu-Yousef MM, Wiese JA, Shamma AR. The "to-and-from" sign: duplex Doppler evidence of femoral artery pseudoaneurysm. AJR Am J Roentgenol 1988;150:632–634
4. Helvie MA, Rubin JM, Silver TM, Kresowik TF. The distinction between femoral artery pseudoaneurysms and other causes of groin masses: value of duplex Doppler sonography. AJR Am J Roentgenol 1988;150:1177–1180
5. Katzenschlager R, Ugurluoglu A, Ahmadi A, et al. Incidence of pseudoaneurysm after diagnostic and therapeutic angiography. Radiology 1995;195:463–466
6. O'Malley CM, Paulson EK, Kliewer MA, et al. Color Doppler sonographic appearance of patent needle tracts after femoral arterial catheterization. Radiology 1995;197:163–165
7. Johns JP, Pupa LE Jr, Bailey SR. Spontaneous thrombosis of iatrogenic femoral artery pseudoaneurysms: documentation with color Doppler and two-dimensional ultrasonography. J Vasc Surg 1991;14:24–29
8. Allen BT, Munn JS, Stevens SL, et al. Selective non-operative management of pseudoaneurysms and arteriovenous fistulae complicating femoral artery catheterization. J Cardiovasc Surg (Torino) 1992;33:440–447
9. Paulson EK, Hertzberg BS, Paine SS, Carroll BA. Femoral artery pseudoaneurysms: value of color Doppler sonography in predicting which ones will thrombose without treatment. AJR Am J Roentgenol 1992;159:1077–1081
10. Fellmeth BD, Roberts AC, Bookstein JJ, et al. Postangiographic femoral artery injuries: nonsurgical repair with US-guided compression. Radiology 1991;178:671–675
11. Coley BD, Roberts AC, Fellmeth BD, et al. Postangiographic femoral artery pseudoaneurysms: further experience with US-guided compression repair. Radiology 1995;194:307–311
12. Paulson EK, Kliewer MA, Hertzberg BS, et al. Ultrasonographically guided manual compression of femoral artery injuries. J Ultrasound Med 1995;14:653–659
13. Paulson EK, Nelson RC, Mayes CE, Sheafor DH, Sketch MH Jr, Kliewer MA. Sonographically guided thrombin injection of iatrogenic femoral pseudoaneurysms. Further experience of a single institution. AJR Am J Roentgenol 2001;177:309–316
14. Paulson EK, Sheafor DH, Kliewer MA, et al. Treatment of iatrogenic femoral arterial pseudoaneurysms: comparison of US-guided thrombin injection with compression repair. Radiology 2000;215:403–408
15. Lemaire J-M, Dondelinger RF. Percutaneous coil embolization of iatrogenic femoral arteriovenous fistula or pseudo-aneurysm. Eur J Radiol 1994;18:96–100
16. Meissner M, Paun M, Johansen K. Duplex scanning for arterial trauma. Am J Surg 1991;161:552–555
17. Frykbert ER, Crump JM, Dennis JW, Vines FS, Alexander RH. Nonoperative observation of clinically occult arterial injuries: a prospective evaluation. Surgery 1991;109:85–96
18. Roubidoux MA, Hertzberg BS, Carroll BA, Hedgepeth CA. Color flow and image-directed Doppler ultrasound evaluation of iatrogenic arteriovenous fistulas in the groin. J Clin Ultrasound 1990;18:463–469
19. Igidbashian VN, Mitchell DG, Middleton WD, Schwartz RA, Goldberg BB. Iatrogenic femoral arteriovenous fistula: diagnosis with color Doppler imaging. Radiology 1989;170:749–752
20. Morton M, Charboneau JW, Banks PM. Internal lymphadenopathy simulating a false aneurysm on color flow Doppler sonography. Am J Radiol 1988;151:115–116
21. Middleton MA, Middleton WD. Femoral hernia simulating a pseudoaneurysm on color Doppler sonography. Am J Radiol 1993;160:1291–1292

4 Carotid Arteries in Patients with Transient Ischemic Accidents, Stroke, or Carotid Bruits

Joseph F. Polak

The results of multicenter trials have shown that carotid endarterectomy benefits a group of patients with significant carotid artery stenoses. These results apply to patients with or without symptoms.[1-3] The determination of what represents a significant carotid artery lesion is based on the results of the North American Symptomatic Carotid Endarterectomy Trial (NASCET) study where the benefit of carotid artery surgery was shown when the intervention is done for a stenosis of ≥ 50% diameter narrowing.[4] However, carotid surgery is not the only intervention that can be offered to patients with severe carotid artery stenoses. Carotid stenting is emerging as a viable alternative to carotid surgery in selected patients.[5]

This chapter reviews data on the incidence of ischemic stroke and the linkage to carotid artery disease. Emphasis will be given to certain pathological aspects of atherosclerotic plaque growth and the way that ultrasound can be used to identify carotid lesions that are more likely to cause neurovascular events.

Link of Stroke and Transient Ischemic Attacks to Carotid Artery Disease

Cerebrovascular events, stroke, and transient ischemic attack (TIA) can have different causes. Strokes can be classified as hemorrhagic or ischemic. In young subjects, neurological events are likely due to subarachnoid hemorrhage caused by an aneurysm rupture or due to emboli from a cardiac source or patent foramen ovale. In older individuals, strokes can be due to diseased intracranial arteries or to atheroembolism from outside the cerebral circulation. Another major cause of ischemic events is lacunar strokes. These are believed to be caused by small vessel disease with lesions affecting the smaller branches of the middle cerebral arteries. Because this chapter focuses on carotid ultrasound, the atheroembolic process is emphasized.

Embolic phenomena account for most cases of stroke in the United States. Cardioembolic events tend to be associated with atrial fibrillation, with embolization of thrombi forming in the left atrium, embolization of thrombi forming on prosthetic valves, or left ventricular thrombi developing in severely diseased and aneurysmal left ventricles. This linkage is supported by the detection of presumed embolic events with transcranial Doppler sonography. These signals, called *high intensity transient events*, are believed to represent emboli. Their event rates are much greater in patients with prosthetic valves and atrial fibrillation than in patients without either.[6]

Atheroembolism is the likely etiology of most strokes in patients with large carotid artery plaque deposits. This linkage is also supported by transcranial Doppler signal detection of high-intensity transitory signals (HITS). The event rate of HITS increases as the severity of carotid plaques increases.[7] This does not exclude the possibility that carotid stenoses can progress and cause significant enough narrowing of the artery to cause an ischemic stroke by simply reducing blood flow to the brain. This hypoperfusion syndrome affects the watershed area between the middle and the posterior and anterior circulations of the brain and is a much less common source of acute symptoms than embolic events from atherosclerotic plaque.

Differential Diagnosis

In the patient presenting with a suspected stroke, the clinical decision algorithm seeks, first, to distinguish ischemic from hemorrhagic strokes. The therapeutic options seem broader in the group of patients with ischemic stroke because the inciting event often has an extracranial origin. Hemorrhagic strokes are often linked to intracranial pathologies, aneurysms, or tumors, or to hypertensive episodes and small vessel rupture. Once a neurological event has been classified as being ischemic, the role of sonography is better defined because it is used to identify lesions that are directly associated with the presenting symptoms.

Ultrasound can be successfully applied to the evaluation of these patients if the technique has proven its efficacy at three levels: (1) identifying the type of lesion that causes ischemic stroke and defining its appearance on ultrasound images, (2) establishing the diagnostic accuracy of ultrasound imaging and Doppler evaluation of blood flow in patients with and without neurological symptoms or carotid bruits, and (3) linking the results of specific ultrasound findings with clinical outcomes.

Diagnostic Evaluation

Ultrasound Imaging

Appearance of Carotid Plaque and Association with Ischemic Stroke

Examination of pathological specimens removed during carotid endarterectomy has shown that plaque hemorrhage is associated with the presence of TIAs and with stroke.[8] Subsequent studies have further suggested that areas of intraplaque hemorrhage correspond to hypoechoic zones seen with B-mode sonography.[9,10] Based on these observations, it would seem possible that sonography might be used to identify specific plaque characteristics that are indicative of an increased risk for subsequent stroke.

Studies have shown that the baseline appearance of carotid plaque is linked to the severity of carotid stenosis.[11,12] The sonographic appearance of carotid artery plaque changes as the severity of disease progresses: large plaques (causing greater degrees of stenosis) are more likely to be heterogeneous and contain hypoechoic areas.[11] The hypoechoic areas seen on ultrasound images can correspond to zones of intraplaque hemorrhage, but can also represent areas where there are higher concentrations of smooth muscle cells, lipid, or thrombus.[13] As such, the ultrasound appearance of echolucent areas is nonspecific and cannot be linked to a specific type of tissue. The value of plaque characterization is further placed in doubt by pathological studies which have shown that the presence of intraplaque hemorrhage need not be associated with any symptoms.[14,15] However, others have shown that as the degree of sonolucency increases from homogeneous to heterogeneous (class 4 to class 1), the percentage of patients with cerebral infarction proven with computed tomography (CT) also increases significantly from 10.5 to 66%.[16]

Surface irregularities in the atherosclerotic plaque are believed to serve as the nidus for the formation of platelet aggregates that can then embolize. Carotid plaque ulceration seen during arteriography seems to be associated with a high likelihood for stroke.[17] This observation may be relevant to symptomatic individuals with high-grade (≥ 70%) stenoses. By itself, however, the arteriographic appearance of carotid plaque does not appear to directly correspond to the findings seen in pathological samples.[9,17,18] Similarly, sonographic detection of carotid ulceration is poor when pathological specimens are used as a gold standard.[19,20]

The one characteristic of atherosclerotic plaque that consistently correlates with the risk of incident stroke is the severity of the internal carotid artery narrowing. The more the internal carotid artery is narrowed, the higher the likelihood for incident stroke. The positive relationship between incident stroke and internal carotid artery disease has also been shown in patients where carotid artery stenosis severity has been measured by Doppler-derived blood flow velocities.[3,21,22]

Although the large endarterectomy trials, Asymptomatic Carotid Atherosclerosis Study (ACAS), European Carotid Surgery Trial (ECST), and NASCET, did not offer any evaluation of plaque characteristics, a study of carotid stenting did include the evaluation of the gray-scale texture of plaque.[23] Plaques with more echolucent components were associated with procedure-related events.[23] In epidemiological studies, echolucent plaques are also associated with the risk of incident stroke.[24,25]

Technique

A high-frequency transducer (above 5 MHz) is typically used to visualize the carotid arteries because they are superficial. Doppler imaging is used to determine if a lesion causes a severe stenosis. Color Doppler imaging is first used to look for areas of turbulence, seen as mosaic patterns, or a zone of increased blood flow velocities, seen as aliasing of the color Doppler signal. This helps identify the area of greatest stenosis. Doppler spectral analysis is then used to determine the peak systolic velocity and the end diastolic velocity of the internal carotid artery by sampling the region of increased blood flow velocity. Measurements are also made of the peak systolic velocity and end diastolic velocity of the unobstructed common carotid artery, usually 2 cm proximal to the bulb. Ratios can be measured of peak systolic and end diastolic velocities.

Evaluation of carotid plaques is then made in both the transverse and the sagittal projections by high-resolution gray-scale, often without color Doppler imaging (**Fig. 4–1**). The combined use of color Doppler images does, however, permit the visualization of plaques that are mostly echolucent or have echolucent components near their surface.

Accuracy of Ultrasound for Evaluating Carotid Artery Disease

Hemodynamically significant stenoses are, by definition, associated with a pressure drop as blood flows across the stenosis. This will typically take place when a plaque causes at least a 50% narrowing of the lumen diameter. The velocity of blood flow increases as the lumen narrows and is the greatest at the point of maximal stenotic narrowing. This phenomenon can be used to determine stenosis severity with continuous-wave Doppler waveform analysis (nonimaging),[26] pulsed-Doppler waveform analysis,[27] and

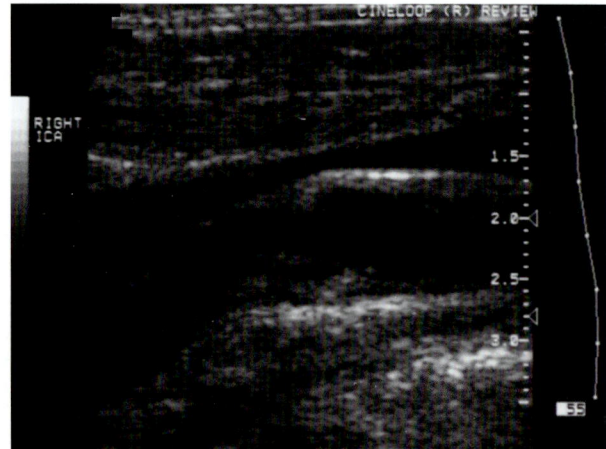 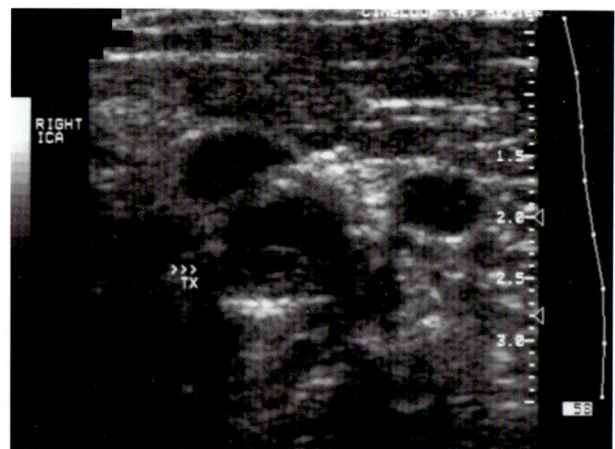

Figure 4–1 (A) Sagittal and (B) transverse images of heterogeneous or type II plaque. Note the presence of a well-defined focal hypoechoic area within the plaque, which is more than 50% of the plaque volume.

color flow imaging.[28,29] The zone of increased velocity that is established at the point of maximal stenosis can continue as a stenotic jet, typically extending 1 to 2 cm distal to the stenosis.[30]

Color Doppler imaging is used in combination with pulsed Doppler waveform analysis to detect and grade the severity of internal carotid artery stenoses.[28] Stenosis severity can also be estimated directly from the color Doppler or power Doppler image by measuring the size of the color channel (**Fig. 4–2**) that corresponds to the residual lumen of the artery.[29,31,32] Direct measurements of residual lumen require that the color and power Doppler sensitivity be set high enough to minimize bleeding of the color Doppler or power Doppler signals outside of the artery walls or into a plaque. Mean velocity estimates can also be made from the color Doppler map by determining the point where the color signals alias,[33] or by selecting a velocity "tag."[29,34] These direct measurements are not possible when the calcified portions of a plaque are sufficiently large to mask the artery lumen by acoustic shadowing of any Doppler information from the artery lumen.[31] However, because the flow disturbances associated with a stenosis extend, this limitation does not extend to Doppler waveform analysis because the flow disturbances associated with a stenosis extend for at least 1 cm, and possibly 2 cm downstream to the lesion.[30,35] The stenotic jet can still be sampled and graded with Doppler waveform analysis (**Fig. 4–3**). Although this can limit the accuracy of grading

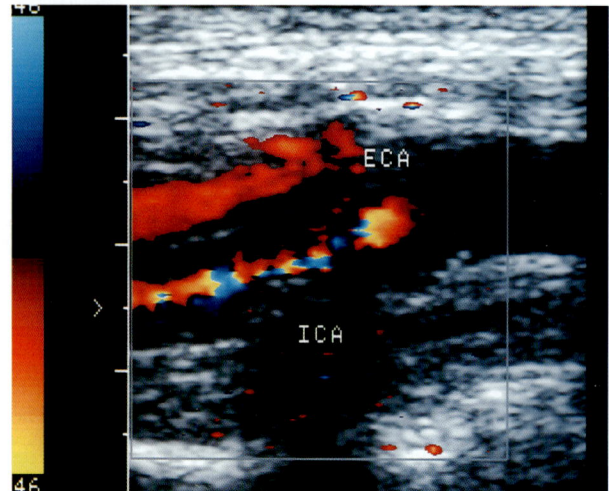 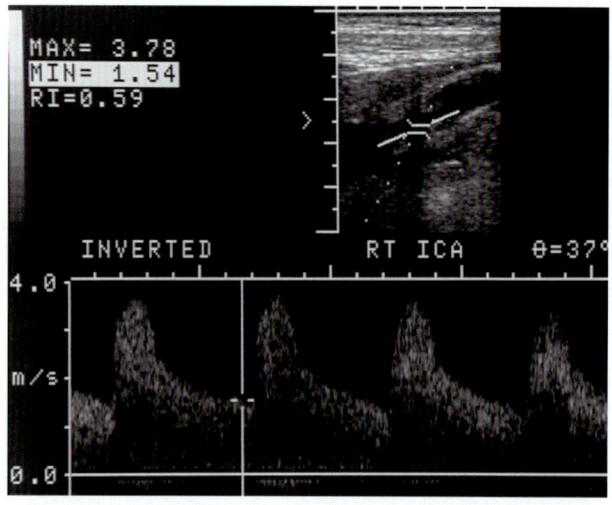

Figure 4–2 This color flow image shows a long stenosis of the internal carotid artery. (A) The actual size of the color flow lumen cannot be used to grade the severity of the lesion because some of the color signals likely "bleed" into the diseased carotid wall. (B) The high-grade lesion is confirmed by analysis of the Doppler waveform. Marked elevations of the peak systolic and end-diastolic velocities are consistent with a greater than 80% stenosis.

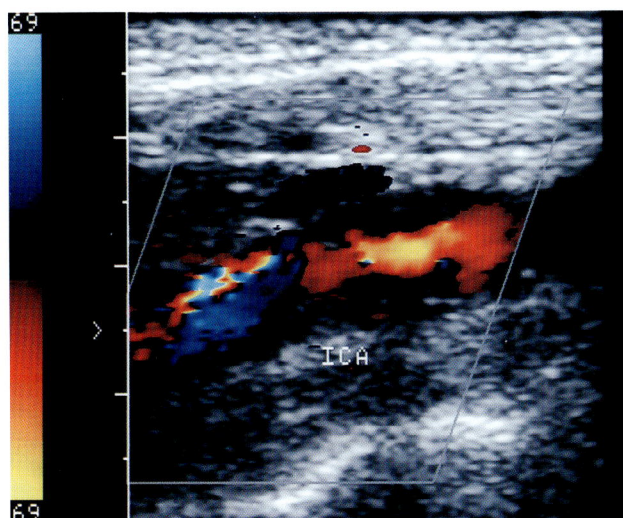 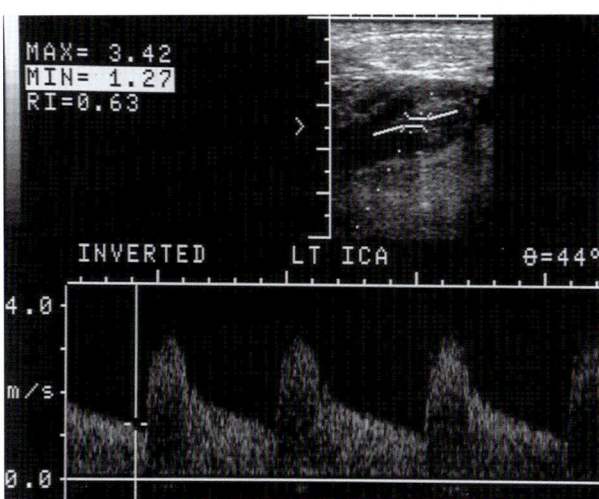

Figure 4–3 This color Doppler image shows aliasing of the color flow signals. **(A)** Beyond the stenosis, the jet impacts on the outer wall of the internal carotid artery while a zone of flow reversal (blue) forms to the side and below. **(B)** The high-grade stenosis is confirmed by Doppler waveform analysis showing marked elevations in the peak-systolic and end-diastolic velocities.

stenosis severity, it does permit the identification of a significant stenosis of greater than 50%. There is, therefore, almost complete reliance on Doppler velocity estimates made with pulsed Doppler sonography when detecting the presence of lesions causing at least 50% diameter narrowing. Reported accuracies are close to 90% or higher.[28] Power Doppler sonography has been shown to help in distinguishing stenoses in the range of 50 to 70% and additionally may be used as a screening test.[32,36,37]

Blood flow velocity measurements are made by sampling the Doppler waveform at the site of stenosis and by correcting the frequency shift caused by moving blood with the aid of the Doppler equation. This requires that the sonographer estimate the direction of motion of blood. Errors made in determining the angle between the Doppler ultrasound beam and the direction of flowing blood increase at angles above 60 degrees. The angle-corrected velocity measurements, therefore, become progressively less reliable as the angle between blood flow and the ultrasound beam increases above 60 degrees. Ambiguity in determining this angle is also a major source of intersonographer variability.

Stenosis Grading

Grading stenosis severity has become an important issue since the results of several randomized controlled trials have demonstrated net benefits of carotid endarterectomy. The first NASCET[38] report has shown an absolute reduction in risk of 16.5% over a 2-year period for symptomatic patients with at least a 70% stenosis. A more recent NASCET report[4] of symptomatic patients with a 50 to 69% stenosis found an absolute risk reduction of 10.1% at 5 years, but no benefit for those with less than 50% stenosis. The ECST trial report documented an absolute risk reduction of 11.6% at 3 years in symptomatic patients with stenosis of 60% or greater as measured by the NASCET method. The ECST trial also showed that patients who had less than a 40% stenosis (by the NASCET method) who underwent surgery had significantly poorer outcomes at 2 or 3 years than those treated medically.[39] Lastly, the ACAS[3] study showed an absolute reduction of 5.9% in the 5-year risk of ipsilateral stroke or any perioperative stroke or death for surgical intervention of asymptomatic patients who had a greater than 60% stenosis. These studies have now reemphasized the importance of using accurate noninvasive ways to identify patients with flow-limiting stenoses.

The carotid endarterectomy trials also changed the method used to measure the degree of stenosis severity on contrast angiograms. In the past, lumen diameter narrowing was measured by comparing the residual lumen of the internal carotid artery with a "best guess" of the diameter of the internal carotid artery at the same level (**Fig. 4–4**). This was originally used in the ECST trial.[2] The approach adopted by the NASCET and ACAS studies[3,38] was to compare the residual diameter of the artery with that of the distal internal carotid artery beyond the stenosis (**Fig. 4–5**). The arteriograms acquired as part of the ECST trial were subsequently reanalyzed and stenosis graded in the NASCET fashion.[40] Results similar to the NASCET results were observed, with benefit for surgery for stenoses above 50%, no benefit for stenoses between 30 and 50% diameter narrowing, and increased morbidity for surgery performed for stenoses of < 30%.[40,41]

With the acceptance of the NASCET method of grading stenosis severity comes the need of standardizing criteria for Doppler evaluation of stenosis severity. With this in mind, a consensus panel reviewed the diagnostic criteria published in the literature and made recommendations with regard to parameters that offer a consistent

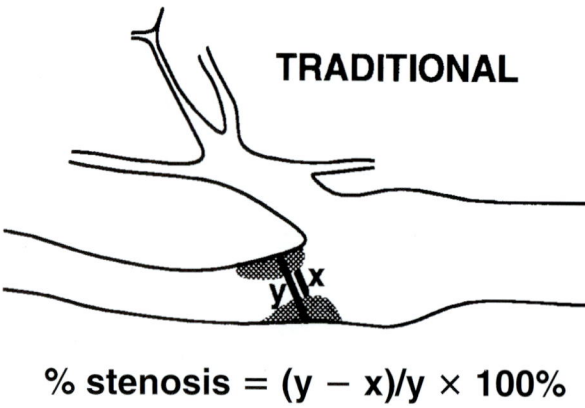

Figure 4–4 This diagram depicts the method of measuring stenosis severity as it has traditionally been performed.

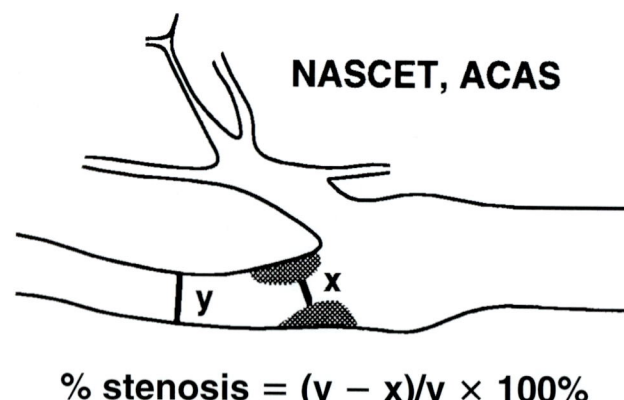

Figure 4–5 This diagram shows the current approach for determining stenosis severity based on the appearance of the distal internal carotid artery. ACAS, Asymptomatic Carotid Atherosclerosis Study; NASCET, North American Symptomatic Carotid Endarterectomy Trial.

way of using Doppler parameters to grade stenosis severity.[42]

A diagnostic cut-point of 125 cm/s in the peak-systolic velocity detects ≥ 50% stenosis when stenosis severity is graded with respect to the distal internal carotid artery.[28] Similarly, a peak-systolic velocity above 230 cm/s is used to identify a 70% diameter stenosis.[43] An internal carotid artery to common carotid artery peak-systolic velocity ratio of 4.0[44] or an end-diastolic velocity of 100 cm/s[45] has also been used for detecting a 70% or greater stenosis. These consensus values were derived after an extensive review of the literature. All of these measurements of stenosis severity are made by relating the severity of carotid lumen diameter at the lesion to the internal carotid artery distal to the lesion (**Table 4–1**), at a presumed normal diameter.[38] Although these values have shown the test of time, a laboratory where carotid ultrasound examinations are done should choose the velocity measurements that correspond with their ability to identify the correct degree of stenosis as compared with local findings at angiography and surgery. If an alternate table has been used successfully in the past, the consensus conference participants did not recommend mandatory switching to the new table.

Determining the relation between sonographic measurements of stenosis severity and outcomes is different than simply correlating the degree of stenosis on ultrasound with estimates made by arteriography. The ACAS study included sonographic evaluations of disease severity as part of the enrollment process.[3] At the early phases of the project, qualifying laboratories showed dismal performance in their ability to grade the severity of carotid artery disease.[46] Final outcome of the carotid ultrasound examination showed a specificity of 97%. The experimental design does not permit the determination of the diagnostic sensitivity of the carotid Doppler examination.[3] However, review of the performance of different laboratories has shown that estimates of stenosis severity made by peak-systolic velocity measurements are less subject to interlaboratory differences.[47,48] The diagnostic performance of sonography for detecting significant carotid artery disease in the NASCET study is very poor, with a sensitivity of 68% and specificity of 67%.[49] There are many reasons why such estimates are biased toward poor performance: (1) no standard protocol, (2) lack of color Doppler imaging, and (3) a process that averaged all of the velocity measurements from all laboratories involved without taking into consideration critical stenoses of ≥ 95%.[49]

Table 4–1 Consensus Criteria for Grading the Severity of Carotid Artery Stenosis According to NASCET

Grade	Peak-Systolic Velocity	ICA/CCA Velocity Ratio	End-Diastolic Velocity
Normal; no plaque	< 125 cm/s	< 2.0	< 40 cm/s
Plaque less than 50%	< 125 cm/s	< 2.0	< 40 cm/s
Plaque 50% to 69%	> 125 cm/s but < 230 cm/s	> 2.0 but < 4.0	> 40 cm/s but < 100 cm/s
Plaque 70% to near occlusion	> 230 cm/s	> 4.0	> 100 cm/s
Plaque with occlusion	No flow	No flow	No flow

Sources: Peak systolic velocity > 125 cm/s for > 50% stenosis by NASCET: Polak et al[28]; peak-systolic velocity > 230 cm/s for >70% stenosis by NASCET: Hunink et al[43]; peak-systolic velocity ratio for > 70% stenosis by NASCET: Moneta et al[44]; end-diastolic velocity > 100 cm/s for >70% stenosis by NASCET: Faught et al[45]; peak-systolic velocity > 2.0 and end-diastolic velocity > 40 cm/s for >50% stenosis were reached by consensus without a direct reference in the literature.

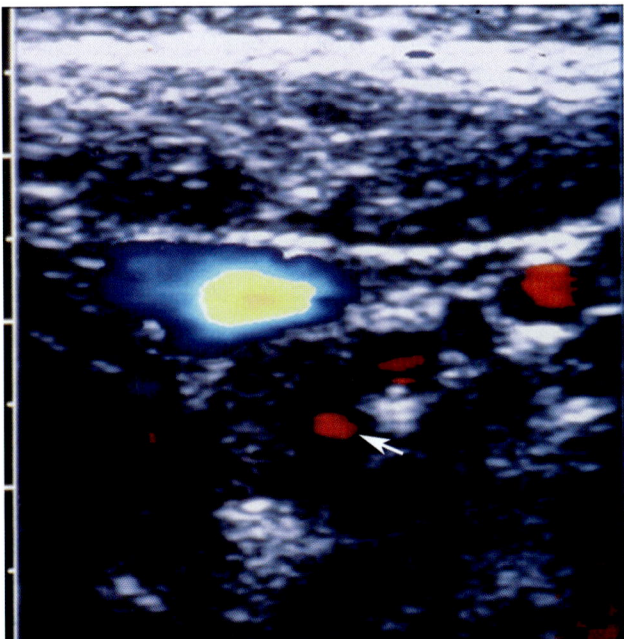

Figure 4–6 This color Doppler image was taken in a transverse plane to better demonstrate the residual lumen of a subtotally occluded internal carotid artery. The arrow points to the residual lumen. The internal carotid artery lies deep to the internal jugular vein (blue).

Total versus Subtotal Occlusions

Very high-grade internal carotid artery lesions may be associated with a decrease in blood flow velocity rather than an increase.[26] The stenosis reaches such a level of severity that volume blood flow decreases, thereby causing the velocities measured at the stenosis to decrease. This type of lesion can be difficult to evaluate with duplex sonography alone. The Doppler gate must be positioned over the very small residual lumen in the internal carotid artery. The hypoechoic elements of the stenosing plaque can obscure the normal residual lumen and mimic a stenosis of lesser severity. Alternatively, the residual lumen may be so small that it can be missed by duplex sonography alone. Color Doppler images, alternatively acquired in the longitudinal and the transverse planes, may help detect this very narrow residual lumen (**Fig. 4–6**). Once a patent lumen is identified, it can be directly interrogated with pulsed Doppler, and waveform analysis is then possible. The color Doppler map can also be used to follow the course of the internal carotid to the point just downstream to the stenosis where blood flow signals are often distorted and of low amplitude. Doppler waveform analysis can then confirm patency of the internal carotid distal to the subtotal occlusion (**Fig. 4–7**). The accuracy of duplex sonography alone for distinguishing total from subtotal occlusions has been poor: ~50% in the early days of carotid Doppler sonography.[50] Color Doppler imaging appears to be more accurate than duplex ultrasound alone.[28,51,53] More recently, some authors have reported very high discriminating power with carotid ultrasound as compared with operative exploration.[42] It is hoped that when ultrasound contrast agents are available and routinely used in studying this type of patient, it will be easier to differentiate total versus severe subtotal occlusions because the residual lumen will be more easily and more reliably seen.

Contralateral Stenosis

A critical stenosis on one side of the neck has a variable effect on the contralateral carotid system. There is a statistically significant increase in the measured velocity on the

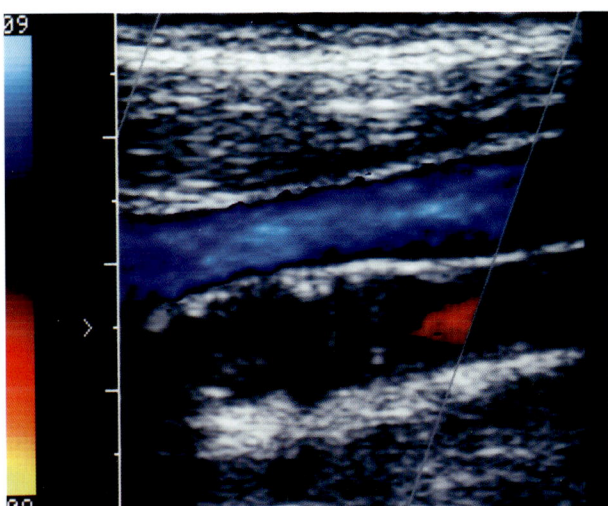
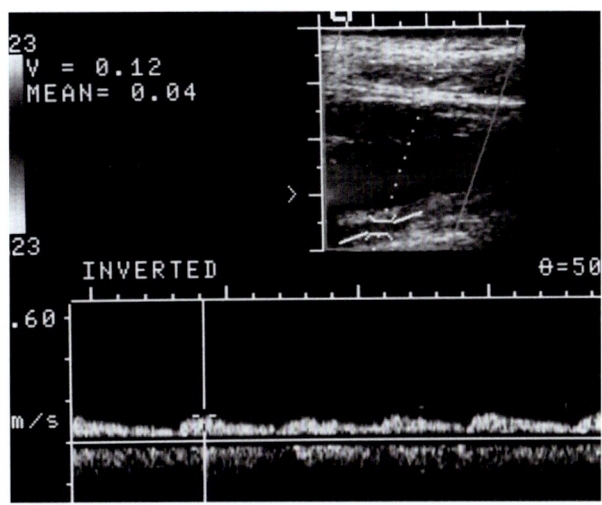

Figure 4–7 This subtotal occlusion is difficult to appreciate on a longitudinal image of the internal carotid artery. **(A)** Only faint color flow signals are seen proximal to the portion of the internal carotid artery that contains echogenic material. **(B)** Flow signals beyond the echogenic material are markedly altered, showing low amplitude and a low resistive index. This pattern is seen in the segment beyond the subtotally occluded internal carotid artery.

side contralateral to a high-grade stenosis or total occlusion.[53] This may lead to overestimation of the severity of stenosis on the side contralateral to a high-grade stenosis.[54] There is no reliable way of predicting which patient will manifest this artificial increase in blood flow velocity. However, by paying careful attention to the correlation of the color or power image on transverse and sagittal sections, and correlating with the velocity measurements obtained, errors of overestimation can be avoided.

Plaque Characterization

Several different classification schemes exist to characterize plaque. The homogeneous and heterogeneous descriptions have been popularized in the United States,[10,55,56] whereas in Europe a grading system is being used.[57] Both classification systems describe similar findings and, as a result, can be translated and in some cases interchanged.

Homogeneous plaque is relatively uniform in texture compared with the soft tissues surrounding the vessel wall. It has a smooth surface. Heterogeneous plaque has a complex echo pattern that contains at least one well-defined focal sonolucent area (**Fig. 4–8**). For plaque to be considered heterogeneous, the degree of sonolucency must be greater than 50% of the plaque volume. The intimal surface of the plaque can be smooth or irregular. To characterize plaque successfully, scanning must be performed in the sagittal and transverse planes. Alternatively, plaque can be classified into types I, II, III, and IV, with type I the most echolucent and type IV the most echogenic. Several studies have linked the presence of heterogeneous, or type I or II, plaques with developing new neurological events as well as ipsilateral CT brain infarcts.[16,24,25,58]

To develop a more reproducible and standardized method of plaque characterization and avoid the pitfalls of operator dependence, a new method has been developed to "normalize" different images by performing digital image processing. This has been successful in decreasing the variability in plaque characterization.[59,60] This has been carried to a further level by having the gray-scale distribution of plaques partitioned into different groups.

Echolucent Plaque

Color Doppler imaging is useful in evaluating lesions causing less than 50% diameter narrowing. Echolucent (hypoechoic) plaque that is not easily perceived on gray-scale image can be quite readily depicted with color Doppler imaging[29,61] and power Doppler imaging.

Ulcerated Plaque

Gray-scale imaging performs poorly in detecting ulcerated carotid plaque.[19,20,27] Color Doppler offers some diagnostic assistance in this regard. A localized zone of flow reversal or stagnation of blood flow on a color Doppler image can be seen in the ulcer crater.[62,63] This sign is specific, but not sensitive for detecting the presence of ulceration in

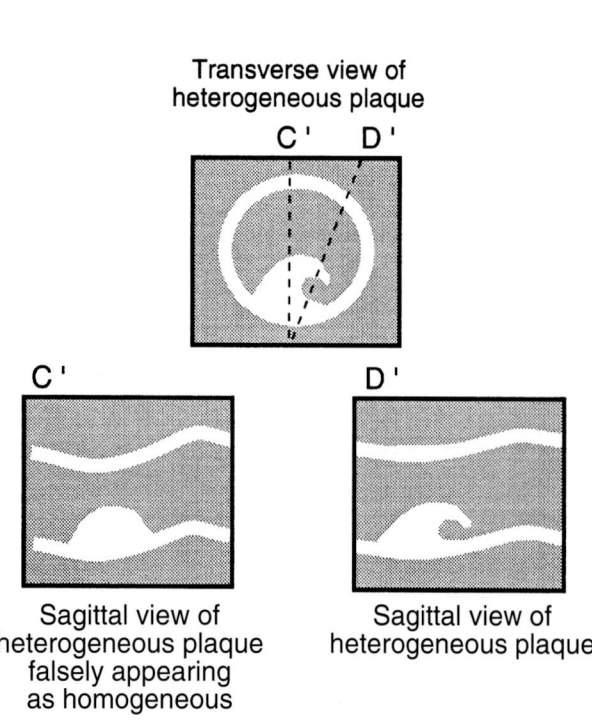
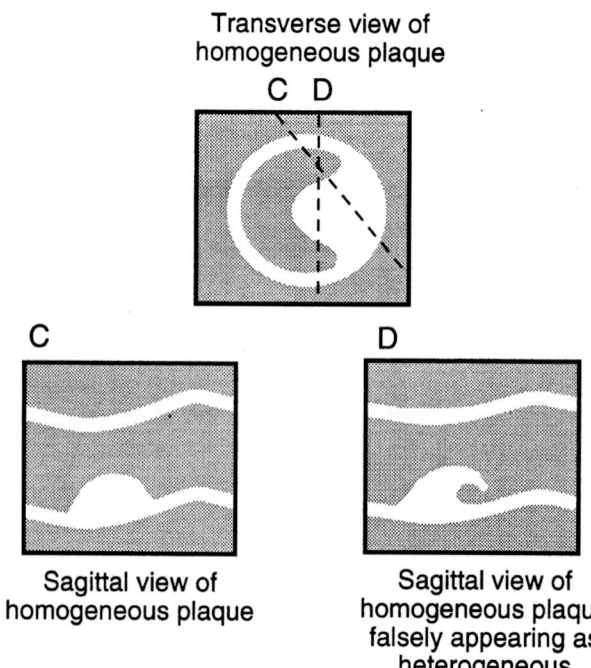

Figure 4–8 Line diagram showing the value of obtaining both transverse and sagittal images when characterizing plaque. In the sagittal plane, images can be obtained that would falsely simulate **(A)** homogeneous plaque (line C prime) or **(B)** heterogeneous plaque (line D). Correlation in both planes is necessary to be certain that the plaque is characterized correctly. (From Bluth E. Evaluation and characterization of carotid plaque. Semin US, CT, MRI 1997; 18:58. Reprinted with permission.)

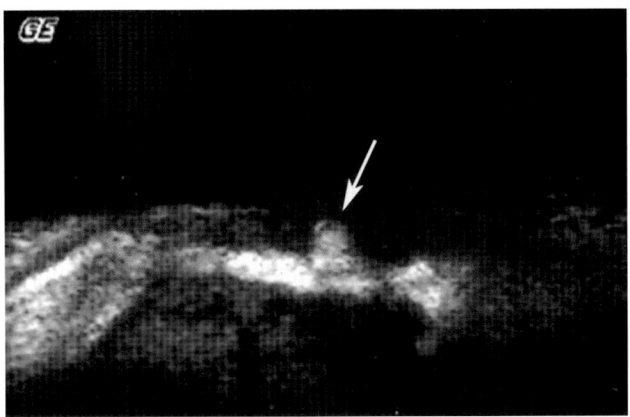

Figure 4–9 This B-flow image outlines the flow channel of a stenotic lesion of the internal carotid artery. An ulcer protrudes into the plaque (arrow).

lesions.[29] However, the presence of smaller irregularities in the contour of the plaque surface on color flow images appears to correlate with the presence of symptoms.[62] These irregularities in plaque contour may be better delineated using an imaging technique that emphasizes the signal of moving blood with a technique referred to as B-flow imaging (**Fig. 4–9**).

Is Carotid Ultrasound Indicated in Patients with Stroke or Transient Ischemic Attacks?

Should carotid sonography be done in patients presenting with stroke or TIAs? The current recommendations from an American Heart Association task force view carotid sonography as a secondary modality: "diagnostic studies aimed at establishing a likely etiology of acute ischemic stroke, including ultrasound or other imaging of intracranial or extracranial vessels, can, in some circumstances, be helpful in making decisions about treatment."[64]

A broader view suggests that ultrasound is an atraumatic way of determining whether a carotid lesion is possibly responsible for the patient's symptoms. The examination, conducted in the early stages of patient presentation, is done at a time when a TIA cannot be distinguished from a stroke. Operative intervention, in the early stages of a TIA or stroke, may carry a higher risk and degree of morbidity than interventions done later.[65,66]

Once a carotid stenosis of clinical significance is identified by ultrasound imaging, additional imaging tests are sometimes done before the patient is subjected to carotid artery surgery. Additional preoperative imaging with arteriography is considered the "gold standard." This strategy carries, however, a higher risk of stroke (1.2% in the ACAS study) than previously thought. One way to overcome this morbidity is to supplement sonography with magnetic resonance angiography (MRA) of the carotid arteries.[67] Cases with conflicting results between MRA and sonography can then be sent to arteriography. Such a strategy is more cost-effective than arteriography for symptomatic patients with ≥ 70% diameter stenosis of the internal carotid artery.[68] This strategy assumes a complete MRA examination consisting of two-dimensional (2-D) as well as three-dimensional (3-D) time-of-flight sequences. The accuracy of sonography is slightly greater than 2-D time-of-flight MRA, whereas it may be slightly less than 3-D time-of-flight techniques.[69] Meta-analysis of the diagnostic performance of magnetic resonance imaging also shows evidence that diagnostic performance is greater for high-grade carotid artery stenosis than for moderate to severe stenoses.[70] For asymptomatic patients, the lower cut-point of 60% stenosis would favor the sole use of carotid ultrasound as a cost-effective strategy to identify individuals for intervention.[71] These strategic approaches are very dependent on the morbidity of the surgical procedure and assume rates of less than 5%.[68,71]

A full evaluation of the carotid artery system from the aorta to the intracranial arteries is easily achieved with the introduction of gadolinium contrast-enhanced MRA. The frequency of unrecognized origin stenoses is estimated at 0.6%, and the more significant ones likely cause perturbations in the downstream Doppler waveform in the carotid branches.[72] The intracranial vessels can also be evaluated if there is a need. The presence of tandem lesions that could possibly be missed with this diagnostic strategy likely does not affect the outcome of subsequent carotid endarterectomy. It appears, in fact, that the number of clinical risk factors might be a better predictor of a negative perioperative outcome.[73] Use of MRA of the origins of the carotid arteries has become more routine because it helps in the planning of catheter access for carotid stenting.

Is Carotid Ultrasound Useful in Patients with Carotid Bruits?

Patient selection based on carotid bruits is an interesting strategy. The presence of a carotid bruit is an insensitive and nonspecific indicator of carotid artery disease. In addition, the presence of a carotid bruit, although it is associated with an increased incidence of neurological events, need not predict an event on the same side as the bruit. The carotid bruit serves as a nonspecific marker of atherosclerotic disease.[74] Often, the bruit may be due to a lesion in the external carotid artery or be transmitted from a more proximal lesion. As a screening strategy, increased blood flow velocities by carotid ultrasound have much better sensitivity and specificity than the presence of a carotid bruit by physical examination.[75]

The finding of an internal carotid artery stenosis in an asymptomatic patient with a carotid bruit can lead to an interesting dilemma. If the findings from the ACAS study are to be believed, then an individual should undergo carotid endarterectomy if the stenosis causes a ≥ 60% narrowing in the diameter of the proximal internal carotid artery. With this apparent indication for carotid surgery, the patient may well be managed cost-effectively with carotid sonography as the sole preoperative diagnostic test.[71] However, because the ACAS results do not apply equally to men and women or to individuals aged 68 years or less, many surgeons consider a stenosis of ≥ 80% as the best cut-point for surgery in the asymptomatic patient. Further study of this important issue is necessary.

This line of reasoning does not yet apply to decisions concerning the use of carotid stenting. Carotid stenting is considered a viable option in symptomatic individuals, especially in those with excess risk for carotid artery surgery.[5]

Estimating the Risk of Atheroembolism Based on the Findings of the Carotid Ultrasound Examination

Prevalent stroke is linked to stenosis severity in the internal carotid artery, but the stroke need not be on the same side as the more severely diseased carotid artery.[76] The relationship between carotid artery lesions and incident stroke is a bit clearer: the greater the severity of internal carotid artery stenosis measured by arteriography, the larger the risk of an incident stroke. In NASCET, for example, there is a positive dose response curve between stenosis severity and the likelihood of incident stroke in symptomatic patients with ≥ 70% diameter stenosis. Sonographic estimates of disease severity do not appear to relate as nicely with stroke risk in the NASCET study.[49] There are many possible explanations for the poor association between estimated carotid artery stenosis severity by Doppler ultrasound and incident stroke in the NASCET study. One likely explanation is the lack of a standardized carotid ultrasound imaging protocol. The lack of a standardized protocol has been shown to affect overall accuracy of the velocity estimates made with Doppler sonography.[46] Correcting these deficiencies dramatically improves the diagnostic performance of carotid sonography.[3]

As discussed previously, the morphology of internal carotid artery plaque also appears to be associated with stroke and TIA. The sonographic appearance of the carotid lesion correlates with symptoms and may be a predictor of subsequent stroke. This area remains somewhat controversial. The situation has, in fact, become less clear with the conclusion of the NASCET and ACAS studies. Most of the emphasis has now shifted to estimating internal carotid artery stenosis as lumen diameter narrowing. Presence or absence of ulceration or areas of plausible intraplaque hemorrhage have taken less importance. New studies looking at the impact of plaque characteristics on subsequent neurological events are therefore needed. A study showing that hypoechoic plaque seen on a carotid artery ultrasound can predict subsequent strokes[24] has been supported by findings from other studies.[25] Increased research is focused on applying this knowledge to routine clinical practice.

Summary

Although MRA is increasingly being considered as a possible screening test for carotid artery disease, it is unlikely to replace duplex sonography. MRA complements duplex sonography, and both techniques serve as a substitute for traditional contrast arteriography.

Color Doppler imaging and duplex sonography are cost-effective screening techniques. Use as the sole preoperative examination preceding carotid endarterectomy in a symptomatic population is possible given the right clinical scenario. Adoption of a strategy where carotid sonography is the sole preoperative test requires careful attention to the technical aspects of the examination with quality control procedures taking on great importance.

In the era of carotid stenting, carotid ultrasound offers a reliable first step to identifying patients with severe disease without subjecting them to an invasive procedure. Therapy can then be planned and the intervention tailored to the findings seen on carotid sonography. However, MRA can be very useful in these cases because it helps visualize the origins of the large arteries and can also be used to evaluate the intracranial branches.

References

1. North American Symptomatic Carotid Endarterectomy Trial Collaborators. Beneficial effect of carotid endarterectomy in symptomatic patients with high-grade stenosis. N Engl J Med 1991;325:445-453
2. European Carotid Surgery Trialists collaborative group. MRC European Carotid Surgery Trial: interim results for symptomatic patients with severe (70-99%) or with mild (0-29%) carotid stenosis. Lancet 1991;337:1235-1243
3. Executive committee for the Asymptomatic Carotid Atherosclerosis Study. Endarterectomy for asymptomatic carotid artery stenosis. JAMA 1995;273:1421-1428
4. Barnett HJM. Final results for the North American Symptomatic Carotid Endarterectomy Trial (NASCET). Stroke 1998;29:286
5. Yadav JS, Wholey MH, Kuntz RE, et al. Protected carotid-artery stenting versus endarterectomy in high-risk patients. [see comment] N Engl J Med 2004;351:1493-1501
6. Georgiadis D, Grosset DG, Kelman A, Faichney A, Lees KR. Prevalence and characteristics of intracranial microemboli signals in patients with different types of prosthetic cardiac valves. Stroke 1994;25:587-592
7. Markus HS, Droste DW, Brown MM. Detection of asymptomatic circulating cerebral emboli signals in patients with potential emboli sources. Lancet 1994;343:1011-1012
8. Lusby RJ, Ferrell LD, Ehrenfeld WK, Stoney RJ, Wylie EJ. Carotid plaque hemorrhage: its role in production of cerebral ischemia. Arch Surg 1982;117:1479-1488
9. O'Donnell TF, Erdoes L, Mackey WC, et al. Correlation of B-mode ultrasound imaging and arteriography with pathologic findings at carotid endarterectomy. Arch Surg 1985;120:443-449
10. Bluth EI, Kay D, Merritt CR, et al. Sonographic characterization of carotid plaque: detection of hemorrhage. AJR Am J Roentgenol 1986;146:1061-1065

11. Polak JF, O'Leary DH, Kronmal RA, et al. Sonographic evaluation of carotid artery atherosclerosis in the elderly: relationship of disease severity to stroke and transient ischemic attack. Radiology 1993; 188:363–370
12. Lennihan L, Kupsky W, Mohr J, Hauser W, Correll J, Quest D. Lack of association between carotid plaque hematoma and ischemic cerebral symptoms. Stroke 1987;18:879–881
13. Widder B, Paulat K, Hackspacher J, et al. Morphological characterization of carotid artery stenoses by ultrasound duplex scanning. Ultrasound Med Biol 1990;16:349–354
14. Svindland A, Torvik A. Atherosclerotic carotid disease in asymptomatic individuals: a histological study of 53 cases. Acta Neurol Scand 1988;?? :506–517
15. Bassiouny HS, Davis H, Massawa N, Gewertz BL, Glagov S, Zarins CK. Critical carotid stenoses: morphologic and chemical similarity between symptomatic and asymptomatic plaques. J Vasc Surg 1989;9:202–212
16. Geroulakos G, Domjan J, Nicolaides A, et al. Ultrasonic carotid artery plaque structure and the risk of cerebral infarction on computed tomography. J Vasc Surg 1994;20:263–266
17. Eliasziw M, Streifler J, Fox A, Hachinski V, Ferguson G, Barnett H. Significance of plaque ulceration in symptomatic patients with high-grade carotid stenosis. North American Symptomatic Carotid Endarterectomy Trial. Stroke 1994;25:304–308
18. Imparato AM, Riles TS, Mintzer R, Baumann FG. The importance of hemorrhage in the relationship between gross morphologic characteristics and cerebral symptoms in 376 carotid artery plaques. Ann Surg 1983;197:195–203
19. O'Leary DH, Holen J, Ricotta JJ, Roe S, Schenk EA. Carotid bifurcation disease: prediction of ulceration with B-mode US. Radiology 1987;162:523–525
20. Bluth EI, McVAy LV III, Merritt CRB, Sullivan MA. The identification of ulceratue plaque with high resolution duplex carotid scanning.
21. Chambers BR, Norris JW. Outcome in patients with asymptomatic neck bruits. N Engl J Med 1986;315:860–865
22. Longstreth WT Jr, Shemanski L, Lefkowitz D, O'Leary DH, Polak JF, Wolfson SK Jr. Asymptomatic internal carotid artery stenosis defined by ultrasound and the risk of subsequent stroke in the elderly. The Cardiovascular Health Study. Stroke 1998;29:2371–2376
23. Biasi GM, Froio A, Diethrich EB, et al. Carotid plaque echolucency increases the risk of stroke in carotid stenting: the Imaging in Carotid Angioplasty and Risk of Stroke (ICAROS) study. Circulation 2004;110:756–762
24. Polak JF, Shemanski L, O'Leary DH, et al. Hypoechoic plaque at US of the carotid artery: an independent risk factor for incident stroke in adults aged 65 years or older. Radiology 1998;208:649–654
25. Gronholdt ML, Nordestgaard BG, Schroeder TV, Vorstrup S, Sillesen H. Ultrasonic echolucent carotid plaques predict future strokes. Circulation 2001;104:68–73
26. Spencer MP, Reid JM. Quantitation of carotid stenosis with continuous-wave (C-W) Doppler ultrasound. Stroke 1979;10:326–330
27. Bluth EI, Stavros AT, Marich KW, Wetzner SM, Aufrichtig D, Baker JD. Carotid duplex sonography: a multicenter recommendation for standardized imaging and Doppler criteria. Radiographics 1988; 8:487–506
28. Polak JF, Dobkin GR, O'Leary DH, Wang AM, Cutler AS. Internal carotid artery stenosis: accuracy and reproducibility of color-Doppler-assisted duplex imaging. Radiology 1989;173:793–798
29. Steinke W, Kloetzsch C, Hennerici M. Carotid artery disease assessed by color Doppler flow imaging: correlation with standard Doppler sonography and angiography. AJR Am J Roentgenol 1990; 154:1061–1068
30. Baxter GM, Polak J. Variance mapping in colour flow imaging: what does it measure? Clin Radiol 1994;49:262–265
31. Erickson SJ, Newissen MW, Foley WD, et al. Stenosis of the internal carotid artery: assessment using color Doppler imaging compared with angiography. AJR Am J Roentgenol 1989;152:1299–1305
32. Bluth EI. Power Doppler imaging to evaluate flow-limiting stenoses. Radiology 2001;221:557–558
33. Hallam MJ, Reid JM, Cooperberg PL. Color-flow Doppler and conventional duplex scanning of the carotid bifurcation: prospective, double-blind, correlative study. AJR Am J Roentgenol 1989;152: 1101–1105
34. Landwehr P, Schindler R, Heinrich U, Dolken W, Krahe T, Lackner K. Quantification of vascular stenosis with color Doppler flow imaging: in vitro investigations. Radiology 1991;178:701–704
35. Vattyam HM, Shu MC, Rittgers SE. Quantification of Doppler color flow images from a stenosed carotid artery model. Ultrasound Med Biol 1992;18:195–203
36. Griewing B, Morgenstern C, Driesner F, Kallwellis G, Walker ML, Kessler C. Cerebrovascular disease assessed by color-flow and power Doppler ultrasonography: comparison with digital subtraction angiography in internal carotid artery stenosis. Stroke 1996; 27:95–100
37. Muller M, Ciccotti P, Reiche W, Hagen T. Comparison of color-flow Doppler scanning, power Doppler scanning, and frequency shift for assessment of carotid artery stenosis. J Vasc Surg 2001;34: 1090–1095
38. North American Symptomatic Carotid Endarterectomy Trial (NASCET) Steering Committee. North American Symptomatic Carotid Endarterectomy Trial. Methods, patient characteristics, and progress. Stroke 1991;22:711–720
39. Randomised trial of endarterectomy for recently symptomatic carotid stenosis: final results of the MRC European Carotid Surgery Trial (ECST). Lancet 1998;351:1379–1387
40. Rothwell PM, Gutnikov SA, Warlow CP. European Carotid Surgery Trialist's C Reanalysis of the final results of the European Carotid Surgery Trial. Stroke 2003;34:514–523
41. Rothwell PM, Eliasziw M, Gutnikov SA, et al. Analysis of pooled data from the randomised controlled trials of endarterectomy for symptomatic carotid stenosis. Lancet 2003;361:107–116
42. Grant EG, Benson CB, Moneta GL, et al. Carotid artery stenosis: gray-scale and Doppler US diagnosis—Society of Radiologists in Ultrasound Consensus Conference. Radiology 2003;229:340–346
43. Hunink MGM, Polak JF, Barlan MM, O'Leary DH. Detection and quantification of carotid artery stenosis: efficacy of various Doppler velocity parameters. AJR Am J Roentgenol 1993;160:619–625
44. Moneta GL, Edwards JM, Chitwood RW, et al. Correlation with North American Symptomatic Carotid Endarterectomy Trial (NASCET) angiographic definition of 70% to 99% internal carotid artery stenosis with duplex scanning. J Vasc Surg 1993;17:152–157
45. Faught WE, Mattos MA, van Bemmelen PS, et al. Color-flow duplex scanning of carotid arteries: new velocity criteria based on receiver operator characteristic analysis for threshold stenoses used in the symptomatic and asymptomatic carotid trials. J Vasc Surg 1994;?? :818–828
46. Howard G, Chambless LE, Baker WH, et al. A multicenter study of Doppler ultrasound versus angiography. J Stroke Cerebrovasc Dis 1991;1:166–173
47. Howard G, Baker WH, Chambless LE, Howard VJ, Jones AM, Toole JF. An approach for the use of Doppler ultrasound as a screening tool for hemodynamically significant stenosis (despite heterogeneity of Doppler performance): a multicenter experience. Stroke 1996;27: 1951–1957

48. Kuntz KM, Polak JF, Whittemore AD, Skillman JJ, Kent KC. Duplex ultrasound criteria for the identification of carotid stenosis should be laboratory specific. Stroke 1997;28:597–602
49. Eliasziw M, Rankin RN, Fox AJ, et al. Accuracy and prognostic consequences of ultrasonography in identifying severe carotid artery stenosis. Stroke 1995;26:1747–1752
50. Zwiebel WJ, Austin CW, Sackett JF, Strother CM. Correlation of high resolution, B mode and continuous wave Doppler sonography with arteriography in the diagnosis of carotid stenosis. Radiology 1983; 149:523–532
51. Hetzel A, Eckenweber B, Trummer B, Wernz M, von Reutern GM. Color-coded duplex ultrasound in pre-occlusive stenoses of the internal carotid artery [in German]. Ultraschall Med 1993;14:240–246
52. Berman SS, Devine JJ, Erdoes LS, Hunter GC. Distinguishing carotid artery pseudo-occlusion with color-flow Doppler. Stroke 1995;26: 434–438
53. Hayes AC, Johnston W, Baker WH, et al. The effect of contralateral disease on carotid Doppler frequency. Surgery 1988;103:19–23
54. Spadone DP, Barkmeier LD, Hodgson KJ, Ramsey DE, Sumner DS. Contralateral internal carotid artery stenosis or occlusion: pitfall of correct ipsilateral classification—a study performed with color flow imaging. J Vasc Surg 1990;11:642–649
55. Reilly LM, Lusby RJ, Hughes L, Ferrell LD, Stoney RJ, Ehrenfeld WK. Carotid plaque histology using real-time ultrasonography: clinical and therapeutic implications. Am J Surg 1983;146:188–193
56. Gray-Weale AC, Graham JC, Burnett JR, Byrne K, Lusby RJ. Carotid artery atheroma: comparison of preoperative B-mode ultrasound appearance with carotid endarterectomy specimen pathology. J Cardiovasc Surg (Torino) 1988;29:676–681
57. de Bray JM, Baud JM, Delanoy P, et al. Reproducibility in ultrasonic characterization of carotid plaques. Cerebrovasc Dis 1998;8: 273–277
58. Sterpetti AV, Schultz RD, Feldhaus RJ, et al. Ultrasonographic features of carotid plaque and the risk of subsequent neurologic deficits. Surgery 1988;104:652–660
59. Sabetai MM, Tegos TJ, Nicolaides AN, et al. Hemispheric symptoms and carotid plaque echomorphology. J Vasc Surg 2000;31:39–49
60. Tegos TJ, Sabetai MM, Nicolaides AN, et al. Comparability of the ultrasonic tissue characteristics of carotid plaques. J Ultrasound Med 2000;19:399–407
61. Gronholdt ML, Nordestgaard BG, Wiebe BM, Wilhjelm JE, Sillesen H. Echolucency of computerized ultrasound images of carotid atherosclerotic plaques are associated with increased levels of triglyceride-rich lipoproteins as well as increased plaque lipid content. Circulation 1998;97:34–40
62. Steinke W, Hennerici M, Rautenberg W, Mohr JP. Symptomatic and asymptomatic high-grade carotid stenoses in Doppler color-flow imaging. Neurology 1992;42:131–138
63. Furst H, Hartl WH, Jansen I, Liepsch D, Lauterjung L, Schildberg FW. Color-flow Doppler sonography in the identification of ulcerative plaques in patients with high-grade carotid artery stenosis. AJNR Am J Neuroradiol 1992;13:1581–1587
64. Adams HP Jr, Brott TG, Crowell RM, et al. Guidelines for the management of patients with acute ischemic stroke: a statement for healthcare professionals, from a special writing group of the Stroke Council, American Heart Association. Circulation 1994;90: 1588–1601
65. Gasecki AP, Ferguson GG, Eliasziw M, et al. Early endarterectomy for severe carotid artery stenosis after a nondisabling stroke: results from the North American Symptomatic Carotid Endarterectomy Trial. J Vasc Surg 1994;20:288–295
66. Ricco JB, Bouin-Pineau MH, Demarque C, et al. The role of polyester patch angioplasty in carotid endarterectomy: a multicenter study. Ann Vasc Surg 2000;14:324–333
67. Polak JF, Kalina P, Donaldson MC, O'Leary DH, Whittemore AD, Mannick JA. Carotid endarterectomy: preoperative evaluation of candidates with combined Doppler sonography and MR angiography. Radiology 1993;186:333–338
68. Kent KC, Kuntz KM, Patel MR, et al. Perioperative strategies for carotid endarterectomy: an analysis of morbidity and cost-effectiveness in symptomatic patients. JAMA 1995;274:888–893
69. Patel MR, Kuntz KM, Klufas RA, et al. Preoperative assessment of the carotid bifurcation: can magnetic resonance angiography and duplex ultrasonography replace contrast arteriography? Stroke 1995;26:1753–1758
70. Westwood ME, Kelly S, Berry E, et al. Use of magnetic resonance angiography to select candidates with recently symptomatic carotid stenosis for surgery: systematic review. BMJ 2002;324:198
71. Kuntz KM, Skillman JJ, Whittemore AD, Kent KC. Carotid endarterectomy in asymptomatic patients: is contrast angiography necessary? A morbidity analysis. J Vasc Surg 1995;22:706–716
72. Akers DL, Markowitz IA, Kerstein MD. The value of aortic arch study in the evaluation of cerebrovascular insufficiency. Am J Surg 1987;154:230–232
73. Mattos MA, van Bemmelen PS, Hodgson KJ, Barkmeier LD, Ramsey DE, Sumner DS. The influence of carotid siphon stenosis on short- and long-term outcome after carotid endarterectomy. J Vasc Surg 1993;17:902–910
74. Heyman A, Wilkinson WE, Heyden S, et al. Risk of stroke in asymptomatic persons with cervical arterial bruits: a population study in Evans County, Georgia. N Engl J Med 1980;302:838–841
75. Ingall TJ, Homer D, Whisnant JP, Baker HL, O'Fallon WN. Predictive value of carotid bruit for carotid atherosclerosis. Arch Neurol 1989;46:418–422
76. Norris JW, Zhu CZ. Silent stroke and carotid stenosis. Stroke 1992;23:483–485

5 Arm Swelling

Janis G. Letourneau and Thomas R. Beidle

In the upper extremity, several mechanisms can produce swelling, a general term used to indicate the accumulation of extracellular fluids. Increased capillary permeability, decreased oncotic pressure, increased intracapillary hydrostatic pressure, and increased lymphatic pressure are basic mechanisms that lead to swelling. A complete history and physical examination should help identify generalized edema, which is commonly caused by congestive heart failure, renal insufficiency, or nephrotic syndrome.[1] Swelling isolated to the arm implies a localized process, such as venous stasis, stenosis, or thrombosis (occlusive or nonocclusive), lymphatic obstruction, cellulitis, or angioneurotic edema. The patient's history will often provide some clues to the most likely underlying causes of arm swelling.[2]

Differential Diagnosis

Cellulitis is often caused by a penetrating injury or by the use of nonsterilized needles by intravenous drug abusers. The swelling of cellulitis is often localized, but it can involve the entire arm. If a focal area of the arm is particularly swollen, then an abscess should be considered, and ultrasound can be used to determine whether a fluid collection is present (**Fig. 5–1**). These collections can be aspirated, diagnostically or therapeutically, and drained under ultrasound guidance. It is important to note that intravenous drug abuse can lead to thrombophlebitis, which can produce swelling and can also coexist with cellulitis.

Treatment of breast cancer with axillary dissection and radiation therapy causes arm swelling in as many as 25% of patients; in many of these patients arm swelling develops several years after surgery and radiation therapy.[3] The pathophysiology of swelling in these patients is controversial. In 1938, Veal[4] stated that 90% of instances of postmastectomy arm swelling were due to venous obstruction. Subsequently, however, Lobb and Harkins[5] showed that axillary vein resection did not increase the incidence of arm swelling. Lymphangiographic studies have shown anatomical abnormalities of the lymphatic channels after surgery and radiotherapy,[6] but these abnormalities were also seen in patients without arm swelling.[7] However, by using color and duplex Doppler sonography, Svensson et al[8] showed that 57% of women with arm swelling after breast cancer treatment had evidence of venous outflow obstruction.

Venous thrombosis has been shown to occur after radiation therapy alone.[9] Thus, venous thrombosis, as well as lymphatic obstruction, should be considered as a possible cause of arm swelling in these patients (**Fig. 5–2**), particularly because, as will be described, venous thrombosis can lead to significant complications: venous thrombosis is often directly treatable, whereas lymphatic obstruction is

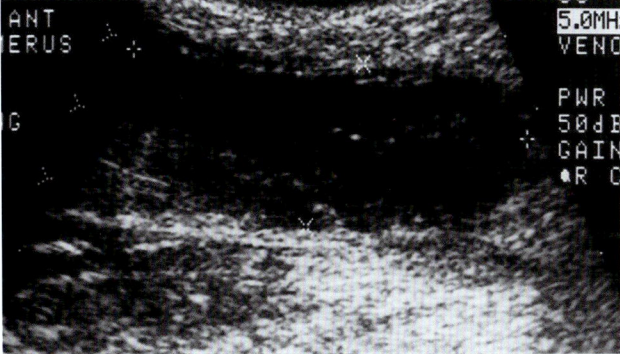

Figure 5–1 Single gray-scale ultrasound image of upper arm of patient with cellulitis and history of intravenous drug abuse shows a cystic structure that contains debris and septations. Purulent material was aspirated, confirming the diagnosis of abscess.

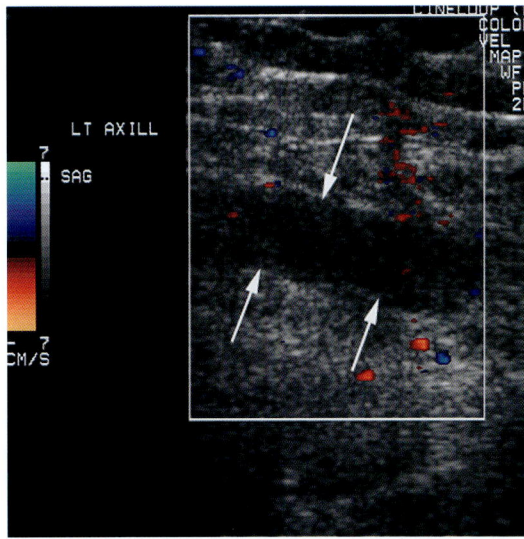

Figure 5–2 Color Doppler flow image demonstrates low-level echogenic material filling the lumen of the left axillary vein (arrows) of a patient who had undergone left axillary dissection for breast carcinoma. Image shows that no flow is present within the vein. Note that pulse repetition frequency has been lowered to detect any slow flow that may be present.

not. Other causes of lymphatic obstruction would include trauma or diseases such as elephantiasis, which is more common in the legs and is rarely seen in the Western world.[1]

Another cause of extremity swelling, angioneurotic edema, is usually well demarcated and localized. It involves only the deep layers of the skin and adjacent subcutaneous tissue. During physical examination, it can be distinguished from other causes of swelling because it is nonpitting; venous stasis and lymphatic obstruction tend to result in pitting edema.[10] Angioedema is frequently caused by an allergic reaction and is often self-limiting.

Venous stasis in the upper extremity is almost always caused by a venous outflow obstruction that results from partial or complete thrombosis of the axillary, subclavian, or innominate veins, or superior vena cava (SVC); underlying venous stenosis may also be a factor. Unlike the situation in the legs, this form of venous stasis is more likely to result from a central venous process than a peripheral, arm vein pathology. Venous outflow obstruction can also be precipitated by extrinsic compression from an adjacent node, mass, or hypertrophied muscle; such extrinsic conditions can also lead to venous thrombosis, one example being effort thrombosis (Paget-Schroetter syndrome),[11] caused by external compression of the subclavian vein usually by hypertrophied scalene muscles; prompt diagnosis of this condition with rapid initiation of thrombolytic treatment followed by surgical correction is recommended to prevent the rather consistent complication of chromic fibrous obliteration of the subclavian vein.[12]

Current or previous placement of a central venous catheter or peripherally inserted central catheter (PICC) or pacemaker wire through the subclavian vein or internal jugular vein (IJV) and underlying malignancy are the most common predisposing factors for thrombosis; there is some evidence to suggest that the incidence of catheter-related, upper extremity deep vein thrombosis in cancer patients is dependent in part on the location of the catheter tip in the brachiocephalic venous system.[13] However, some investigators also believe that a hypercoagulable state is an underrecognized risk factor for developing upper extremity deep vein thrombosis.[14-20] Moreover, there is increasing evidence to support that upper extremity deep vein thrombosis is associated with significant risk of pulmonary embolism and a high rate of 1 month and 3 month mortality.[16] Because the incidence of thrombosis in patients with indwelling catheters is so high,[21] the diagnosis of venous thrombosis should be ruled out in any of these patients who develop arm swelling. Bilateral findings raise the possibility of an obstruction of the SVC caused by either luminal caval stenosis or extrinsic compression from an adjacent tumor, such as lung carcinoma or lymphoma.

Arm swelling is only one of several symptoms that can occur as a result of venous outflow obstruction. Other signs include a poorly functioning catheter; local hyperemia; fever; pain; elevated white blood cell count; appearance of superficial varicosities in the arm, neck, and chest; and facial and neck swelling. However, these clinical signs and symptoms (including arm swelling) are nonspecific. The sensitivity of clinical diagnosis is also very low; thrombosis has been shown to be asymptomatic in 50% of patients with indwelling catheters.[22] Prompt diagnosis is important because thrombosis can lead to permanent venous insufficiency, thrombophlebitis, and pulmonary embolism. Venous thrombosis of the upper extremity is associated with pulmonary embolism in up to 16% of cases.[17,23,24]

Diagnostic Evaluation

History and physical examination are important in determining the cause of arm swelling. Diagnostic tests are used to identify or exclude venous outflow obstruction because it is potentially treatable and can lead to complications. Imaging procedures are required to identify venous obstruction; noninvasive imaging studies represent the most attractive diagnostic alternatives, with venography increasingly limited to the context of minimally invasive treatments.[25-27]

Contrast venography has been the gold-standard for making this determination. However, venography is an invasive procedure that can cause pain, a phlebitic reaction, or skin necrosis, particularly in patients with thrombosis.[28] In addition, the potential for allergic or nephrotoxic reactions exists, and the procedure may be contraindicated in patients with renal failure.

Contrast material–enhanced computed tomography (CT) of the chest is accurate for detection of intrinsic and extrinsic obstruction of the SVC. Although accuracy has not been documented, subclavian venous obstruction can be identified using sophisticated CT technologies.[29,30] However, CT has the same drawbacks as venography because ipsilateral venous contrast material injection is needed to identify thrombosis, and high volumes of contrast medium are often required for diagnostic studies.

Radionuclide venography has been used to assess patency of the upper extremity veins and indwelling catheters, but is used less commonly. False-positive and false-negative results can result from poor venous access, indwelling catheter, or collateral veins being mistaken for the subclavian vein.[31,32] Advantages of nuclear imaging are its low cost, relative noninvasiveness, and ability to assess catheter patency.

All of these imaging techniques focus on the subclavian vein, but are inherently unable to evaluate the IJV. Kroger et al[33] demonstrated that there is a high incidence of IJV thrombosis in patients with subclavian vein thrombosis. Extensive thrombosis of the IJV can lead to dural sinus thrombosis and possible cerebral venous infarction.

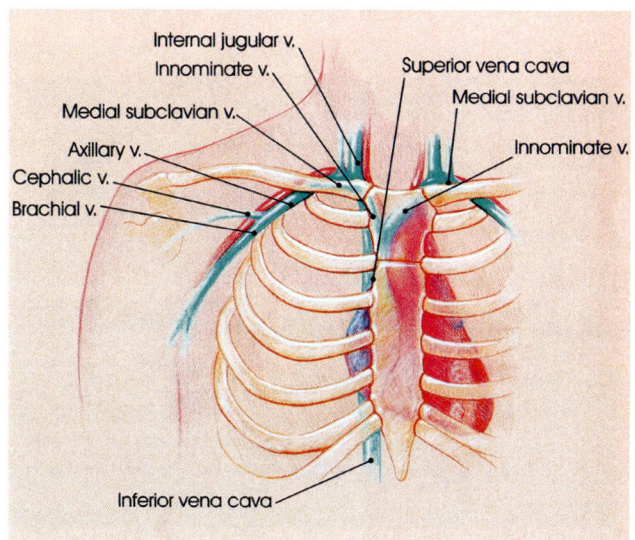

Figure 5–3 Anatomical drawing of the upper extremity and thoracic inlet veins shows normal relationships of the internal jugular, innominate, subclavian, axillary, brachial, and cephalic veins.

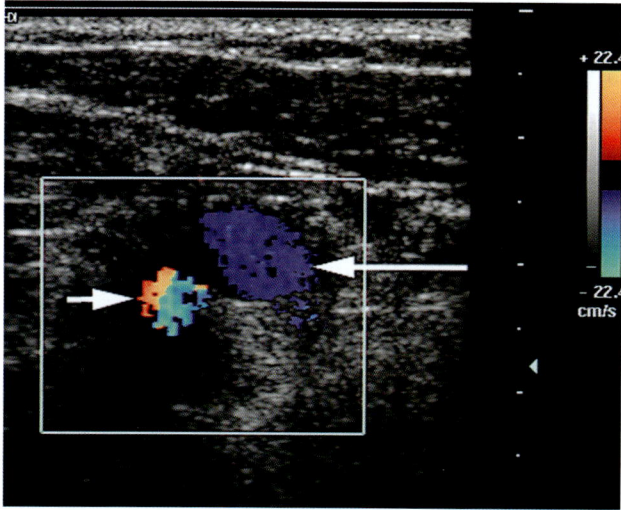

Figure 5–4 Color Doppler image obtained with a linear transducer in a plane axial to the vessel lumina. Note the normal relationship of the axillary vein (long arrow) anterior to the axillary artery (short arrow). Color pulse repetition frequency is set low to visualize flow in the vein. As a result, higher velocity in the artery causes aliasing.

Magnetic resonance (MR) angiography is capable of imaging the IJV as well as the subclavian vein, innominate vein, and SVC. Two-dimensional time-of-flight MR angiography is accurate and can image the extent of thrombus more completely than venography.[34,35] MR angiography has also been used to evaluate occlusion of the subclavian vein in patients with thoracic outlet syndrome.[36]

Ultrasound Imaging

Ultrasound is an attractive alternative to other imaging modalities because it is noninvasive, portable, inexpensive, and capable of fully evaluating the IJV, as well as assessing the peripheral veins to establish extent of the process and to provide information on peripheral venous access to the interventional radiologist. However, the test can be challenging to perform and interpret.

Sonography of the thoracic inlet veins requires knowledge of the regional anatomy. The basilic and brachial veins merge at the lateral margin of the pectoralis minor muscle to form the axillary vein, which lies medial and inferior to the axillary artery (**Fig. 5–3**).[37] As it courses medially past the lateral margin of the first rib, the axillary vein becomes the subclavian vein, which lies anterior and inferior to the subclavian artery. If a vein becomes occluded, collateral veins enlarge and are often oriented parallel to the subclavian and axillary veins.

Part of the sonographic examination involves verifying the close anatomical relationship between the subclavian artery and vein by scanning in a plane perpendicular to the course of the vessels to ensure that a large collateral vessel is not misidentified as the subclavian or axillary (**Fig. 5–4**). The subclavian vein courses over the first rib and posterior to the clavicle before turning inferiorly and merging with the IJV to form the innominate vein. The right innominate vein is shorter and more vertically oriented than the left innominate vein, and the junction of these veins behind the sternal manubrium forms the SVC. In dehydrated patients, visualization of the thoracic inlet veins may be difficult due to lack of venous distention. This situation can be remedied by placing the patient in the supine position with the head flat on the examining table, and elevating the legs if necessary.

A complete ultrasound examination of the upper extremity and the thoracic inlet veins includes bilateral evaluation of the IJVs, innominate veins, subclavian veins, and axillary veins. The cephalad portion of the SVC can be visualized in some patients (**Fig. 5–5**). If thrombosis of the axillary vein is present, the distal extent of thrombus can be documented by examining the brachial vein and its tributaries. Unless the patient is an IV drug abuser, has had trauma or surgery in the arm, or has a dialysis fistula, isolated thrombosis of an arm vein is rare. In addition, unless a dialysis fistula is present, isolated thrombosis of an arm vein is usually not symptomatic and is of less importance than a more proximal thrombosis because of the presence of a large number of potential collateral veins; however, in the face of thrombosis in the context of peripheral dialysis access, central subclavian stenosis should be considered.

Gray-scale ultrasound, color Doppler imaging, and pulsed Doppler imaging are all essential for sonographic evaluation of the upper extremity veins.[38] A high frequency (7 to 12 MHz) linear transducer is usually optimal for visualizing and compressing the peripherally located portions of the subclavian veins and IJVs, as well as the axillary vein

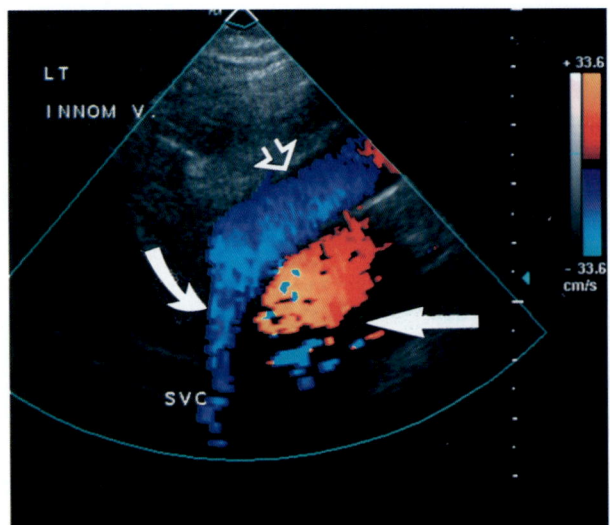

Figure 5-5 Color Doppler images of the central thoracic veins in a normal patient. **(A)** Coronal image obtained through the left supraclavicular fossa with a phased-array 7 to 4 MHz transducer shows the central portion of the left innominate vein (open arrow) turning into the superior vena cava (SVC) (curved arrow) over the aortic arch (arrow). **(B)** Coronal image with the transducer angled more to the right and slightly twisted to visualize the SVC bifurcation. The right innominate vein (arrow) joins the left innominate vein (arrowhead) to form the SVC (open arrow). The edge of the aortic arch (curved arrow) is also visualized.

and veins of the upper arm (**Fig. 5–6, Fig. 5–7**). Overlying osseous structures render visualization of the more centrally located veins more difficult.

Because of the greater ease with which the sonographer can angle the scan plane, a small footprint phased-array or sector transducer (4 to 8 MHz) aids in visualization of the inferior IJV, the medial half of the subclavian vein, the innominate vein, and the SVC. Proper positioning of the probe is essential for imaging these vessels. The junction of the subclavian and jugular veins is best visualized with the probe positioned in the supraclavicular fossa, angling medially, inferiorly, and slightly anteriorly (**Fig. 5–8, Fig. 5–9**). Note that the veins in this region are located anterior to the arteries. A small footprint 8 MHz transducer can be used in thin patients to view the superior portion of the innominate veins. A 4 MHz small footprint transducer is sometimes required in large patients and for evaluating the lower innominate veins and SVC (**Fig. 5–5**).

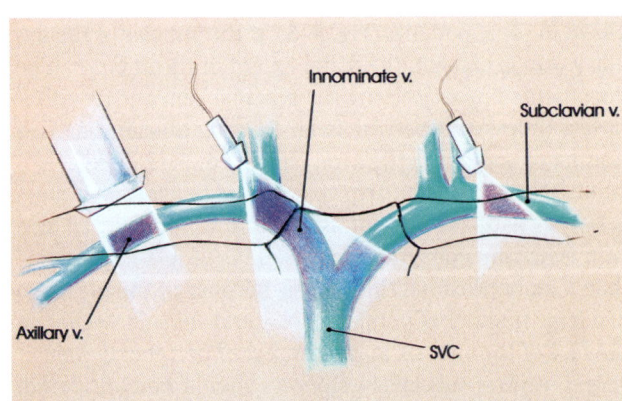

Figure 5-6 Drawing demonstrates probe positioning for sonographic evaluation of the thoracic inlet veins. The linear transducer can be used peripherally in the axillary vein and internal jugular vein. A small-footprint phased-array transducer is placed in the supraclavicular notch and angled medially to visualize the innominate veins and superior vena cava (SVC). The probe is angled more laterally to visualize the remaining portion of the subclavian vein.

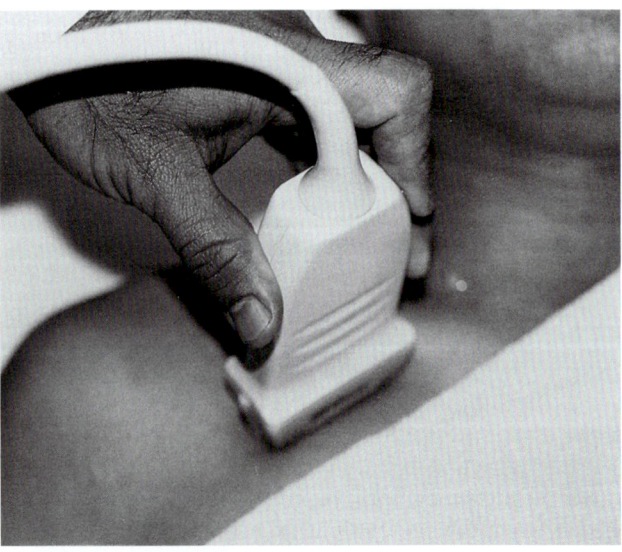

Figure 5-7 A 7 MHz linear transducer is used to visualize the axillary vein, inferior to the clavicle. The transducer should be turned 90 degrees to perform compression and confirm a normal relationship of the axillary vein to the axillary artery, to avoid mistaking a collateral vein for the axillary vein.

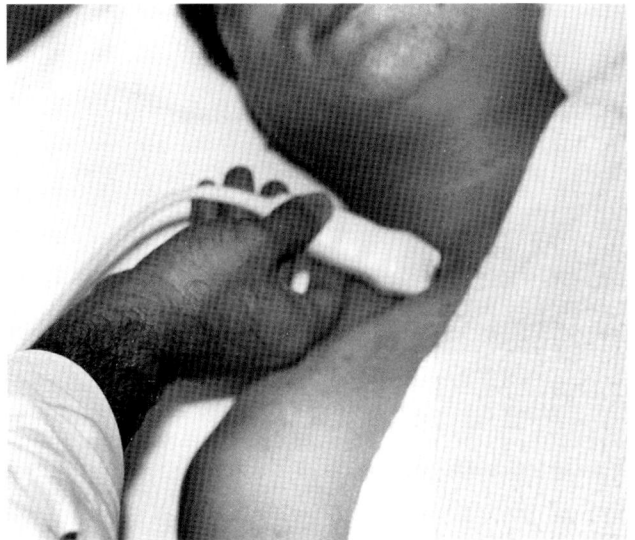

Figure 5–8 Positioning of small-footprint probe to visualize the right innominate vein and superior vena cava (SVC). Anterior view shows that the probe should be positioned in the supraclavicular fossa and angled medially. On the left side, greater medial angulation may be required, and, in some patients, sliding the probe toward the suprasternal notch may allow better visualization of the SVC (see **Fig. 5–5**).

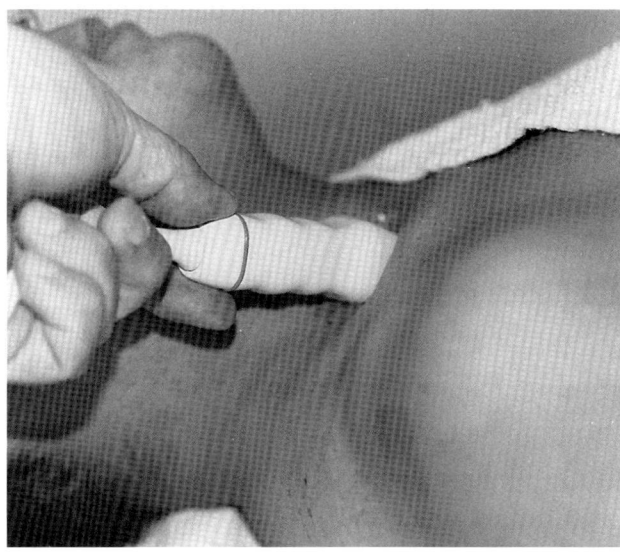

Figure 5–9 Lateral photograph shows the probe in a coronal plane positioned to visualize the right innominate vein and superior vena cava. In some patients more anterior angulation may be required.

The surface of the transducer should be kept in the same location, but angled laterally and inferiorly to visualize the midportion of the subclavian vein, which lies immediately posterior to the clavicle (**Fig. 5–6**). Additionally, in very symptomatic patients who are uncomfortable in the supine position for the duplex examination because of venous engorgement, the entire study can be performed with a small-footprint probe; this usually allows for a more rapid examination, even though the compression component of the protocol is not performed under ideal circumstances.

The entire lumen of a normal upper extremity vein is typically anechoic. With gray-scale sonography, thrombus is often apparent as variably echogenic material within the lumen (**Fig. 5–10**). Thrombosis can also result in expansion of the venous lumen. However, thrombus can be relatively or completely anechoic or difficult to appreciate in obese patients due to decreased resolution and increased acoustic scatter. Additionally, intravascular linear thrombus can mimic retained catheter fragments following catheter removal.[39] If pressure is applied with the transducer, a normal vein will completely collapse if no thrombus is present; a thrombosed segment of vein will not be completely compressible because the intraluminal filling defect prohibits complete coaptation of the vessels walls by virtue of it space-occupying nature (**Fig. 5–11**). Compression should be consistently applied to the more peripherally located veins and is best performed with a linear transducer. Because of the overlying clavicle, first rib, and sternum, compression is not feasible in the medial half of the subclavian vein, the inferior IJV, the innominate vein, or the SVC. Other gray-scale features have been described for the central upper extremity veins, but have been used less in interpretation of sonographic studies recently; in particular, the normal subclavian vein will decrease in diameter during a sniffing maneuver and increase in diameter during the Valsalva maneuver, both findings observable with real-time imaging.[40]

Color Doppler sonography is an important component of the examination of the upper extremity veins. It can aid

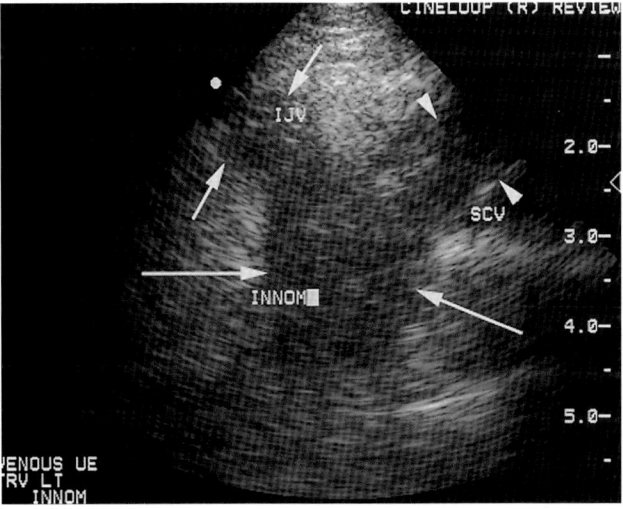

Figure 5–10 Gray-scale coronal ultrasound image of the left thoracic inlet shows material of midlevel echogenicity filling the lumens of the innominate vein (long arrows), internal jugular vein (IJV) (short arrows), and medial subclavian vein (arrowheads).

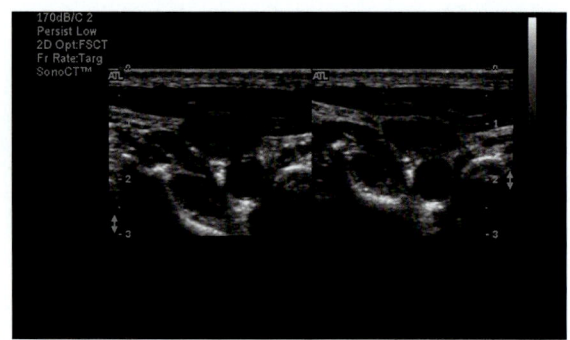
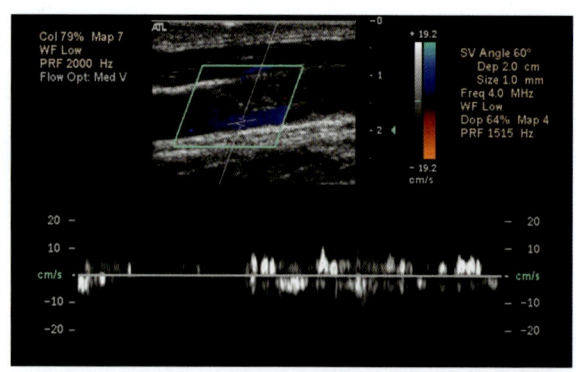

Figure 5-11 Thrombosis of the internal jugular vein. (A) Scanning with compression in a plane transverse to the course of the internal jugular vein reveals minimally echogenic thrombus and lack of coaptation of the walls of the vessel. (B) Color Doppler image of the superior aspect of the extracranial internal jugular vein shows that some flow is present (nonocclusive thrombosis) and there are dampened waveforms with loss of expected cardiac pulsatility and respiratory phasicity and slow flow velocities (~10 cm/s).

in the identification of major vessels that may be difficult to specifically characterize with standard sonography. The direction of flow can be quickly and easily ascertained. Color Doppler sonography is crucial for localization and evaluation of the more centrally located veins that are not amenable to compression.[22] Although pulsed Doppler imaging findings can confirm the presence of flow, a nonocclusive thrombus can still be present. Therefore, color Doppler flow imaging is used to confirm that the vessel completely fills with color. Any portion that does not fill may contain a thrombus that may not have been visible at gray-scale sonography. Because color Doppler imaging can help identify small channels of flow through a thrombus that appears to completely fill the venous lumen, it aids in distinguishing between an occlusive and a nonocclusive thrombus (**Fig. 5-12**). Color Doppler sonography can also facilitate identification of venous stenosis, which is characterized by luminal narrowing and color aliasing, indicating high velocity (**Fig. 5-13**). In addition, color Doppler imaging allows easy identification of collateral venous channels that arise as a result of venous obstruction (**Fig. 5-14**).[41] These collaterals may occur in the thoracic inlet region, in the axilla, or in the neck.

Even if optimal sonographic technique is employed, the innominate vein and medial subclavian vein can be difficult to evaluate in some patients, and the junction of the innominate veins is sometimes not visualized.[42] Therefore, the analysis of venous waveforms obtained with duplex sonography is geared toward identification of a centrally located venous obstruction that may not be directly visualized.

Normally, waveforms within centrally located veins demonstrate respiratory phasicity resulting from decreased intrathoracic pressure that occurs during inspiration (**Fig. 5-15**). Cardiac pulsatility is also present and results from retrograde transmission of the changing right-atrial pressure during the cardiac cycle. A small retrograde component is often present, making the waveform biphasic. Waveforms are less phasic and pulsatile when obtained further away from the thoracic inlet. If a similar degree of phasicity and pulsatility is not present in waveforms obtained from a corresponding location on the opposite side, then venous obstruction should be suspected (**Fig. 5-16, Fig. 5-17**).[43,44] Therefore, even if symptoms are unilateral, Doppler interrogation should always be performed bilaterally.[45] A complete bilateral examination is needed because asymmetry in peripheral waveforms can help identify a central, unilateral obstructing lesion that may be overlooked initially using gray-scale or color Doppler sonography. In addition, although a collateral vein can be mistaken for a patent subclavian vein (**Fig. 5-17**),[41] the waveform obtained from a collateral vein will often differ from the unaffected subclavian vein on the opposite side, prompting a search for the ipsilateral thrombosed subclavian vein. Additionally, abnormally elevated venous velocities can occur

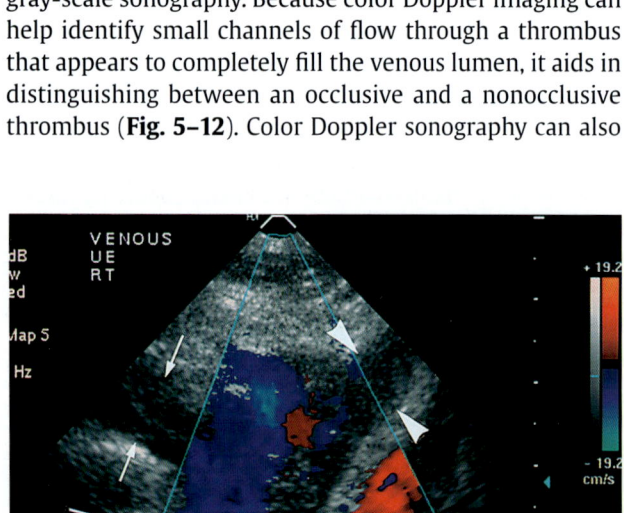

Figure 5-12 Thrombus is present throughout the right subclavian vein (short arrows), internal jugular vein (arrowheads), and innominate vein (long arrows). Blue color indicates a patent channel within the lateral portion of the innominate vein. The medially located vessel with red color is the caudal portion of the right common carotid artery.

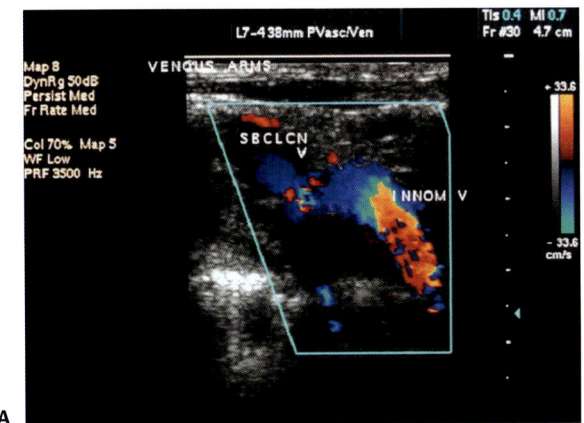
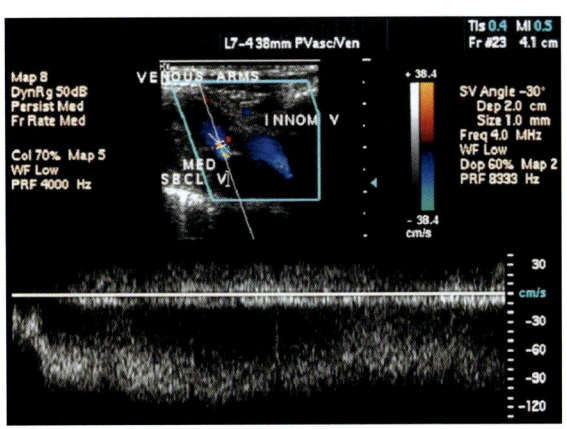
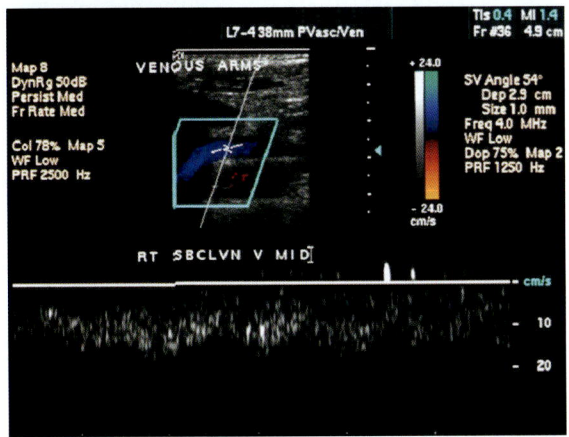
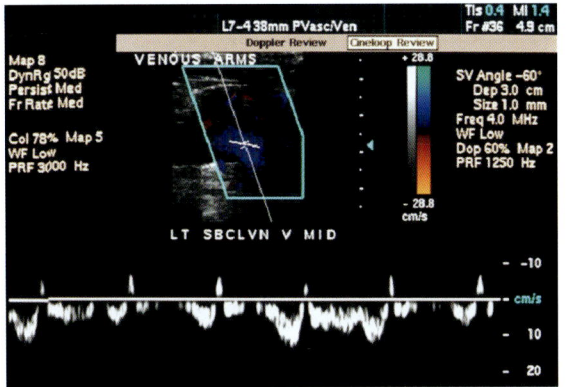

Figure 5–13 Kinking of the right subclavian vein following insertion and subsequent removal of a large-bore dialysis catheter with consequent functional stenosis of the vessel. **(A)** Luminal narrowing and angulation of the course of the medial aspect of the subclavian vein is seen as it joins with the innominate vein, causing a small amount of turbulence, expressed as color mixing on the color Doppler image. **(B)** Very high velocities (approximating 120 cm/s) are seen at the level of the venous narrowing with loss of the expected transmitted cardiac pulsatility. Some respiratory phasicity persists. **(C)** Distal flow in the midaspect of the subclavian vein is characterized by dampened flow and slow flow velocities. **(D)** In contrast the mid-left subclavian vein has a normal spectral waveform and can be used as a comparison.

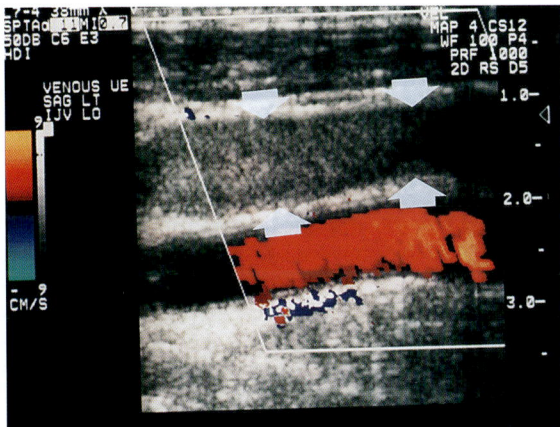
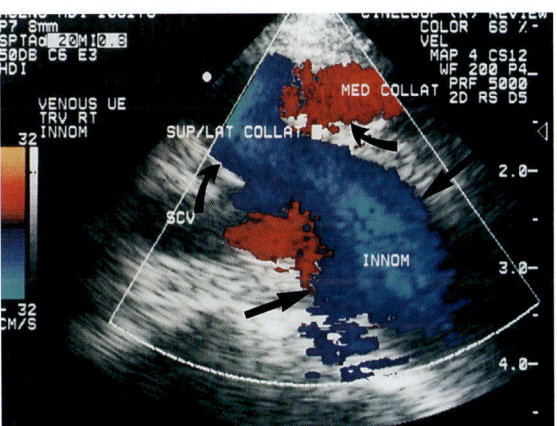

Figure 5–14 **(A)** Sagittal color Doppler flow image of the left internal jugular vein (IJV) demonstrates thrombus filling the lumen (arrows). No color signal is present in the IJV, indicating a complete occlusion. **(B)** Color Doppler flow image from the right supraclavicular region in the same patient shows large collateral veins (curved arrows) connecting to the innominate vein (straight arrows).

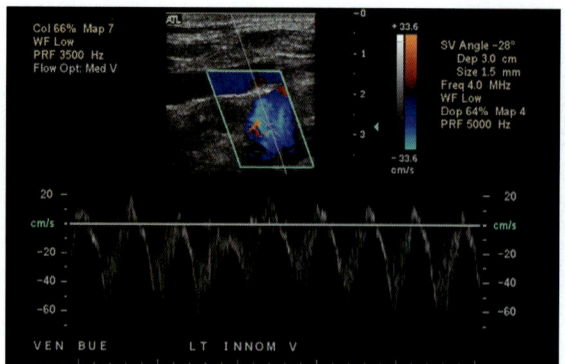

Figure 5–15 Color duplex ultrasound image of the left innominate vein shows a normal central vein waveform. Note respiratory phasicity with change in peak velocity, cardiac pulsatility with flow accentuated in concert with cardiac cycle, and small retrograde component of flow.

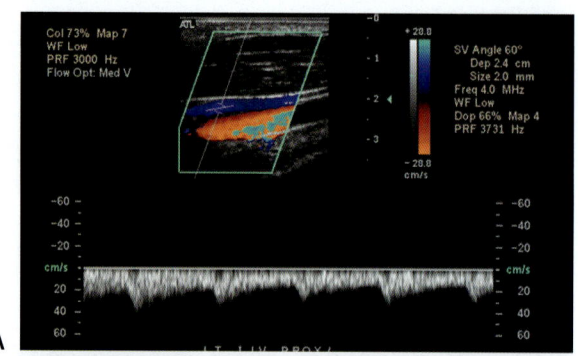
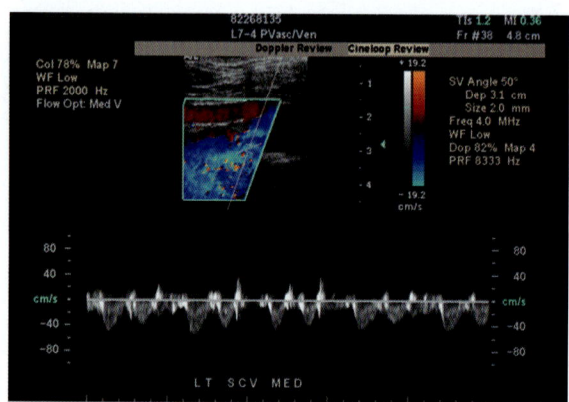
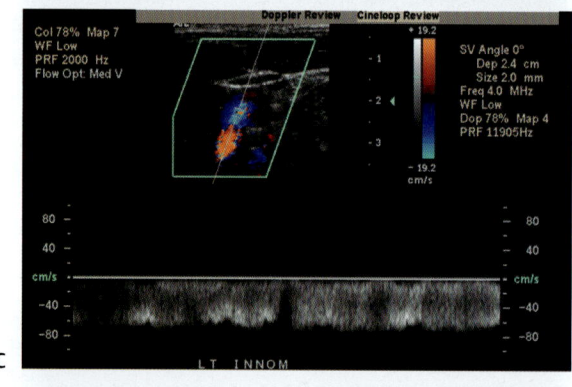
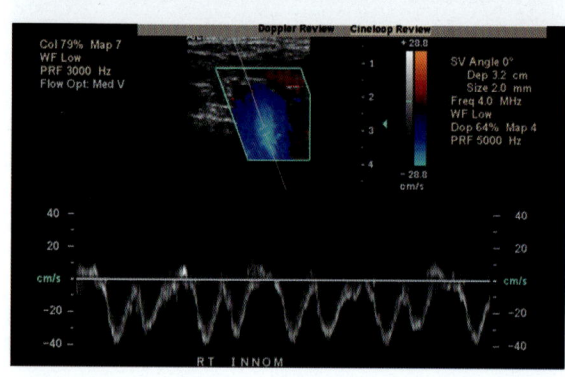
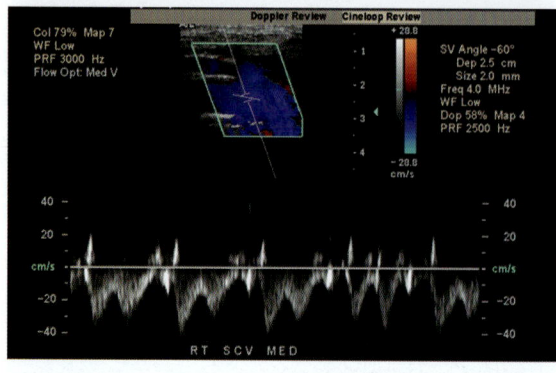

Figure 5–16 Unilateral left innominate vein stenosis. **(A)** Slightly dampened flow characteristics are seen in the left internal jugular vein. **(B)** Similarly dampened flow characteristics are seen in the left subclavian vein. **(C)** A strikingly flat, abnormal waveform is present in the left innominate vein. **(D)** In comparison, a normal waveform is seen in the right innominate vein and **(E)** in the right subclavian vein.

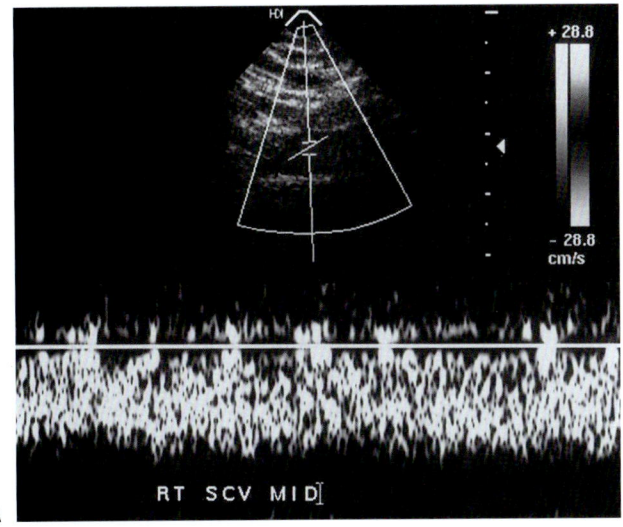
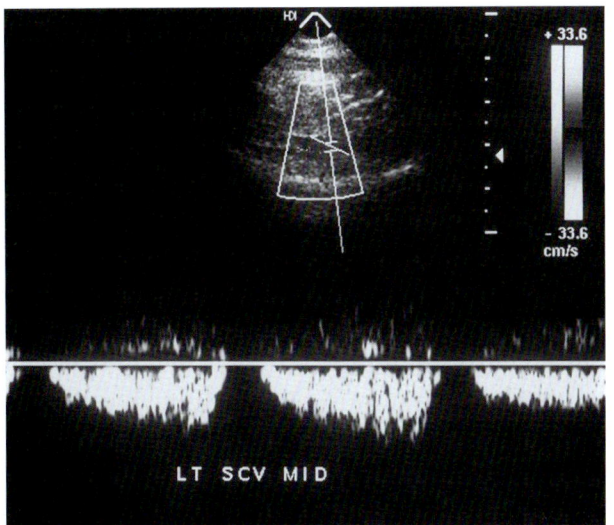
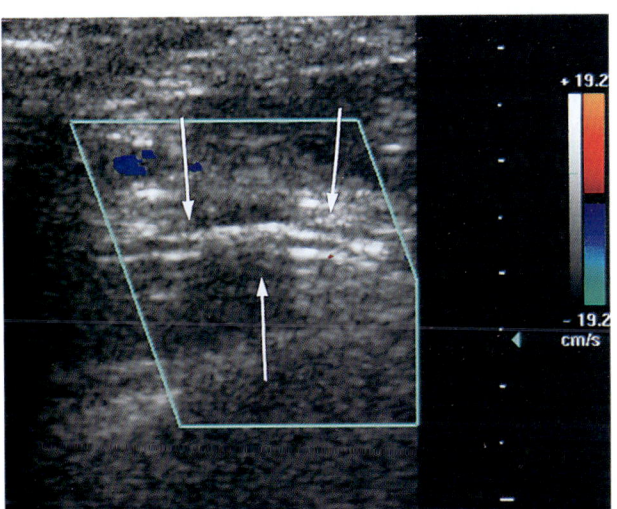
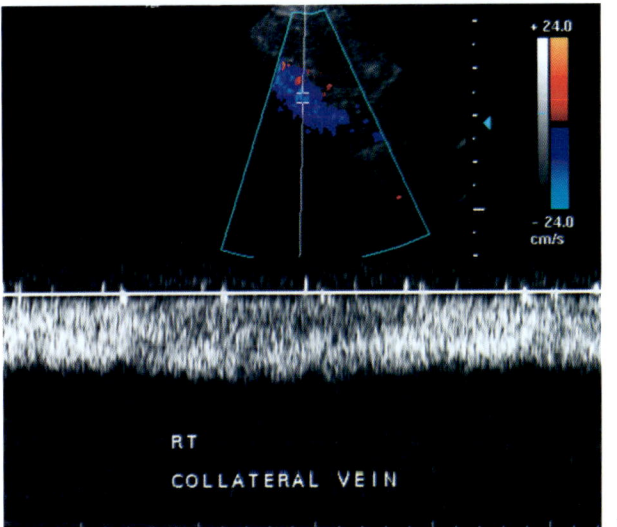
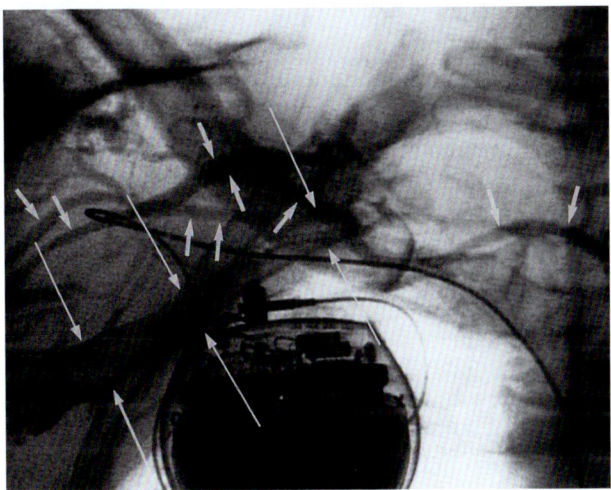

Figure 5–17 Patient with indwelling right subclavian cardiac pacing wire presented with right arm swelling and underwent ultrasound that was initially interpreted as normal. **(A)** Ultrasound waveform obtained was labeled as right subclavian vein. **(B)** Ultrasound waveform from left subclavian vein. Upon further review by a second radiologist, the right subclavian waveform **(A)** was thought to lack respiratory phasicity compared with the left subclavian waveform **(B)**. The technologist stated that the entire right subclavian vein was identified, but the cardiac pacing wire was not visualized. A second ultrasound was performed. **(C)** Color Doppler image shows no flow in the right subclavian vein containing pacing wire (arrows). **(D)** Coronal color duplex image obtained from the medial right supraclavicular fossa shows a collateral vein oriented similar to the right medial subclavian vein. Note dampening of the venous waveform, as on the previous examination. **(E)** Venogram confirms thrombus filling the right axillary and subclavian vein (long arrows). Multiple collateral veins are also identified (short arrows).

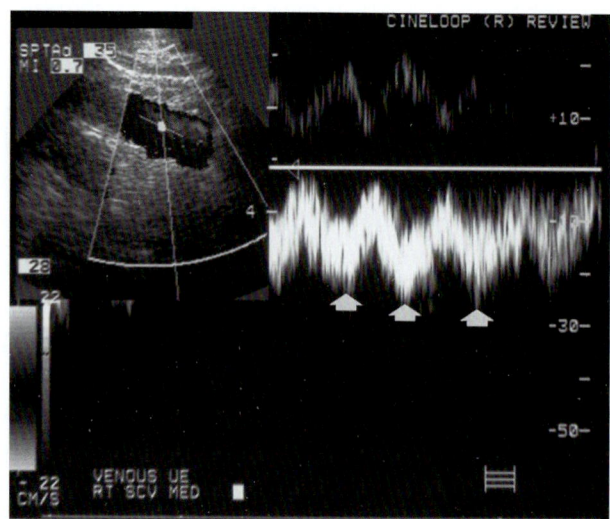 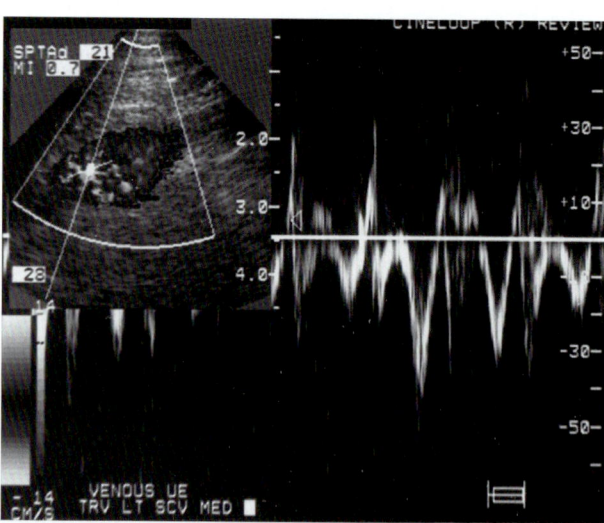

Figure 5–18 (A) Although velocity is not elevated, high-intensity spectral broadening in this duplex ultrasound scan indicates increased flow in the right subclavian vein of this patient with an ipsilateral dialysis fistula. Also note transmitted arterial pulsatility (arrows). **(B)** Left subclavian vein in the same patient has a normal ultrasound waveform.

at a site of narrowing; narrowing may be caused by a nonocclusive thrombus or a stenosis resulting from a previous thrombosis or cannulation-related trauma or even vessel kinking (**Fig. 5–13**).[44,46]

Additional maneuvers may be needed if thoracic outlet compression of the subclavian vein is suspected. In the majority of cases, thoracic outlet syndrome is caused by compression of the brachial plexus, and arm swelling from vascular compromise is not usually present.[47] However, the subclavian vein can be compressed at the thoracic outlet between the scalene muscles and the first rib. Compression of this vein can result in intermittent arm swelling and other symptoms of thoracic outlet syndrome. Repeated compression of the subclavian vein, often during strenuous exercise, can lead to the Paget-Schroetter syndrome (also known as effort thrombosis).[48,49] If thrombosis is present, it should be detectable sonographically, employing the technique already described. If thrombosis is not identified, then a more extensive ultrasound examination may help to determine whether compression of the subclavian vein occurs during arm abduction. Color Doppler and pulsed Doppler imaging should be used to evaluate the subclavian vein with the arm abducted at 90, 135, and 180 degrees, as well as in any position that reproduces symptoms. Thoracic outlet compression may be present if cessation of flow or dampening of the venous waveform occurs.[50] However, some dampening has been shown to occur in a small percentage of asymptomatic individuals.[50]

Benefits of Ultrasound

Accuracy of Ultrasound

Determination of the accuracy of ultrasound of the thoracic inlet and upper extremity veins is complicated because of the variety of sonographic methods used to diagnose venous obstruction. Koksoy et al[22] used color and duplex ultrasound and contrast venography to study 44 patients with subclavian venous catheters. They concluded that the most useful combination of parameters included visualization of thrombus, absence of spontaneous flow, and absence of respiratory phasicity. In their study, sonography had a sensitivity of 94% and a specificity of 96% for depiction of thrombus; its positive predictive value was 94%, and its negative predictive value was 96%.

One potential weakness of this study is that it was limited to patients with subclavian venous catheters, a group of patients recognized to have a high incidence of venous complications. However, this study does demonstrate the accuracy of ultrasound in patients with a history of indwelling catheter, a group that comprises the vast majority of cases of upper extremity venous thrombosis in a hospital setting. Knudson et al[42] reported a larger study with a more diverse population of 91 patients, but imaging correlation was available for only 22 of these patients. Sensitivity of ultrasound was 78%, and specificity was 92%. All four of the false-negative color Doppler examinations involved the innominate vein or SVC.

This result is not unexpected because analysis of pulsed Doppler waveforms was not included as part of the sonographic technique. Baxter et al[51] compared color Doppler sonography with venography in 19 patients and found a sensitivity of 89% and a specificity of 100%. The accuracy of ultrasound for detecting innominate or SVC obstruction was not documented. Patel et al[44] reported a sensitivity of 100%, specificity of 100%, positive predictive value of 100%, and negative predictive value of 100% for diminished or absent cardiac pulsatility as a sign of central venous thrombosis, with somewhat lower statistics for combined use of the signs of diminished respiratory phasicity and

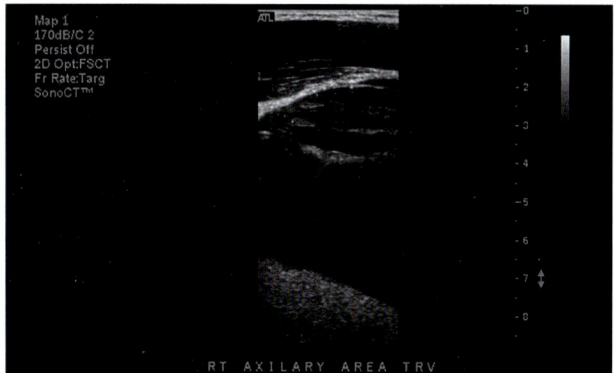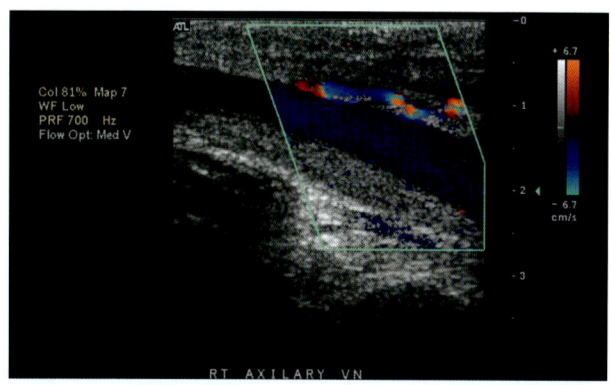
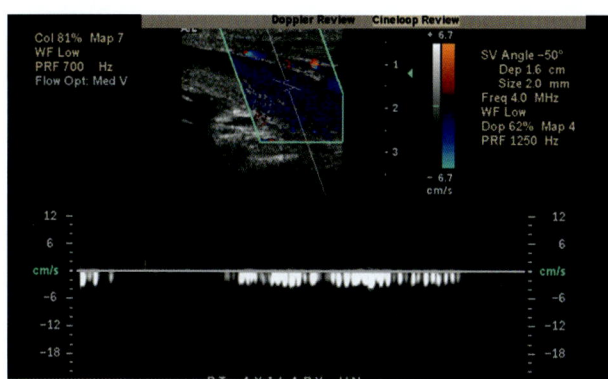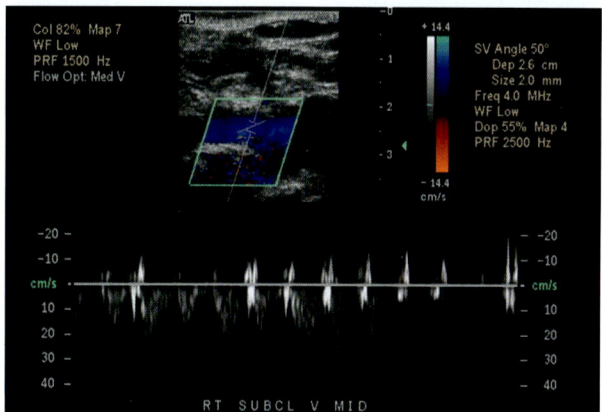

Figure 5–19 **(A)** A sonographically complex mass is seen in the right axilla following lymph node biopsy in a patient infected with human immunodeficiency virus. **(B)** Nonocclusive, mural-based thrombus is present in the lumen of the adjacent axillary vein, which is also displaced by the presence of the axillary mass. **(C)** Very dampened flow characteristics are present in the right axillary vein, associated with slow flow velocities (< 5 cm/s). **(D)** In contrast, the normal waveform of the proximal aspect of the medial subclavian vein supports the thesis that the venous pathology is all situated more peripherally in relationship to the perivascular mass causing extrinsic mass effect with secondary segmental venous thrombosis.

diminished or absent cardiac pulsatility. Although large studies comparing sonography with contrast venography are unavailable, most investigators have concluded that ultrasound is a useful test for detection of venous obstruction of the upper extremity veins.[11,22,28,41,42,44,45,51]

Limitations of Ultrasound

Because of the overlying osseous structures, upper extremity venous ultrasound is a technically demanding study and can be difficult to interpret. Most of the inaccurate results in the aforementioned studies involved the innominate veins and SVC, which might not be easily visualized. Therefore, reliance on waveform analysis is often necessary to suggest a centrally located obstruction. The central portion of the subclavian vein, located posterior to the clavicle, can also be difficult to visualize. A nonocclusive thrombus in this region can be overlooked.[52] In addition, because of overlying skeletal structures, the entire subclavian vein and adjacent artery cannot be tracked continuously with the probe oriented perpendicularly to the vessel course, increasing the likelihood of mistaking a collateral vein for the subclavian vein.[41] Bilateral waveform analysis may help prevent this potential pitfall because flow within a collateral vein may be dampened when compared with the normal subclavian vein on the opposite side (**Fig. 5–17**).

Because the study is technically demanding, experience performing and interpreting these examinations probably increases accuracy. Use of color Doppler technology is particularly important for direct visualization of the lower innominate veins and SVC. A 4 to 8 MHz sector-type probe with a small footprint is essential for direct visualization of the SVC in several patients. Nonocclusive thrombus can be missed if we are forced to rely solely on waveform analysis.

Several other pitfalls must be avoided when obtaining and interpreting pulsed Doppler waveforms. Excessive pressure applied to the ultrasound transducer can narrow the vessel lumen and lead to increased velocity, decreased velocity, or dampening of the waveform. Large-bore indwelling catheters may cause turbulent flow or dampening of the Doppler waveform, although small-caliber catheters do not cause this phenomenon.[53] The presence of a hemodialysis fistula may lead to increased flow volumes and velocities and spectral broadening in the thoracic inlet

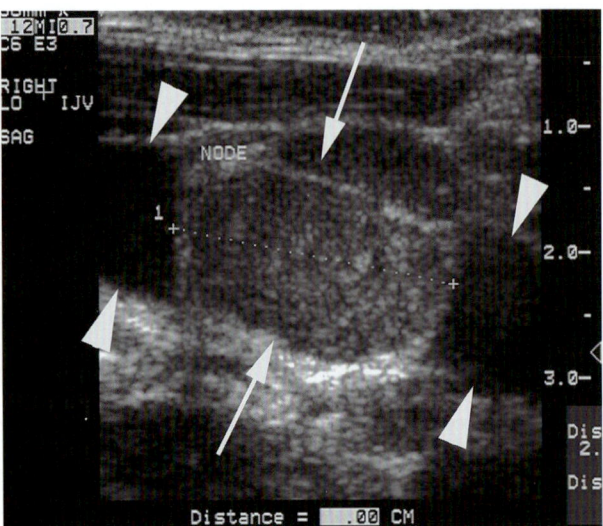

Figure 5–20 (A) Sagittal gray-scale ultrasound image shows enlarged lymph node (arrows) that appears to be a thrombus expanding the right internal jugular vein (IJV) (arrowheads). **(B)** Axial color Doppler flow image shows that the node (arrows) is compressing the IJV (arrowheads) medially. No color-filling defects are present in the IJV lumen.

veins of the ipsilateral arm (**Fig. 5–18**).[41] Dialysis patients are at risk for central venous obstruction, especially when they have a history of previous central lines placement.

As mentioned previously, lymphadenopathy can cause extrinsic compression of a thoracic inlet vein (**Fig. 5–19**), resulting in high velocity and peripheral waveform dampening. Evaluation for thrombosis may be more difficult in these patients. Occasionally, an enlarged node can simulate an intraluminal thrombus (**Fig. 5–20**).

Role of Ultrasound in Diagnostic Evaluation

Color duplex sonography should be used as the initial imaging modality for detection of venous outflow obstruction in patients with arm swelling. Although large studies with complete correlation are still unavailable, multiple investigators have concluded that ultrasound is sufficiently accurate to be used as an initial screening test.[17,22,41,42,45,51] Ultrasound is also noninvasive, inexpensive, often readily available, and portable, allowing it to be used with critically ill patients in intensive care. Ultrasound is most sensitive for the depiction of thrombosis of the axillary, subclavian, and jugular veins because of our ability to directly visualize these veins and to use compression techniques with them. It is somewhat less useful for the identification of obstruction of the innominate veins and SVC, but the presence of this condition is often suggested by waveform analysis, prompting further evaluation with other imaging modalities.

As mentioned previously, optimal technique and modern probe technology will allow sonographic evaluation of the SVC bifurcation in some patients. However, if an obstruction of the SVC is clinically suspected, CT or MR imaging may be used as the initial imaging test. Otherwise, CT, MR angiography, and contrast venography can be used as secondary imaging modalities in a few groups of patients. These groups would include patients without evidence of thrombus at gray-scale or color Doppler sonography, but with abnormal duplex findings that suggest a centrally located obstruction, patients with normal ultrasound findings in whom thrombosis still seems likely on the basis of clinical information, and patients in whom surgical or radiological intervention is planned.

There are several treatment options for patients with upper extremity venous thrombosis.[54,55] If a central venous catheter is present, removal of the catheter combined with anticoagulant therapy may relieve symptoms and prevent pulmonary embolism.[56] However, persistent morbidity including pain and swelling persists in a significant number of patients; morbidity rates vary depending on etiology of thrombosis and study population.[57,58] Percutaneous thrombolysis is more invasive, but produces long-term symptomatic relief.[59] Success of therapy and follow-up can be evaluated with sonography. Percutaneous recanalization and thrombolysis is also effective in reestablishing central venous access for parenteral therapy or nutrition.[60] Surgical decompression of the subclavian vein with first rib resection is usually reserved for patients with Paget-Schroetter syndrome who are shown to have thoracic outlet compression of the subclavian vein.[12,61] Sonography can also be used to follow these patients after treatment.

Summary

Venous outflow obstruction involving the thoracic inlet veins is a common and treatable cause of arm swelling that can lead to life-threatening complications; moreover, it is associated with high rates of 1 and 3 month mortality. Ultrasound can be used as the primary imaging modality for identifying patients with thrombosis, venous stenosis, or extrinsic venous compression, and its use is associated with acceptable statistics for diagnostic sensitivity, specificity, and accuracy when combined use of gray-scale, color Doppler, and pulsed Doppler modalities is applied. The ultrasound examination of the upper extremity veins requires knowledge of regional vascular anatomy and ideally, use of linear, as well as phased-array or sector, transducers to visualize vessels behind the sternum and clavicle. However, very symptomatic patients may need to be studied with small-footprint probes alone. With careful imaging technique, it is possible to visualize the SVC in some patients.

Frequently, ultrasound is able to help confirm or rule out the existence of thrombosis, and no further evaluation is needed. Even if the innominate veins are not completely visualized, central venous outflow obstruction can still be suggested on the basis of pulsed Doppler waveform analysis. Additional imaging with CT, MR, or contrast venography can be used to help confirm the diagnosis.

References

1. Braunwald E. Edema. In: Kasper DL, Braunwald E, Fauci AS, Hauser SL, Longo DL, Jameson JL, eds. Harrisons' Principles of Internal Medicine. 16th ed. New York: McGraw-Hill; 2005:212–216
2. Hingorani A, Ascher E. Acute upper extremity deep vein thrombosis. In: Ascher E, ed. Haimovici's Vascular Surgery. 5th ed. Malden, MA: Blackwell; 2004:1091–1096
3. Kissin MW, Querci della-Rovere G, Easton D, Westbury G. Risk of lymphoedema following the treatment of breast cancer. Br J Surg 1986;73:580–584
4. Veal JR. The pathological basis for swelling of the arm following radical amputation of the breast. Surg Gynecol Obstet 1938;67: 752–760
5. Lobb AW, Harkins HN. Postmastectomy swelling of the arm with a note on the effect of segmental resection of the axillary vein at the time of radical mastectomy. Western J Surg Obstet Gynaecol 1949; 57:550–557
6. McIvor J, O'Connell D. The investigation of postmastectomy oedema of the arm by lymphography and venography. Clin Radiol 1978;29:457–462
7. Danese C, Howard JM. Postmastectomy lymphedema. Surg Gynecol Obstet 1965;120:797–802
8. Svensson WE, Mortimer PS, Tohno E, Cosgrove DO. Colour Doppler demonstrates venous flow abnormalities in breast cancer patients with chronic arm swelling. Eur J Cancer 1994;30:675–660
9. Wilson CB, Lambert HE, Scott RD. Subclavian and axillary vein thrombosis following radiotherapy for carcinoma of the breast. Clin Radiol 1987;38:95–96
10. Austen KF. Allergies, anaphylaxis, and systemic mastocytosis. In: Kasper DL, Braunwald E, Fauci AS, Hauser SL, Longo DL, Jameson JL, eds. Harrisons' Principles of Internal Medicine. 16th ed. New York: McGraw-Hill, 2005:1947–1956
11. Grassi CJ, Polak JF. Axillary and subclavian venous thrombosis: follow-up evaluation with color Doppler flow US and venography. Radiology 1990;175:651–654
12. Molina JE. Need for emergency treatment in subclavian vein effort thrombosis. J Am Coll Surg 1995;181:414–420
13. Luciani A, Clement O, Halimi P, et al. Catheter-related upper extremity deep venous thrombosis in cancer patients: a prospective study based on Doppler US. Radiology 2001;220:655–660
14. Druy EM, Trout HH, Giordano JM, Hix WR. Lytic therapy in the treatment of axillary and subclavian vein thrombosis. J Vasc Surg 1985;2:821–827
15. Warden GD, Wilmore DW, Pruitt BA. Central venous thrombosis: a hazard of medical progress. J Trauma 1973;13:620–626
16. Hingorani A, Ascher E, Hanson J, et al. Upper Extremity versus lower exremity venous thrombosis. Am J Surg 1997;174:214–217
17. Hingorani A, Ascher E, Lorenson E, et al. Upper extremity deep venous thrombosis and its impact on morbidity and morality rates in a hospital based population. J Vasc Surg 1997;26:853–860
18. Hingorani A, Ascher E, Yorkovich W, et al. An upper extremity deep venous thrombosis: an under recognized manifestation of a hyper coagulable state. Vasc Surg 2000;14:421–426
19. Prandoni P, Polistena P, Bernardi E, et al. Upper extremity deep vein thrombosis: risk factors, diagnosis, and complications. Arch Intern Med 1997;157:57–62
20. Martinelli I, Cattaneo PM, Panzeri D, Taioli E, Mannucci M. Risk factors for deep venous thrombosis of the upper extremities. Ann Intern Med 1997;126:707–711
21. Balestreri L, DeCicco M, Matovic M, Coran F, Morassut S. Central venous catheter-related thrombosis in clinically asymptomatic oncologic patients: a phlebographic study. Eur J Radiol 1995;20: 108–111
22. Koksoy C, Kuzu A, Kutlay J, et al. The diagnostic value of colour Doppler ultrasound in central venous catheter related thrombosis. Clin Radiol 1995;50:687–689
23. Horattas MC, Wright DJ, Fenton AH, et al. Changing concepts of deep venous thrombosis of the upper extremity: report of a series and review of the literature. Surgery 1988;104:561–567
24. Monreal M, Raventos A, Lerma R, et al. Pulmonary embolism in patients with upper extremity DVT associated to venous central lines–a prospective study. Thromb Haemost 1994;72:548–550
25. Dymarkowski S, Bosmans H, Marchal G, Bogaert J. Three-dimensional MR angiography in the evaluation of thoracic outlet syndrome. AJR Am J Roentgenol 1999;173:1005–1008
26. Shinde T, Lee V, Rofsky N, Krinsky G, Weinreb J. Three-dimensional gadolinium-enhanced MR venographic evaluation of patency of central veins in the thorax initial experience. Radiology 1999;213: 555–560
27. Thornton M, Ryan R, Varghese J, Farrell M, Lucey B, Lee M. A three dimensional gadolinium-enhanced MR venography technique for imaging central veins. AJR Am J Roentgenol 1999;173:999–1003
28. Svensson WE, Mortimer PS, Tohno E, et al. The use of colour Doppler to define venous abnormalities in the swollen arm following therapy of breast carcinoma. Clin Radiol 1991;44:249–252
29. Tello R, Scholz E, Finn JP, Costello P. Subclavian vein thrombosis detected with spiral CT and three-dimensional reconstruction. AJR Am J Roentgenol 1993;160:33–34
30. Qanadli S, El Hajjam M, Bruckert F, et al. Helical CT phlebography of the superior vena cava; diagnosis and evaluation of venous obstruction. AJR Am J Roentgenol 1999;172:1327–1333
31. Fielding JR, Nagel JS, Pomeroy O. Upper extremity DVT correlation of MR and nuclear medicine flow imaging. Clin Imaging 1997;21: 260–263
32. Podoloff DA, Kim EE. Evaluation of sensitivity and specificity of upper extremity radionuclide venography in cancer patients with indwelling central venous catheters. Clin Nucl Med 1992;17:457–462
33. Kroger K, Gocke C, Schelo C, Hinrichs A, Rudofsky G. Association of subclavian and jugular vein thrombosis: color Doppler sonographic evaluation. Angiology 1998;49:189–191

34. Finn JP, Zisk JH, Edelman RR, et al. Central venous occlusion: MR angiography. Radiology 1993;187:245–251
35. Chang YC, Dai MH, Wang TC, Su CT, Chiu LC. 2-D time-of-flight (TOF) MRA of thrombophlebitis of upper extremity and subclavian veins. Angiology 1996;47:1019–1022
36. Esposito MD, Arrington JA, Blackshear MN, Murtagh FR, Silbiger ML. Thoracic outlet syndrome in a throwing athlete diagnosed with MRI and MRA. J Magn Reson Imaging 1997;17:598–599
37. Woodburne RT. Essentials of Human Anatomy. 7th ed. New York: Oxford University Press; 1983
38. Practice ACR. Guidelines for the performance of peripheral venous ultrasound examination. www.acr.org
39. Konen O, Daneman A, Traubici J, Epelman M. Intravascular linear thrombus, after catheter removal: sonographic appearance mimicking retained catheter fragment. Pediatr Radiol 2004;34: 125–129
40. Hightower DR, Gooding GA. Sonographic evaluation of the normal response of subclavian veins to respiratory maneuvers. Invest Radiol 1985;20:517–520
41. Nazarian GK, Foshager MC. Color Doppler sonography of the thoracic inlet veins. Radiographics 1995;15:1357–1371
42. Knudson GJ, Wiedmeyer DA, Erickson SJ, et al. Color Doppler sonographic imaging in the assessment of upper-extremity deep venous thrombosis. AJR Am J Roentgenol 1990;154:399–403
43. Pucheu A, Evans J, Thomas D, Scheuble C, Pucheu M. Doppler ultrasonography of normal neck veins. J Clin Ultrasound 1994;22: 367–373
44. Patel M, Berman L, Moss H, McPherson S. Subclavian and internal jugular veins at Doppler US: abnormal cardiac pulsatility and respiratory phasicity as a predictor of complete central occlusion. Radiology 1999;211:579–583
45. Longley DG, Finlay DE, Letourneau JG. Sonography of the upper extremity and jugular veins. AJR Am J Roentgenol 1993;160:957–962
46. Criado E, Marston WA, Jaques PF, Mauro MA, Keagy BA. Proximal venous outflow obstruction in patients with upper extremity arteriovenous dialysis access. Ann Vasc Surg 1994;8:530–535
47. Pollak W. Thoracic Outlet Syndrome: Diagnosis and Treatment. Mount Kisko, NY: Futura; 1986
48. Smith-Behn J, Althar R, Katz W. Primary thrombosis of the axillary/subclavian vein. South Med J 1986;79:1176–1178
49. Thompson RW, Schneider PA, Nelken NA, Skioldebrand CG, Stoney RJ. Circumferential venolysis and paraclavicular thoracic outlet decompression for effort thrombosis of the subclavian vein. J Vasc Surg 1992;16:723–732
50. Longley DG, Yedlicka JW, Monila EJ, et al. Thoracic outlet syndrome: evaluation of the subclavian vessels by color duplex sonography. AJR Am J Roentgenol 1992;158:623–630
51. Baxter GM, Kincaid W, Jeffrey RF, et al. Comparison of colour Doppler ultrasound with venography in the diagnosis of axillary and subclavian vein thrombosis. Br J Radiol 1991;64:777–781
52. Haire WD, Lynch TG, Lund GB, Lieberman RP, Edney JA. Limitations of magnetic resonance imaging and ultrasound-directed (duplex) scanning in the diagnosis of subclavian vein thrombosis. J Vasc Surg 1991;13:391–397
53. Burbidge SJ, Finlay DE, Letourneau JG, Longley DG. Effects of central venous catheter placement on upper extremity duplex US findings. J Vasc Interv Radiol 1993;4:399–404
54. Sharafuddin M, Sun S, Hoballah J. Endovascular management of venous thrombotic diseases of the upper torso and extremities. J Vasc Interv Radiol 2002;13:975–990
55. Thorpe P, Osse F. Endovascular intervention for venous occlusion compared with surgical reconstruction. In: Vascular Surgery: Basic Science and Clinical Correlations. 2nd ed. Malden, MA: Blackwell Futura; 2005:587–607
56. Haire WD. Arm vein thrombosis. Clin Chest Med 1995;16:341–351
57. AbuRahma AF, Short YS, White JF. Treatment alternatives for axillary-subclavian vein thrombosis: long-term follow-up. Cardiovasc Surg 1996;4:783–787
58. Becker DM, Philbrick JT, Walker FB. Axillary and subclavian venous thrombosis. Arch Intern Med 1991;151:1934–1943
59. Beygui RE, Olcott C, Dalman RL. Subclavian vein thrombosis: outcome analysis based on etiology and modality of treatment. Ann Vasc Surg 1997;11:247–255
60. Ferral H, Bjarnason H, Wholey M, et al. Recanalization of occluded veins to provide access for central catheter placement. J Vasc Interv Radiol 1996;7:681–685
61. Adelman MA, Stone DH, Riles TS, et al. A multidisciplinary approach to the treatment of Paget-Schroetter syndrome. Ann Vasc Surg 1997;11:149–154

6 Hypertension and Bruit
Laurence Needleman

The vast majority of patients with hypertension have essential hypertension; only a minority has renovascular hypertension (RVH). Despite this fact, the impetus to identify this minority exists because there is a possibility of curing their disease.

It is impractical to screen all hypertensive patients; therefore, it is important to identify the subset of patients who are at higher risk for RVH and might benefit from screening. It is equally important to identify the imaging tests that can be applied consistently and safely to this group.

Renal artery stenosis (RAS) is the most common cause of RVH. RAS is also associated with renal insufficiency.[1-4] Interest in applying diagnostic tests and therapeutic interventions to this risk group is growing.[5] It is clear that renal artery stenosis is associated with excess morbidity and mortality. Those with renal artery stenosis are at high risk for cardiovascular death; it is less established that renal interventions provide long-term benefit.[6]

Differential Diagnosis

Goldblatt and coworkers[7] were the first to prove that a renal lesion could cause hypertension by showing that renal artery constriction in a dog was followed by hypertension and renal atrophy. In the years that followed, understanding of the renin–angiotensin system has led to an understanding of RVH. Although RAS produces RVH, the two entities are not equivalent. RAS may not produce hypertension or it may coexist with essential hypertension. Processes other than RAS, such as Page kidney or dissecting aneurysm of the renal artery may also produce RVH. Other etiologies of secondary hypertension include renal disease, hyperaldosteronism, pheochromocytoma, Cushing's syndrome, sleep apnea syndrome, and coarctation of the aorta. Renal aneurysms may be associated with hypertension.[8]

The diagnosis of RVH is established retrospectively after the patient undergoes treatment: those whose hypertension responds to revascularization of RAS have RVH. The absence of a response to revascularization may be due to a variety of factors: technical failure of the intervention, incidental RAS in a patient with essential hypertension, or irreversible renal disease superimposed on RAS or RVH. There may be no way to distinguish these groups, so it may not be possible to find a gold standard that establishes the presence or absence of RVH.

Most tests used to evaluate the hypertensive patient are anatomical—they detect RAS. A physiological test for RVH is one that bases its diagnosis on the determination of whether the renal blood flow is abnormal. Physiological tests are theoretically more likely to predict the response to therapy, and therefore, RVH.

The prevalence of RVH is quite variable, but only represents around 0.5 to 5% of the hypertensive population.[9,10] Suggestive clinical clues may raise the likelihood of RVH to 5 to 15%.[9] Certain groups will have even greater incidence of RVH. For example, 31% of patients with accelerated hypertension may have RVH.[9]

The Cooperative Study of Renovascular Hypertension evaluated clinical features that might distinguish RVH from essential hypertension. The study compared 175 patients with RVH (91 cases of arteriosclerotic stenosis and 84 cases of fibromuscular dysplasia) that had been cured by surgery to 339 patients with essential hypertension.[11] Fibromuscular dysplasia was shown to be a disease of younger, predominantly female patients with no family history of hypertension. Arteriosclerotic patients were profiled as older, with higher systolic blood pressure, and often showed evidence of arterial disease at sites other than the kidney.

Although this study showed differences between the groups, no criteria were sufficiently sensitive or specific to distinguish the groups completely (**Table 6–1**). For instance, although a bruit was more often associated with RVH, a bruit is heard as frequently in essential hypertension. This is true because, although a lower percentage of patients with essential hypertension have bruits, essential hypertension is much more common than RVH. Still, this and other studies do point out some characteristics of patients that suggest RVH.

Mann and Pickering produced indexes of clinical suspicion that can guide the evaluation of patients with hypertension.[9] Those with borderline, low, or moderate hypertension and no clinical clues have a low index of suspicion and do not require a workup. For patients with a high index of suspicion, diagnostic testing is indicated. Angiography may be the appropriate first diagnostic imaging test. They identified patients at high risk, including those with (1) severe hypertension and either progressive renal insufficiency or lack of response to therapy, (2) accelerated or malignant hypertension, (3) grade 3 or 4 retinopathy, (4) hypertension with recent unexplained elevation of serum creatinine, (5) hypertension with elevation of serum creatinine reversibly induced by angiotensin-converting en-

Table 6–1 Clinical Characteristics of 131 Matched Cases of Essential and Renovascular Hypertension

	Hypertension	
	Essential (%)	Renovascular (%)
Duration of hypertension		
Less than 1 year	12	24
Greater than 10 years	15	6
Age of onset > 50	9	15
Family history of hypertension	71	46
Grade 3 or 4 fundi	7	46
Bruit		
Abdomen	9	46
Flank	1	12
Both	9	48
BUN > 20 mg/100 mL	8	15
Serum K < 3.4 mEq/L	8	15
Serum CO_2 > 30 mEq/L	8	16
Urinary casts	9	20
Proteinuria (a trace or more)	32	46

Note: 131 cases in each group matched by age, sex, race, and blood pressure. Only statistically significant differences are noted. (From Detection, evaluation, and treatment of renovascular hypertension: final report of the working group on renovascular hypertension. Arch Intern Med 1987;147:820–829. Reprinted with permission.)

zyme inhibitor, or (6) moderate or severe hypertension with asymmetrical renal size.

The workup of those with moderate risk such as those with refractory hypertension or moderate hypertension with a bruit or occlusive vascular disease elsewhere may require additional testing. Noninvasive tests may be helpful in this group if they identify patients for angiography.

The Dutch Renal Stenosis Intervention Cooperative (DRASTIC) study is a large multicenter Dutch study looking at RVH.[12] Angiography was performed in those who did not respond to two-drug therapy in 2 months. Up to 25% of persistently hypertensive patients had RAS.[13] The investigators concluded that drug resistance is a simple and useful clinical criterion to identify patients for angiography. A more recent multicenter trial that used the DRASTIC model showed that those with abdominal bruit, atherosclerotic disease, body mass index < 25 kg/m[2], renal function < 60 mL/min, and age greater than 58 years were significantly linked to RAS.[14] In this study no variable or combination of variables predicted RAS, but the absence of all five variables excluded RAS with a probability of 98%.

Although clinical criteria may determine some characteristics that suggest RVH, using a noninvasive screening test (such as imaging) to identify a subgroup with an even higher likelihood of a positive angiogram is another widely utilized strategy. Noninvasive tests must be applied to a subset of hypertensives with a greater likelihood of RVH. No matter how accurate the noninvasive screening test is, it will be ineffective if it is used on an unselected population of hypertensives. For example, suppose a test is quite accurate—100% sensitive and 95% specific. If this is applied to all hypertensives (3% incidence of RVH), the predictive value for RVH is only 6%. Only six of 100 angiograms will demonstrate RAS. If the population is preselected to have more RVH, the predictive value is higher. If applied to a population with 25% RVH, the test will have a predictive value of 87%; this will increase to 93% if 40% of patients have RVH. Indices of clinical suspicion are necessary to define a population that would reasonably benefit from screening.

The clinician's view about therapy also affects the workup. The results of revascularization are not entirely clear-cut in favor of subjecting patients to this treatment. In the absence of consensus, the diagnostic workup and referrals for treatment vary. The arguments made for repair of RAS cite the potential for removing or reducing a lifetime dependency on medication and for stopping or slowing the development of renal failure and other complications of hypertension. The argument against repair cites the morbidity and mortality of the procedures, the absence of long-term proven benefit, and the view that modern medical treatment may effectively treat many patients.[13,15]

Those who favor medical therapy may see no need to put patients through tests that will not alter their therapy. Those who favor revascularization are more aggressive in their efforts to detect RAS. Dean[16] has all operative candidates with diastolic blood pressure above 105 mm Hg evaluated for secondary hypertension.

Diagnostic Evaluation

Nonimaging Evaluation

Peripheral plasma renin activity and its evaluation after captopril (captopril test) are nonimaging screening tests used to determine whether hypertension is renin dependent. These tests do not localize the disease.

Vaughan's group advocates that all patients at high risk for RVH receive an ambulatory plasma renin activity level test[17] to determine the functional impact of an anatomical lesion that might be found. They find that low plasma renin activity levels are rare in untreated patients who do not have renal disease. The reported usefulness of plasma renin levels varies widely in other studies, probably due to such factors as patient preparation, medications, and assay techniques.[18,19]

Another blood test is provocative testing with captopril to elicit a hyperreninemic response. A wide range of sensitivities (34 to 100%) and specificities (72 to 95%) has been reported.[13,18,19] To perform the test correctly patients should discontinue antihypertensive medications and have an adequate amount of salt intake. Renal insufficiency, bilateral disease, and restrictive conditions make the test difficult to perform correctly. Derkx et al reported sensitivity of 84% and specificity of 93%, but the test was performed in the hospital.[13]

Renal vein determinations can be done with or without captopril stimulation. These invasive tests showed excellent results in early studies and results that are more modest on follow-up.[19]

Imaging Other than Ultrasound

Scintigraphy

Captopril renal scintigraphy (CRS) is the most widely studied noninvasive imaging test for RVH. It is used in suspected RVH, not as a general screening study. Captopril inhibits angiotensin-converting enzyme, thereby blocking angiotensin II conversion. This, in turn, prevents postglomerular efferent arteriolar vasoconstriction and decreases the glomerular filtration rate (GFR) in the stenotic kidney. The contralateral normal kidney shows an increase in GFR. This disparity in renal function can be detected by scintigraphy. Most studies have used diethylenetriaminepentaacetic acid (DPTA), but some have also evaluated radiopharmaceuticals secreted by the tubules.

Prigent has pooled the results of several series of nuclear scans.[19] The sensitivity for RAS of these pooled data was 73%, with specificity of 85% for evaluating differences between baseline and postcaptopril scans. If only the postcaptopril scans are used, the sensitivity rises to 85% and specificity becomes 83%. The value of captopril is questioned by other investigators.[13]

Pooled data also exist on how well captopril predicts a response to revascularization, and, therefore, RVH rather than RAS. Scintigraphy has a sensitivity of 76%, with a specificity of 92%, for the prediction of a cure or improvement.[19] If only postcaptopril scans are evaluated, then the test's ability to detect kidneys that will improve rises, but specificity drops off dramatically to a disappointing 66%.

Captopril renal scintigraphy is less accurate if patients have a small kidney. In the European multicenter trial,[20] abnormal renal function markedly diminished the test's specificity and accuracy (from 93 to 55% and from 90 to 68%, respectively). When this trial removed the results of patients with small kidneys and abnormal renal function, the specificity for response to treatment rose from 82 to 100%.

Magnetic Resonance and Computed Tomographic Angiography

Magnetic resonance angiography (MRA) is being actively investigated as a means of diagnosing RAS.[21-33] A variety of tests is being evaluated, including time-of-flight and

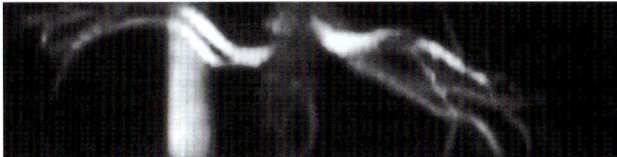

Figure 6–1 Three-dimensional reconstruction of phase-contrast magnetic resonance angiography of normal renal arteries.

phase-contrast techniques (**Fig. 6–1**). Protocols using gadolinium enhancement are also being investigated. Gadolinium has the potential to speed the examination, improve spatial resolution, and diminish artifacts. Results in the various studies have reported sensitivities from 92 to 100% with specificities of 71 to 96%.[22,29,33,34] In a meta-analysis, enhanced three-dimensional MRA and computed tomographic angiography (CTA) outperformed ultrasound and other diagnostic tests, and nonenhanced MRA also outperformed ultrasound.[35] In the multicenter RADISH trial from the Netherlands, enhanced MR demonstrated less than expected sensitivity of 62% (confidence interval [CI] 54 to 71%) and specificity of 84% (CI 81 to 87%).[36]

Some of the poor results were due to inability to detect fibromuscular dysplasia (36% of the patients with RAS), but MRA for atherosclerotic RAS yielded a modestly improved sensitivity of 78% (CI 70 to 87%) and specificity of 88% (CI 86 to 91%). Raising the threshold to diagnose RAS from 50 to 70% did not change the results.

MRA misses accessory vessels and the intrarenal stenoses of fibromuscular dysplasia. In one recent study, gadolinium enhancement did allow detection of more accessory vessels, but did not improve the accuracy of the phase-contrast study for RAS detection.[22]

MR may also be used to evaluate some physiological aspects of RVH similar to nuclear scanning. Ros et al are using the passage of gadopentetate dimeglumine to determine glomerular filtration rate.[37]

CTA using multidetector CT is being evaluated for a variety of abdominal vascular diseases, including RAS.[38-41] CTA produces volumetric data that can produce three-dimensional reconstructions of arterial structures (**Fig. 6–2**). Thin-section axial scans can also be interpreted. A variety of reconstruction schemes are possible. With some thresholding techniques, stenoses may be misinterpreted.[42] The examination takes little time and the collection of data is operator-independent; however, reconstructions take additional time to create and interpret.

Studies using spiral and 16-channel multidetector CTs report high sensitivity ranging from 86 to 100%, and high specificity, ranging from 94 to 100%.[38-40,43] In the RADISH trial, CTA demonstrated less sensitivity and specificity than previous studies, 64% (CI 55 to 73%) and 92% (CI 90 to 95%).[36] Only one of six centers used a multidetector CT (four slice); nonetheless, all scanners yielded similar results. As with MRA, some of the poor results were due to inability to detect fibromuscular dysplasia. CTA for ath-

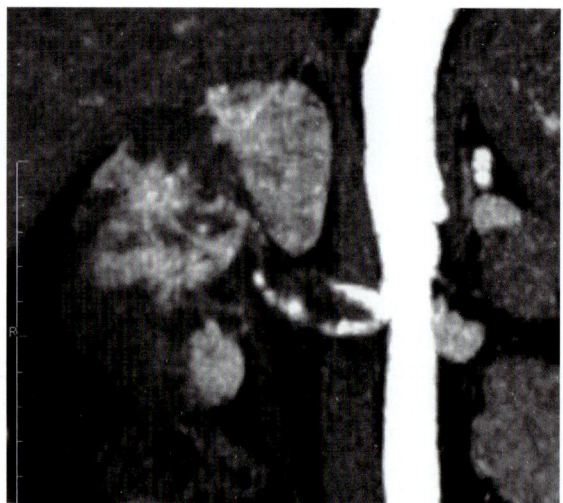

Figure 6–2 Multiplanar coronal reconstruction of multidetector computed tomographic angiogram. There is a right renal artery dissection and multiple renal infarcts. The patient has Ehlers-Danlos syndrome.

erosclerotic RAS yielded a better sensitivity of 77% (CI 67 to 86%).

Olbricht et al found some loss of accuracy when there was impaired renal function, but the numbers were too small for statistical evaluation.[40] Accessory vessels may be missed if they are outside of the acquired volume. A potential drawback to CTA is the requirement of iodinated contrast medium.

Both MRA and CTA are emerging techniques. Clinical trials with newer equipment (e.g., 16 and higher detector CT) and standardization of techniques (particularly for MR) are needed to determine their final place. For those patients whose doctor has a high clinical suspicion, angiography may still be required for a definitive diagnosis, despite a negative scan.

Ultrasound

Kidney atrophy and loss of mass over time are related to RAS.[44] In patients suspected of RVH, kidney size should be measured. In serial studies, it should be determined if there is a loss of renal mass. The demonstration of a small kidney (< 7.5 cm) is important because the shrunken kidney is unlikely to respond to revascularization.[4] Testing should concentrate on detecting a potentially curable lesion in the normal-sized kidney.

The role of Doppler ultrasound in evaluating a patient for RAS is far from clear. Although some investigators have shown superb results with Doppler ultrasound imaging, others have failed to duplicate these results. Successful groups and skeptics all agree the test is technically challenging. Investigations to diagnose Doppler examinations to diagnose RAS have fallen into two broad techniques: those that evaluate the renal arteries directly and those that evaluate the intrarenal vasculature.

Direct Doppler Evaluation of the Renal Artery

In this test, the renal artery is insonated along its course, and spectral Doppler tracings are obtained from the origin of the vessel to their entry into the kidney. Scanning is typically directed by color Doppler scanning (**Fig. 6–3**). For examination of the renal arteries, lower frequency transducers are often preferable, especially those at 2 to 2.5 MHz. Although resolution decreases with lower frequency transducers, attenuation also decreases, and this is the more critical factor. Filter settings should be set low yet high enough to suppress peristalsis, noise, and respiratory movement.

The left renal artery is found behind the left renal vein. The right renal artery originates at a similar level, or it can be found behind the inferior vena cava. Although the vessels travel posteriorly, their origins are typically from the middle, or even the anterior third, of the aorta. In certain patients, a decubitus view is helpful to move bowel out of the way. One can detect the renal origins in a coronal plane (**Fig. 6–4**).

Localization of the site of RAS is based on the detection of a high-velocity jet at the stenosis (**Fig. 6–5**). The velocity is maximal at the site of the tightest stenosis. Distal to the jet, secondary flow disturbances may exist. These include spectral broadening, shift of the distribution of blood velocities toward the baseline and away from the envelope, and simultaneous forward and reverse flow (**Fig. 6–6**). Velocities downstream from the stenotic jet are diminished. In some patients a bruit may be seen or heard. It appears on the spectrum as a low-velocity signal that is symmetrically above and below the baseline (**Fig. 6–7, Fig. 6–8**). Color Doppler may demonstrate a bruit as random color

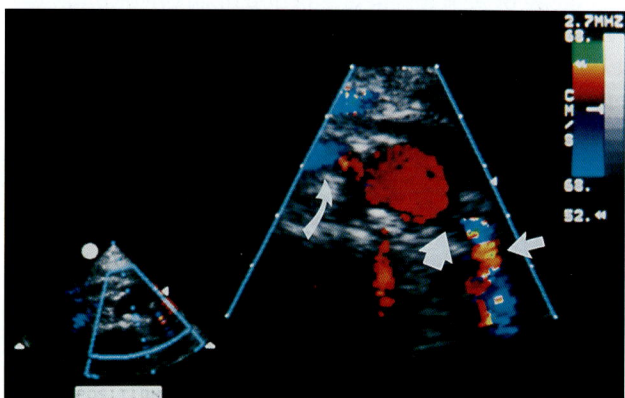

Figure 6–3 Renal color Doppler flow image of left renal artery stenosis shows marked narrowing of origin of the left renal artery (*thick straight arrow*). Red in the left renal artery, just after color is detected, represents aliasing (*thin straight arrow*). Normal right renal artery is also noted (*curved arrow*).

6 Hypertension and Bruit 71

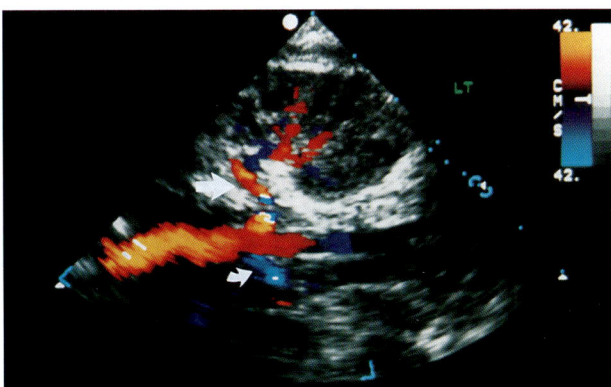

Figure 6–4 Coronal color Doppler flow image of renal artery origins. Left renal artery (*straight arrow*) can be traced in its entirety into the kidney. Proximal right renal artery (*curved arrow*) can also be seen.

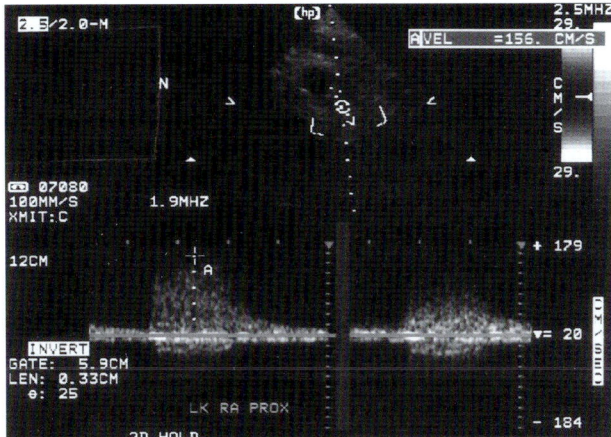

Figure 6–6 Spectral duplex Doppler image demonstrates downstream flow disturbances distal to a site of renal artery stenosis. Edge of the waveform is poorly seen. Whiter shades near the baseline indicate that more blood is moving at the lower velocities. Many different velocities are represented, which produces spectral broadening. Note simultaneous forward and reverse flow, probably the result of vortices and flow in many directions.

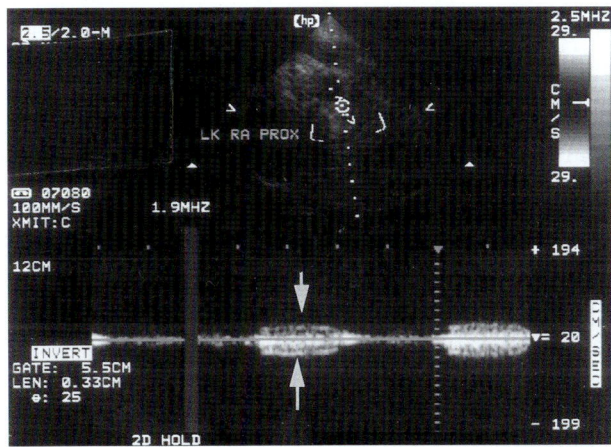

Figure 6–8 Spectral duplex Doppler image demonstrates bruit. Because bruits (*arrows*) travel through tissue, they can be detected even where no blood is flowing, as in this case. Bruits detected with Doppler imaging may not necessarily be auscultated and vice versa.

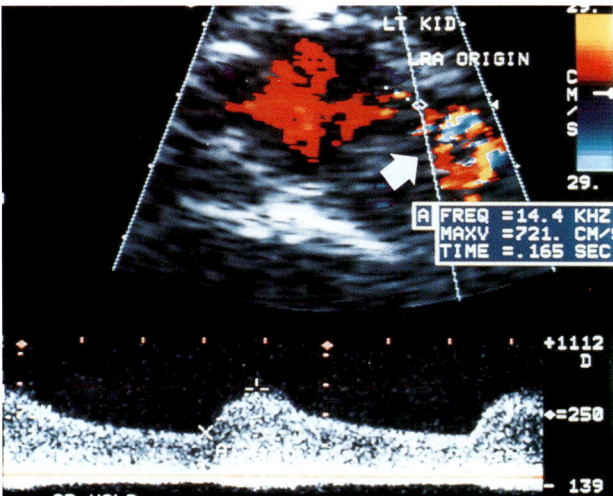

Figure 6–5 Left renal artery stenosis. Spectral color Doppler flow image shows marked narrowing of color column at origin of left renal artery. Sample volume within the narrowing yields a peak systolic velocity of 721 cm/s. Poststenotic dilatation (*arrow*) is seen distal to the narrowing. Note mosaic pattern, a mixture of colors in poststenotic regions that indicates aliasing.

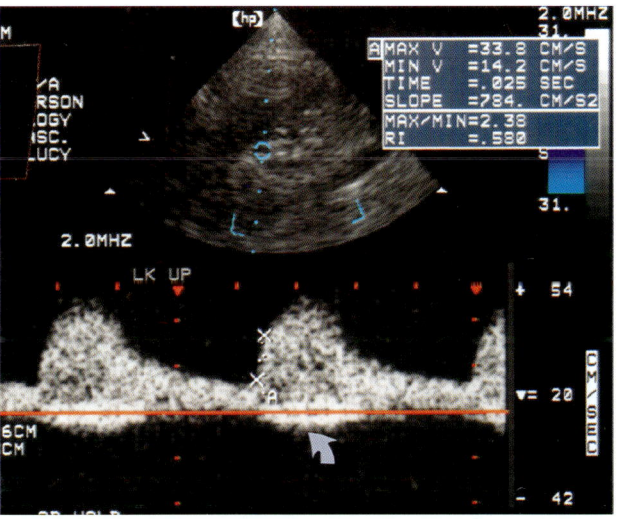

Figure 6–7 Spectral duplex Doppler intrarenal waveform with bruit. A strong, low-frequency symmetric signal above and below the baseline indicates a bruit (*arrow*). The bruit is pansystolic. Early systolic acceleration is measured as the slope in the fastest accelerating part of systole. Its value is 7.8 m/s^2. It is not measured to the peak systolic frequency, which occurs later in systole.

appearing in the adjacent soft tissues. Spectral or color bruits are usually detected in systole.

Color Doppler flow imaging can help detect stenoses as well as show the course of the vessels. Stenoses may be seen as narrowing of the color lumen (**Fig. 6–3, Fig. 6–5**). Poststenotic dilatation may also be appreciated (**Fig. 6–5**). The edge of the color does not exactly correspond to the edge of the flow because it may over- or underestimate the lumen, depending on the unit settings. The high-velocity jet is seen as a change in color that reflects the change in velocity. The jet can be seen as a different intensity of the same color, but more frequently, it is seen as aliased color. Aliasing is produced by an inadequate sampling rate for the velocity that is being sampled. Color aliasing may be seen in a variety of ways: it may appear as a region where flow appears reversed (**Fig. 6–3**), as bands of color changes (an onion-skin appearance), or as a wilder "mosaic" pattern (**Fig. 6–5**).

Because the normal renal artery has no fixed velocity, many investigators have chosen to compare the velocity of the jet to that of the aorta where the renal arteries originate. The diagnosis of RAS is made when the value of the "renal:aortic ratio" (RAR) is elevated. The ratio is calculated by dividing the highest velocity obtained in the renal artery jet by the peak systolic velocity (PSV) of the aorta. A ratio over 3.5 has been correlated to RAS above 60% diameter reduction.[45–47] Other studies have looked at absolute velocities in the renal artery jet. Although earlier studies used lower values,[48] later studies used abnormal values of PSV > 180 cm/s[49,50] or > 200 cm/s with poststenotic flow disturbances to diagnose a stenosis greater than 60%.[46,51]

In an accredited laboratory, using colorflow duplex scanning, receiver operating characteristics (ROC) analysis determined that RAR and PSV had similar accuracy.[52] In this analysis, a PSV of 220 cm/s or greater yielded a sensitivity of 91% and specificity of 85%. The best RAR was 3.2, which yielded a sensitivity of 81% and a specificity of 89%. An RAR of 3.5 yielded a sensitivity of 72% with a specificity of 92%.

In an early prospective evaluation of ultrasound duplex scanning of the main renal artery, Taylor et al[45] found a sensitivity of 84%, specificity of 97%, and positive predictive value of 94%; 12% of scans were technically inadequate.

Olin et al[46] reported detection of 98% of stenoses and occlusions (31/32 cases with stenoses of 60 to 79%, 67/69 cases with stenoses of 80 to 99%, 22/23 cases with occlusions). Specificity was 99%. One hour was allowed for the studies, which were performed by vascular technologists. Because only main renal arteries were reported, the analysis did not evaluate any accessory renal vessels.

Hoffman et al[49] had a 10% failure rate. In this study sensitivity was 92% (44/48 cases with stenoses) but the specificity was only 62% for 60% stenoses. Ten of 11 patients with occlusions were correctly identified.

Hansen, et al[53] showed excellent results for cases where there was one renal artery (sensitivity 93%, specificity 98%). However, only 49% of accessory vessels were detected. When all kidneys were considered, the resultant sensitivity was 88%.

Halpern et al[54] used similar techniques and employed experienced vascular technologists, taking as long as necessary to produce an examination. The sensitivity for the RAR was 71% with a specificity of 91%. This is also identical to the results of Krumme et al,[55] who showed 71% sensitivity and 96% specificity for abnormal PSV greater than 200 cm/s.

Spies et al[56] evaluated 135 consecutive patients using color duplex sonography. Although they had trouble identifying all segments of the renal arteries, in those with adequate scans (75% of patients, 195 arteries), the sensitivity was 93% and specificity 92%. All 12 stenosis above 75% were detected, although one was considered a 50 to 74% stenosis.

A more recent report utilized colorflow and tissue harmonic imaging.[49] Despite these technical advances, bowel gas made arteries in 9% of patients unevaluable and accessory arteries were not seen in 16 of the 19 present. All patients had atherosclerotic RAS. Doppler detected 91% (CI 89 to 93%) of stenoses and had a specificity of 97% (CI 92 to 96%).

Scanning the main renal artery is time consuming and does not reliably detect accessory vessels. Technical failure continues to be a problem because bowel gas can obscure the vessels. An overnight fast and bowel prep can help minimize this.[50,53]

Van der Hulst et al[57] validated the use of PSV and renal artery ratios for RAS. Using a Doppler guidewire, this group compared the renal artery parameters to hemodynamically significant RAS as determined by transstenotic pressure gradients in 30 vessels. This group determined that PSV and velocity ratios did correlate with RAS. Furthermore, the ROC curves produced by absolute velocity measurements were equal to those generated by digital subtraction angiography.

Intrarenal Artery Evaluation

Handa et al[58,59] described abnormal waveforms in vessels downstream from renal stenoses. Handa's group described a series of indices using frequency: the acceleration index, acceleration time, and a comparison of acceleration time in the renal artery compared with the aorta. Several years later Martin et al[60] described successful results with a flank rather than translumbar approach. This Australian group described the initial systolic (the so-called compliance) peak but did not use its appearance to make a diagnosis. The work of Stavros et al[61] resulted in more widespread interest in the technique in the United States. Several European groups were also pursuing intrarenal evaluation at that time.[62–64]

Normal intrarenal signals show a rapid rise during early systole and continuous flow through diastole (**Fig. 6–9, Fig. 6–10**). To be accurate when one measures intrarenal waveforms, the scale should be diminished so the waveform fills the spectrum. The sweep rate should be fast so only one or two waveforms are in the image. Measurement errors are reduced if the size of the spectral display is larger. The highest frequency transducer that can give an adequate signal is used, preferably 3 to 5 MHz. Position and Doppler settings should be optimized to maximize signal to noise. The Doppler angle should be minimized. Doppler parameters such as acceleration are angle-dependent because they

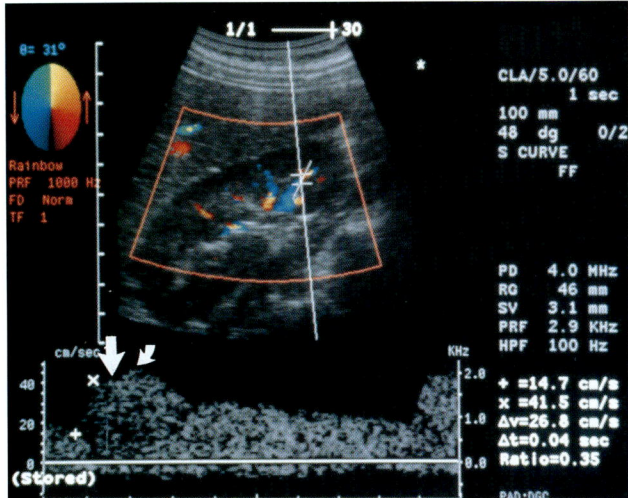

Figure 6–9 Normal intrarenal spectral Doppler waveform. The spectrum has been optimized so that one waveform fills the whole spectrum. Sweep speed is rapid so only one complete cardiac cycle is displayed. Doppler angle is determined by direction of blood flow on the color image. The angle of 31 degrees is acceptably low. Early systolic acceleration is the slope from the + marker to the x marker. In early systole, the fast-moving flow hesitates (*straight arrow*), slows down, then speeds up to peak systole (*curved arrow*). The acute angle at the hesitation marks the early systolic compliance peak/reflective wave complex.

require velocity measurements. One should attempt measurement along the plane of the intrarenal arteries, and angles should be routinely less than 30 degrees.

Intrarenal waveforms are taken from the hilus and from segmental waveforms from the upper, middle, and lower kidney (**Fig. 6–9**). Interlobar or interlobular arteries can be used,[65] although it is not known if the same normal values will apply because waveform shapes can vary along the vessels.[66] Differences in the appearance between segmental waveforms may indicate stenosis of an accessory artery supplying the abnormal segment.[65,67]

In distinction to the main renal artery test, which may take an hour or more, intrarenal scanning usually takes around 20 minutes. Technical failures rarely occur because the kidney can usually be insonated. Martin et al[60] reported a failure rate of 1.5%, although a recent investigation had a 16% failure rate.[68] Patients' inability to hold their breath is the most common cause of technical difficulties. A small kidney or poor flow caused by severe occlusive disease are other causes.

In stenosis, there is a slow rise to the peak velocity distal to the stenosis, the so-called pulsus tardus. The slope (which is the systolic acceleration) of the systolic rise is diminished and the time to the first peak velocity is lengthened (diminished acceleration time) (**Fig. 6–10, Fig. 6–11**). The arterial stenosis "filters" the normally complex arterial pulse. In early systole, this filtering accounts for diminished acceleration. The stenosis evens out the changes between systole and diastole and produces diminished pulsatility. In extreme cases, pulsatility is so diminished that the artery may resemble a vein (**Fig. 6–12**).

Martin et al and others[60,61] have described a normal early systolic compliance peak (ESP), which is an acute angle formed after the early systolic rise (**Fig. 6–9, Fig. 6–10**). ESP was associated with normal upstream vessels and was lost if there was proximal RAS. Halpern et al evaluated this phenomenon with a phantom.[66] Their results suggest the early peak is caused by transmitted systole. Following this the blood slows and may speed up again. It is this region, in the later part of systole, which is the produced by compliance. Furthermore, phantom studies suggested that changes in compliance could significantly affect the appearance of renal waveforms.[66,69]

In Martin et al's study, acceleration time and acceleration index were 87% sensitive and 98% specific.[60] Stavros et

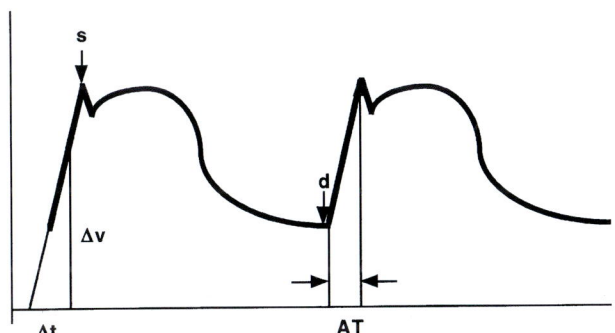
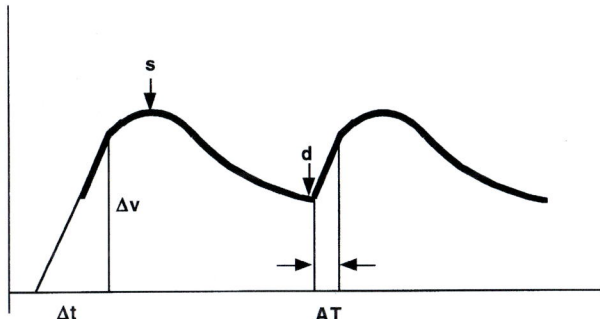

Figure 6–6 Intrarenal waveform parameters in (**A**) a normal and (**B**) abnormal waveform. Early systolic acceleration is the slope of the fastest-moving portion of the systolic component (v/t). It is not the slope of the waveform to peak systole (s) unless there is one continuous straight line to peak systole [as is the case in waveform (**B**) but not waveform (**A**)]. Acceleration time (AT) is the time it takes to get to the first inflection of the waveform (between two arrows). In the normal case (**A**) this is the time to peak systole. In the abnormal waveform (**B**) this is the time to the first inflection, which occurs earlier than peak systole. The early systolic compliance peak/reflective wave complex (ESP) is identified in waveform (**A**) at the acute angle in the waveform just after the first peak (s). The ESP is not present in waveform (**B**). Resistance index is calculated by the (peak systolic velocity − end diastolic velocity)/peak systolic velocity or (s − d)/s. The pulsatility index uses the mean velocity (not shown) as the denominator.

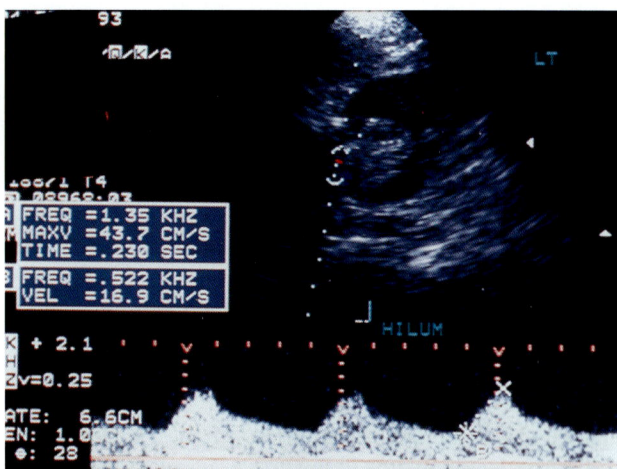

Figure 6–11 Abnormal intrarenal hilar spectral Doppler waveform. The slope of systolic acceleration is diminished, and the time to peak systole is prolonged (0.23 s), indicating proximal stenosis.

al[61] found the acceleration time to be only 78% sensitive and 94% specific, and the acceleration index to be 89% sensitive and 83% specific. Kliewer et al[70] found that the acceleration time and index distinguished normal from abnormal vessels only when the stenosis was severe (80 to 95%), but not when all the stenoses above 50% were considered. The result is not entirely unexpected because 50% diameter-reducing lesions are not hemodynamically significant in the kidneys. Higher-grade lesions of 60 to 75% may actually be necessary to produce downstream changes.[65,71,72] Indirect measures are generally less sensi-

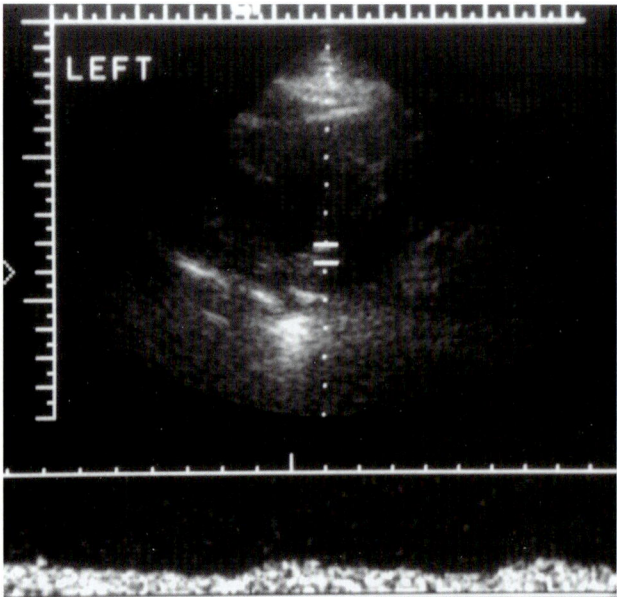

Figure 6–12 Markedly abnormal intrarenal spectral Doppler waveform shows greatly diminished systolic acceleration. Pulsatility is markedly low, to the extent that the artery might be mistaken for a vein. Note loss of the early systolic compliance peak.

tive; Motew et al demonstrated only a sensitivity of 58% using acceleration time for stenoses greater than 60%.[51]

Halpern et al[54] found the best intrarenal test to be early systolic acceleration, which is the slope of the fastest moving part of the early waveform. Early systolic acceleration is not always the slope to the PSV (**Fig. 6–7, Fig. 6–10**). Values of less than 3 m/s^2 were considered abnormal. Minimum early systolic acceleration had 86% sensitivity and 91% specificity. Halpern et al[54] concluded that a slope was better than acceleration time because the onset of acceleration is not precisely defined. Gottlieb et al[73] also determined that difficulty determining the onset of systole was the largest source of error in intrarenal measurements.

Stavros et al[61] found that a visual estimate of an abnormal waveform, as determined by the loss of the ESP, was better than any calculated measure. This loss had a sensitivity of 95% and a specificity of 97%. Because recognition of ESP is a visual parameter that describes the waveform shape, it does not require any calculation. Visual estimates of waveform shape were unsuccessful in the study by Halpern et al,[54] with the exception of a truly blunted waveform, which had a specificity of 100%. Kliewer et al[74] also found the interpretation of waveform morphology to be unsuccessful in predicting the presence or severity of RAS. However, in another study using pattern recognition before and after captopril, Rene et al[75] found this technique useful after captopril. Pattern recognition was only 68% sensitive at baseline, but rose to 100% after captopril.

Accessory vessels were identified as contributing to the misses in several of the studies.[60,70,76] Increased pulsatility in renal vessels is also associated with missed diagnosis,[60,65,77] which may be due to diminished compliance or elevated resistance.[69]

Pulsatility parameters evaluate the shape of a Doppler waveform by evaluating the relationship between peak systolic velocity and end diastolic velocity. Two common indices are the pulsatility index (PI), which is (peak systolic velocity − end diastolic velocity)/mean velocity, and the resistance index (RI), which is (peak systolic velocity − end diastolic velocity)/end diastolic velocity.

Soulen et al[78] showed that the intrarenal RI changed significantly from baseline following angioplasty. Ozbek et al[64] showed there were significant differences in PI and RI between normal kidneys and those with RAS. Bardelli et al[62] used side-to-side PI differences to diagnose unilateral RAS. In initial trials, Schwerk et al[79] determined that a difference of the RI of greater than 5% between the kidneys was 82% sensitive and 92% specific for RAS, while greater than 50% and 100% sensitive and 94% specific for stenoses with greater than 60% diameter reduction. The group conceded the test might not be as good for bilateral stenoses, and they recommended considering bilaterally low indices as suggesting bilateral RAS.

Subsequent studies using pulsatility have not been as encouraging. Burdick et al[80] evaluated acceleration, acceleration time, PI, RI, and side-to-side differences of PI and RI.

This group found acceleration and acceleration time to be superior to any of the pulsatility parameters. Side to side RI differences were only 73% sensitive and 86% specific. Bilateral disease accounted for some of the errors in using RI or PI. Acceleration time was significantly correlated with the degree of narrowing, whereas RI and PI correlated with age rather than RAS. Both acceleration time and pulsatility worked better in those with fibromuscular dysplasia than atherosclerosis. The authors postulated that changes in pulsatility due to age and atherosclerosis reduced the accuracy of the pulsatility parameters. This was probably due to resistance and compliance differences in the older, stiffer vessels. Pedersen et al[81] found a kidney length difference of 1 cm or a PI difference of greater than 0.1 to be only 75% sensitive and 76% specific for stenoses above 50%, and 84% sensitive and 73% specific for stenoses above 70%. Krumme et al[55] had a sensitivity of only 51% for bilateral stenosis.

Doppler to Predict Response to Revascularization

Preprocedural Doppler parameters have shown conflicting results to predict blood pressure or renal function response after revascularization. Pulsatility parameters change after successful revascularization for RVH.[64,65,78] Although Frauchiger et al[82] showed intervention was less successful if diastole was less than 30% of systole, Hansen et al[53] did not find a relationship between end diastolic values and the response of blood pressure or renal function to revascularization. Krumme et al[55] were also unable to show a relationship between preoperative side-to-side differences of RI and blood pressure response after successful treatment.

A prospective trial by Radermacher et al of 131 patients suggested that those with resistive indices above 0.80 were unlikely to improve their hypertension or renal function after balloon angioplasty.[83] More recently, authors have questioned this after revascularization with stents demonstrated better results despite nephrosclerosis.[84] A Doppler study by Garcia-Criado et al also does not support an upper limit of the pulsatility index to withhold revascularization.[85] Their prospective evaluation in 36 patients followed for 23 ± 15 months demonstrated improvement in blood pressure and renal function for some patients with an RI greater than 0.80. More patients showed benefit if the RI was lower, but blood pressure improved in both groups (85% for those with low RI compared with 50% in the high RI group, a significant difference), as did renal function (45% vs 28.5%, not significant). A decline in renal function occurred in 18% of the low RI group compared with 35% in the high RI group ($P = .407$). Larger studies will be necessary to determine if Doppler indices can be used to predict who may or may not benefit from revascularization.[76]

Renal Artery or Intrarenal Evaluation

Van der Hulst et al[57] seriously challenged the validity of all the intrarenal Doppler analyses. In this study using pressure gradients as a gold standard, no intrarenal parameter (acceleration time, acceleration, RI, PI, or loss of ESP) correlated with the presence of RAS. The group also found that the ROC curve of PSV is equal to angiography. This indicates that the direct renal artery study is potentially as accurate as an angiogram. However, in the real world, transabdominal scanning is not as accurate as the Doppler guidewire. The changing Doppler angle, bowel gas, deep position, and diminished signal from flow-reducing lesions all contribute to transabdominal inaccuracies and technical failures.

It is the technical difficulties encountered in certain patients rather than the interpretation of the test that makes direct renal artery duplex difficult. The criteria of an RAR above 3.5 or a PSV of greater than 180 to 200 cm/s is reproducible. In technically adequate examinations, renal artery duplex scanning can reliably detect and exclude main renal artery stenosis. An adequate amount of time must be allowed to perform the study. The experience of the sonographer or vascular technologist is crucial; the more experienced sonographer will make fewer mistakes and produce fewer inadequate examinations. An experienced examiner will also be able to determine if the study is reliable or limited. When color or spectral Doppler evaluation does not demonstrate substantial portions of the renal arteries, the results should be reported as less reliable unless there is unequivocal evidence for RAS in the region seen. Those with limited examinations may need additional testing with another modality.

Intrarenal Doppler parameters are easier to produce, but their significance is more difficult to interpret. The degree of stenosis,[71] etiology of the lesion,[55] resistance and compliance,[66,69] age of the patient, presence of parenchymal disease,[66] and arterial pressure[63]—all affect the final waveform shape. It is unknown if medical therapy itself affects waveform shape. Severe stenoses are correlated with the intrarenal indices, but less severe stenoses are not. Some investigators feel this is because those lesser stenoses are not hemodynamically significant based on some experimental data.[65] The results of van der Hulst et al, appear to refute this concept.[57]

The slope of the early systolic acceleration is more reproducible than acceleration time.[54,73] Acceleration and acceleration time are less accurate in pulsatile renal arteries, presumably due to intrinsic renal disease. Determining if there is loss of ESP is operator dependent[65] and not reproducible.[54,70,74,86] Pulsatility parameters are not accurate enough and miss many bilateral stenoses.

A very blunted waveform[54] or a very long acceleration time (above 0.12 s[68]) have a high predictive value for RAS. Normal intrarenal waveforms and mildly abnormal measurements are less reliable. Direct renal artery evaluation should always be performed if there are normal or equivocal intrarenal results. This is particularly true if there is diminished diastolic flow.

Future research efforts should be made to make direct renal evaluation simpler and to diminish the number of inadequate studies. It is hoped that by increasing the signal from the blood, intravenous microbubble contrast agents can improve the accuracy of renal Doppler. In two initial studies of direct renal artery evaluation,[87] and intrarenal evaluation,[77] contrast enhancement improved the results and shortened the examination time. In a multicenter trial, the number of inadequate scans decreased with contrast, but neither the sensitivity nor the specificity improved.[88]

The etiology of suspected RAS helps determine if Doppler should be performed and how it should be interpreted. Direct renal artery duplex scanning detects RAS in large, typically main vessels. Accessory vessels are routinely missed.[31,48,53,56,89,90] This may be less important in atherosclerotic patients because some investigators feel renal artery stenosis in small accessory vessels rarely causes hypertension in this group.[89] Fibromuscular dysplasia is different—patients may have RVH from main or intrarenal stenoses. In those suspected of fibromuscular dysplasia, the significance of a normal Doppler study is not reassuring because accessory and branch disease may be missed. Patients with suspected fibromuscular dysplasia might require angiography because angiography is currently the only examination that has the resolution to evaluate intrarenal stenoses well.

Other Causes of Abdominal Bruit

Significant stenoses in any vessel may produce a bruit. In the abdomen, common locations for occlusive disease are the celiac axis and superior mesenteric artery. In patients who present with a bruit, and in whom the renal arteries are not stenotic, evaluating the celiac axis and superior mesenteric artery may be worthwhile to determine if they are stenosed (**Fig. 6–13**). Bruits from stenoses in the iliac artery are heard lower in the abdomen than the bruit from upper abdominal vessels. Bruits from arteriovenous fistulas usually have a continuous quality. Epigastric bruits are more common from the celiac axis or superior mesenteric artery, whereas flank bruits are more typical for a renal origin.

Renal arteriovenous fistulas (**Fig. 6–14**) are associated with bruits.[8] They often appear as a cystic mass, typically in a hilar location. Color flow imaging demonstrates flow in these lesions. Arteriovenous fistulas have a typical high-velocity spectral waveform with low pulsatility. Fistulas are often congenital, although they are found in renal carcinoma and after trauma. Parenchymal arteriovenous fistulas may be seen after kidney biopsy.

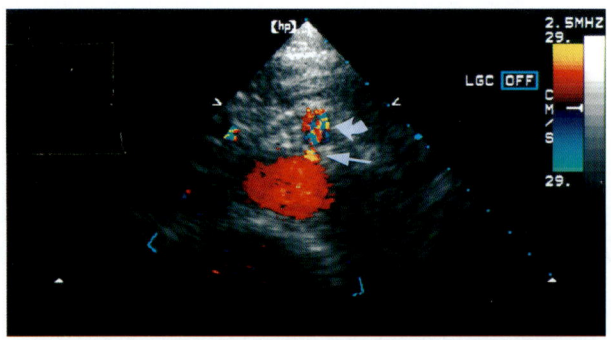

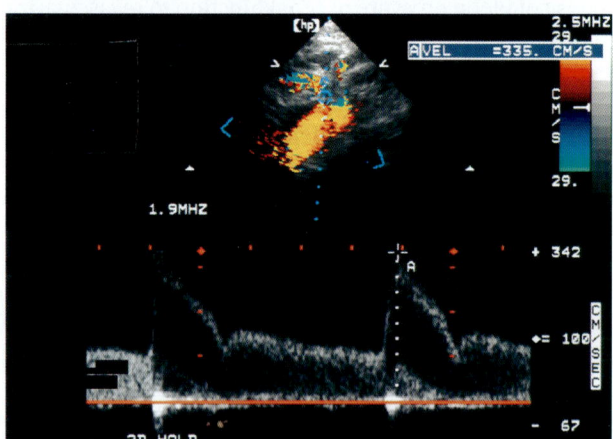

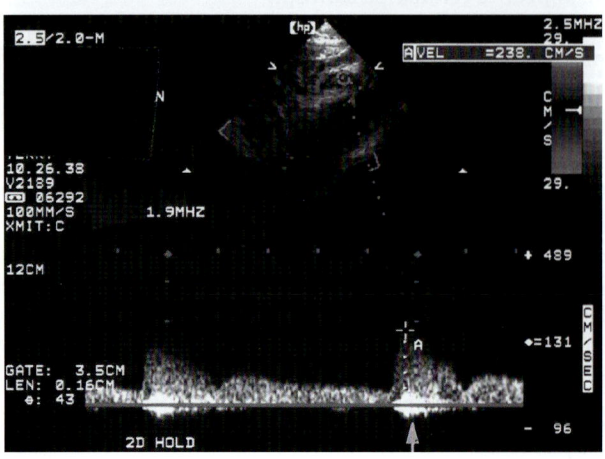

Figure 6–13 Celiac axis stenosis producing abdominal bruit. Patient had a bruit, and a diagnosis of renal artery stenosis had been ruled out. **(A)** Color Doppler flow image shows celiac stenosis with narrowing of color column immediately after the celiac origin (*straight arrow*). Distal to the stenosis, a mosaic pattern of color can be seen (*curved arrow*), which represents aliasing. **(B)** Spectral Doppler image shows celiac stenosis with high-velocity jet (335 cm/s) at origin of the celiac axis. Jet has a well-defined envelope and no spectral broadening because jets have laminar flow. A second, smaller waveform, superimposed on the celiac waveform, is the aortic signal, which is partially in the sample volume. **(C)** Spectral Doppler image shows celiac stenosis with bruit. Downstream from the jet, the velocity diminishes (238 cm/s). Note the spectral broadening. Systolic bruit is shown (*arrow*) as a symmetrical, low-velocity waveform above and below the baseline.

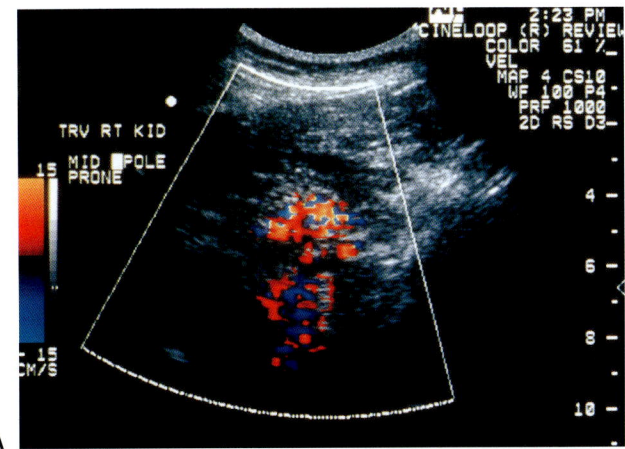

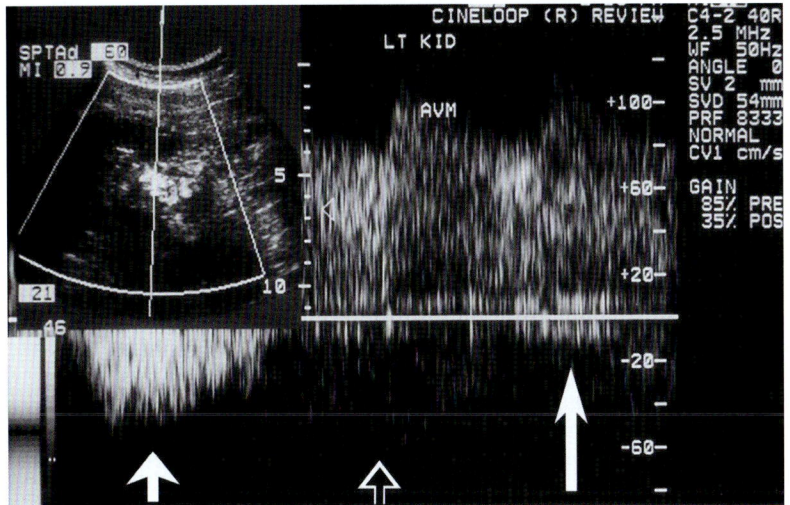

Figure 6–14 Renal arteriovenous fistula. (A) Transverse color Doppler flow image of the right renal hilum shows a large area of color not conforming to normal vessels indicating a vascular malformation. (B) Spectral Doppler image shows an increased velocity and markedly increased diastolic velocity indicating diminished pulsatility from arteriovenous shunting. Systolic acceleration is normal and there is spectral broadening. A continuous bruit can be seen as a symmetrical, low-velocity waveform above and below the baseline (*arrow*). Flow below the baseline is renal vein in the early portion of the spectrum (*from a short arrow*) and disturbed flow in the later portion (*open arrow*). (Case courtesy of Beatrice Madrazo, M.D., William Beaumont Hospital, Royal Oak, MI)

Midaortic syndrome may cause hypertension and bruit. In this case, the aorta is narrowed, possibly affecting the renal, celiac, or superior mesenteric arteries. More commonly, the aorta alone is narrowed. Because the renal arteries are downstream from the stenosis, their waveforms are abnormal, showing diminished pulsatility and systolic upstroke. A jet may be identified in the aorta at the site of the narrowing. Distal flow disturbances such as spectral broadening can be identified in the aorta beyond the narrowing.

Summary

Although clinicians can identify some patients at greater risk for RVH, there is no consensus on who should be tested. A noninvasive test cannot be applied to all hypertensive patients. Clinical criteria are needed to establish a subgroup of patients with a high prevalence of RVH. Part of the reluctance to study patients results from the lack of well-defined criteria for defining who will benefit from revascularization, and from the lack of a clearly effective screening test. Angiography is the standard, but it is invasive and carries some risk. Nuclear scanning after captopril has some appeal because it reflects the pathophysiology of RAS. However, the ability of scintigraphy to predict the outcome after revascularization is not as good as might be expected. Nuclear scanning is not warranted if there is renal insufficiency or a small kidney.

Ultrasound studies show wide variations. Although there are technical failures, direct evaluation is generally accurate if the technical quality of the study is adequate. Intrarenal waveform analysis has not been the panacea it was hoped to be. The use of renal pulsatility indices to predict the results of catheter-based treatments has shown variable results and awaits further study.

MRA and CTA are more accurate than nuclear medicine or ultrasound; however, not all patients are candidates for these tests for reasons such as renal insufficiency, claustrophobia, or allergy. Technical failures also occur with these tests, which are far more expensive than ultrasound.

Outcome analyses incorporating the accuracy, cost, technical success, and complication rates are not available and need to be performed. Various diagnostic pathways should be evaluated, including proceeding straight to angiography, directly to CT or MRA, and using ultrasound. Decision analyses should not simply use positive and negative results but should evaluate technically limited studies to determine how they might be handled.

In high-risk groups, it may not be appropriate to use a screening test. In some patients (for instance, those with suspected fibromuscular dysplasia and normal renal function), it is appropriate to go directly to angiography.

References

1. Schreiber MJ, Pohl MA, Novick AC. The natural history of atherosclerotic and fibrous renal artery disease. Urol Clin North Am 1984; 11:383–392
2. Meyrier A. Renal vascular lesions in the elderly: nephrosclerosis or atheromatous renal disease? Nephrol Dial Transplant 1996;11 (Suppl 9):45–52
3. O'Neil EA, Hansen KJ, Canzanello VJ, Pennell TC, Dean RH. Prevalence of ischemic nephropathy in patients with renal insufficiency. Am Surg 1992;58:485–490
4. Textor SC, Wilcox CS. Renal artery stenosis: a common, treatable cause of renal failure? Annu Rev Med 2001;52:421–442
5. Palmaz JC. The current status of vascular intervention in ischemic nephropathy. J Vasc Interv Radiol 1998;9:539–543
6. Weinrauch LA, D'Elia JA. Renal artery stenosis: "fortuitous diagnosis," problematic therapy. J Am Coll Cardiol 2004;43:1614–1616
7. Goldblatt H, Lynch J, Hanzal RF, Summerville WW. Studies on experimental hypertension, I: The production of persistent elevation of systolic blood pressure by means of renal ischemia. J Exp Med 1934;59:347–378
8. Van Way CW. Renal artery aneurysms and arteriovenous fistulas. In: Rutherford RB, ed. Vascular Surgery. 4th ed. Philadelphia: WB Saunders; 1995:1274–1286
9. Mann S, Pickering T. Detection of renovascular hypertension: state of the art: 1992. Ann Intern Med 1992;117:845–853
10. Detection, evaluation, and treatment of renovascular hypertension: final report of the working group on renovascular hypertension. Arch Intern Med 1987;147:820–829
11. Simon N, Franklin SS, Bleifer KH, Maxwell MH. Clinical characteristics of renovascular hypertension. JAMA 1972;220:1209–1218
12. van Jaarsveld BC, Derkx FH, Krijnen P, et al. Hypertension resistant to two-drug treatment is a useful criterion to select patients for angiography: the Dutch Renal Artery Stenosis Intervention Cooperative (DRASTIC) study. Contrib Nephrol 1996;119:54–58
13. Derkx FH, van Jaarsveld BC, Krijnen P, et al. Renal artery stenosis towards the year 2000. J Hypertens Suppl 1996;14:S167–S172
14. Ducher M, Cerutti C, Marquand A, et al. How to limit screening of patients for atheromatous renal artery stenosis in two-drug resistant hypertension? J Nephrol 2005;18:161–165
15. Textor SC. Pitfalls in imaging for renal artery stenosis. Ann Intern Med 2004;141:730–731
16. Dean RH. Renovascular hypertension: an overview. In: Rutherford RB, ed. Vascular Surgery. 4th ed. Philadelphia: WB Saunders; 1995: 1371–1377
17. Vaughan ED. Pathophysiology of renovascular hypertension. In: Rutherford RB, ed. Vascular Surgery. 4th ed. Philadelphia: WB Saunders; 1995:1377–1390
18. Nally JV. Provocative captopril testing in the diagnosis of renovascular hypertension. Urol Clin North Am 1994;21:227–234
19. Prigent A. The diagnosis of renovascular hypertension: the role of captopril renal scintigraphy and related issues. [see comments] Eur J Nucl Med 1993;20:625–644
20. Fommei E, Ghione S, Hilson AJ, et al. Captopril radionuclide test in renovascular hypertension: a European multicentre study. European Multicentre Study Group. Eur J Nucl Med 1993;20: 617–623
21. Borrello JA, Li D, Vesely TM, et al. Renal arteries: clinical comparison of three-dimensional time-of-flight MR angiographic sequences and radiographic angiography. Radiology 1995;197:793–799
22. De Cobelli F, Mellone R, Salvioni M, et al. Renal artery stenosis: value of screening with three-dimensional phase-contrast MR angiography with a phased-array multicoil. Radiology 1996;201: 697–703
23. Debatin JF, Spritzer CE, Grist TM, et al. Imaging of the renal arteries: value of MR angiography. AJR Am J Roentgenol. 1991;157:981–990
24. Gedroyc WM, Neerhut P, Negus R, et al. Magnetic resonance angiography of renal artery stenosis. Clin Radiol 1995;50:436–439
25. Loubeyre P, Revel D, Garcia P, et al. Screening patients for renal artery stenosis: value of three-dimensional time-of-flight MR angiography. AJR Am J Roentgenol 1994;162:847–852
26. Kim D, Edelman RR, Kent KC, Porter DH, Skillman JJ. Abdominal aorta and renal artery stenosis: evaluation with MR angiography. Radiology 1990;174:727–731
27. Kent KC, Edelman RR, Kim D, et al. Magnetic resonance imaging: a reliable test for the evaluation of proximal atherosclerotic renal arterial stenosis. J Vasc Surg 1991;13:311–318
28. Postma CT, Hartog O, Rosenbusch G, Thien T. Magnetic resonance angiography in the diagnosis of renal artery stenosis. J Hypertens 1993;11(Suppl):S204–S205
29. Rieumont MJ, Kaufman JA, Geller SC, et al. Evaluation of renal artery stenosis with dynamic gadolinium-enhanced MR angiography. AJR Am J Roentgenol 1997;169:39–44
30. Servois V, Laissy JP, Feger C, et al. Two-dimensional time-of-flight magnetic resonance angiography of renal arteries without maximum intensity projection: a prospective comparison with angiography in 21 patients screened for renovascular hypertension. Cardiovasc Intervent Radiol 1994;17:138–142
31. Strotzer M, Fellner CM, Geissler A, et al. Noninvasive assessment of renal artery stenosis: a comparison of MR angiography, color Doppler sonography, and intraarterial angiography. Acta Radiol 1995;36:243–247
32. Yucel EK, Kaufman JA, Prince M, et al. Time of flight renal MR angiography: utility in patients with renal insufficiency. Magn Reson Imaging 1993;11:925–930
33. Bakker J, Beek FJ, Beutler JJ, et al. Renal artery stenosis and accessory renal arteries: accuracy of detection and visualization with gadolinium-enhanced breath-hold MR angiography. Radiology 1998;207:497–504
34. Postma CT, Joosten FB, Rosenbusch G, Thien T. Magnetic resonance angiography has a high reliability in the detection of renal artery stenosis. Am J Hypertens 1997;10(9 Pt 1):957–963
35. Vasbinder GB, Nelemans PJ, Kessels AG, Kroon AA, De Leeuw PW, Van Engelshoven JM. Diagnostic tests for renal artery stenosis in patients suspected of having renovascular hypertension: a meta-analysis. Ann Intern Med 2001;135:401–411
36. Vasbinder GB, Nelemans PJ, Kessels AG, et al, Renal Artery Diagnostic Imaging Study in Hypertension (RADros Inf ServH) Study Group. Accuracy of computed tomographic angiography and magnetic resonance angiography for diagnosing renal artery stenosis. Ann Intern Med 2004;141:674–684; discussion 682

37. Ros PR, Gauger J, Stoupis C, et al. Diagnosis of renal artery stenosis: feasibility of combining MR angiography, MR renography, and gadopentetate-based measurements of glomerular filtration rate. AJR Am J Roentgenol 1995;165:1447–1451
38. Kaatee R, Beek FJA, de Lange EE, et al. Renal artery stenosis: detection and quantification with spiral CT angiography versus optimized digital subtraction angiography. Radiology 1997;205:121–127
39. Elkohen M, Beregi JP, Deklunder G, et al. A prospective study of helical computed tomography angiography versus angiography for the detection of renal artery stenoses in hypertensive patients. J Hypertens 1996;14:525–528
40. Olbricht CJ, Paul K, Prokop M, et al. Minimally invasive diagnosis of renal artery stenosis by spiral computed tomography angiography. Kidney Int 1995;48:1332–1337
41. Zeman RK, Fox SH, Silverman PM, et al. Helical (spiral) CT of the abdomen. AJR Am J Roentgenol 1993;160:719–725
42. Halpern EJ, Wechsler RJ, DiCampli D. Threshold selection for CT angiography shaded surface display of the renal arteries. J Digit Imaging 1995;8:142–147
43. Willmann JK, Wildermuth S, Pfammatter T, et al. Aortoiliac and renal arteries: prospective intraindividual comparison of contrast-enhanced three-dimensional MR angiography and multi-detector row CT angiography. Radiology 2003;226:798–811
44. Guzman RP, Zierler RE, Isaacson JA, Bergelin RO, Strandness DJ. Renal atrophy and arterial stenosis: a prospective study with duplex ultrasound. Hypertension 1994;23:346–350
45. Taylor DC, Kettler MD, Moneta GL, et al. Duplex ultrasound scanning in the diagnosis of renal artery stenosis: a prospective evaluation. J Vasc Surg 1988;7:363–369
46. Olin JW, Piedmonte MR, Young JR, et al. The utility of duplex ultrasound scanning of the renal arteries for diagnosing significant renal artery stenosis. Ann Intern Med 1995;122:833–838
47. Kohler TR, Zierler RE, Martin RL, et al. Noninvasive diagnosis of renal artery stenosis by ultrasonic duplex scanning. J Vasc Surg 1986;4:450–456
48. Desberg AL, Paushter DM, Lammert GK, et al. Renal artery stenosis: evaluation with color Doppler flow imaging. Radiology 1990;177:749–753
49. Hoffmann U, Edwards JM, Carter S, et al. Role of duplex scanning for the detection of atherosclerotic renal disease. Kidney Int 1991;39:1232–1239
50. Nchimi A, Biquet JF, Brisbois D, et al. Duplex ultrasound as first-line screening test for patients suspected of renal artery stenosis: prospective evaluation in high risk group. Eur Radiol 2003;13:1413–1419
51. Motew SJ, Cherr GS, Craven TE, et al. Renal duplex sonography: main renal artery versus hilar analysis. J Vasc Surg 2000;32:462–469;462–471
52. Hua HT, Hood DB, Jensen CC, Hanks SE, Weaver FA. The use of colorflow duplex scanning to detect significant renal artery stenosis. Ann Vasc Surg 2000;14:118–124
53. Hansen KJ, Tribble RW, Reavis SW, et al. Renal duplex sonography: evaluation of clinical utility. J Vasc Surg 1990;12:227–236
54. Halpern EJ, Needleman L, Nack TL, East SA. Renal artery stenosis: should we study the main renal artery or segmental vessels? Radiology 1995;195:799–804
55. Krumme B, Blum U, Schwertfeger E, et al. Diagnosis of renovascular disease by intra- and extrarenal Doppler scanning. Kidney Int 1996;50:1288–1292
56. Spies KP, Fobbe F, El-Bedewi M, et al. Color-coded duplex sonography for noninvasive diagnosis and grading of renal artery stenosis. Am J Hypertens 1995;8(12 Pt 1):1222–1231
57. van der Hulst VP, van Baalen J, Kool LS, et al. Renal artery stenosis: endovascular flow wire study for validation of Doppler US. [see comments] Radiology 1996;200:165–168
58. Handa N, Fukanaga R, Etani H, et al. Efficacy of echo-Doppler examination for the evaluation of renovascular disease. Ultrasound Med Biol 1988;14:1–15
59. Handa N, Fukanaga R, Uehara A, et al. Echo-Doppler velocimeter in the diagnosis of hypertensive patients: the renal artery Doppler technique. Ultrasound Med Biol 1986;12:945–952
60. Martin RL, Nanra RS, Wlodarczyk J, DeSilva A, Bray AE. Renal hilar Doppler analysis in the detection of renal artery stenosis. J Vasc Tech 1991;15:173–180
61. Stavros AT, Parker SH, Yakes WF, et al. Segmental stenosis of the renal artery: pattern recognition of tardus and parvus abnormalities with duplex sonography. [see comments] Radiology 1992;184:487–492
62. Bardelli M, Jensen G, Volkmann R, Aurell M. Noninvasive ultrasound assessment of renal artery stenosis by means of the Gosling pulsatility index. J Hypertens 1992;10:985–989
63. Veglio F, Provera E, Pinna G, et al. Renal resistive index after captopril test by echo-Doppler in essential hypertension. [see comments] Am J Hypertens 1992;5:431–436
64. Ozbek SS, Aytac SK, Erden MI, Sanlidilek NU. Intrarenal Doppler findings of upstream renal artery stenosis: a preliminary report. Ultrasound Med Biol 1993;19:3–12
65. Stavros T, Harshfield D. Renal Doppler: renal artery stenosis, and renovascular hypertension: direct and indirect duplex sonographic abnormalities in patients with renal artery stenosis. Ultrasound Q 1994;12:217–263
66. Halpern EJ, Deane CR, Needleman L, Merton DA, East SA. Normal renal artery spectral Doppler waveform: a closer look. Radiology 1995;196:667–673
67. Hall NJ, Thorpe RJ, MacKechnie SG. Stenosis of the accessory renal artery: Doppler ultrasound findings. Australas Radiol 1995;39:73–77
68. Baxter GM, Aitchison F, Sheppard D, et al. Colour Doppler ultrasound in renal artery stenosis: intrarenal waveform analysis. Br J Radiol 1996;69:810–815
69. Bude RO, Rubin JM, Platt JF, Fechner KP, Adler RS. Pulsus tardus: its cause and potential limitations in detection of arterial stenosis. Radiology 1994;190:779–784
70. Kliewer MA, Tupler RH, Carroll BA, et al. Renal artery stenosis: analysis of Doppler waveform parameters and tardus-parvus pattern. Radiology 1993;189:779–787
71. Lafortune M, Patriquin H, Demeule E, et al. Renal arterial stenosis: slowed systole in the downstream circulation: experimental study in dogs. Radiology 1992;184:475–478
72. Strandness DE Jr. Duplex imaging for the detection of renal artery stenosis. Am J Kidney Dis 1994;24:674–678
73. Gottlieb RH, Snitzer EL, Hartley DF, Fultz PJ, Rubens DJ. Interobserver and intraobserver variation in determining intrarenal parameters by Doppler sonography. AJR Am J Roentgenol 1997;168:627–631
74. Kliewer MA, Tupler RH, Hertzberg BS, et al. Doppler evaluation of renal artery stenosis: interobserver agreement in the interpretation of waveform morphology. AJR Am J Roentgenol 1994;162:1371–1376
75. Rene PC, Oliva VL, Bui BT, et al. Renal artery stenosis: evaluation of Doppler US after inhibition of angiotensin-converting enzyme with captopril. [see comments] Radiology 1995;196:675–679
76. Nazzal MMS, Hoballah JJ, Miller EV, et al. Renal hilar Doppler analysis is of value in the management of patients with renovascular disease. Am J Surg 1997;174:164–168

77. Missouris CG, Allen CM, Balen FG, et al. Noninvasive screening for renal artery stenosis with ultrasound contrast enhancement. J Hypertens 1996;14:519–524
78. Soulen MC, Benenati JF, Sheth S, Merton D, Rothgeb J. Changes in renal artery Doppler indexes following renal angioplasty. J Vasc Interv Radiol 1991;2:457–461
79. Schwerk WB, Restrepo IK, Stellwaag M, Klose KJ, Schade-Brittinger C. Renal artery stenosis: grading with image-directed Doppler US evaluation of renal resistive index. [see comments] Radiology 1994;190:785–790
80. Burdick L, Airoldi F, Marana I, et al. Superiority of acceleration and acceleration time over pulsatility and resistance indices as screening tests for renal artery stenosis. J Hypertens 1996;14:1229–1235
81. Pedersen EB, Egeblad M, Jorgensen J, et al. Diagnosing renal artery stenosis: a comparison between conventional renography, captopril renography and ultrasound Doppler in a large consecutive series of patients with arterial hypertension. Blood Press 1996;5:342–348
82. Frauchiger B, Zierler R, Bergelin RO, Isaacson JA, Strandness DE Jr. Prognostic significance of intrarenal resistance indices in patients with renal artery interventions: a preliminary duplex sonographic study. Cardiovasc Surg 1996;4:324–330
83. Radermacher J Chavan A, Bleck J, et al. Use of Doppler ultrasonography to predict the outcome of therapy for renal-artery stenosis. N Engl J Med 2001;344:410–417
84. Zeller T, Frank U, Muller C, et al. Predictors of improved renal function after percutaneous stent-supported angioplasty of severe atherosclerotic ostial renal artery stenosis. Circulation 2003;108:2244–2249
85. Garcia-Criado A, Gilabert R, Nicolau C, et al. Value of Doppler sonography for predicting clinical outcome after renal artery revascularization in atherosclerotic renal artery stenosis. J Ultrasound Med 2005;24:1641–1647
86. Postma CT, Bijlstra PJ, Rosenbusch G, Thien T. Pattern recognition of loss of early systolic peak by Doppler ultrasound has a low sensitivity for the detection of renal artery stenosis. J Hum Hypertens 1996;10:181–184
87. Melany ML, Grant EG, Duerinckx AJ, Watts TM, Levine BS. Ability of a phase shift US contrast agent to improve imaging of the main renal arteries. Radiology 1997;205:147–152
88. Claudon M, Plouin PF, Baxter GM, et al. Renal arteries in patients at risk of renal arterial stenosis: multicenter evaluation of the echo-enhancer SH U 508A at color and spectral Doppler US. Levovist Renal Artery Stenosis Study Group. Radiology 2000;214:739–746
89. Miralles M, Cairols M, Cotillas J, Gimenez A, Santiso A. Value of Doppler parameters in the diagnosis of renal artery stenosis. J Vasc Surg 1996;23(3):428–435
90. Antonica G, Sabba C, Berardi E, et al. Accuracy of echo-Doppler flowmetry for renal artery stenosis. J Hypertens Suppl 1991;9:S240–S241

7 Acute Scrotal Pain: Diagnosing with Color Duplex Sonography

Thomas A. Stavros and Cynthia L. Rapp

Differential Diagnosis

The differential diagnosis for acute scrotal pain includes testicular torsion (spermatic cord torsion), infection (epididymitis, orchitis, epididymo-orchitis), torsion of the appendix testis, trauma, incarcerated or strangulated inguinal hernia, hemorrhage into or necrosis of a testicular tumor, vasculitis, spermatic cord thrombosis or compression (during inguinal hernia surgery), and complications of vasectomy. The most common causes vary with age, but in all age groups, spermatic cord torsion and infection are the leading causes of acute scrotal pain. In adults, infection is more common than torsion, but in children (including neonates), torsion is more common. Torsion of the appendix testis or appendix epididymis is also relatively common in children. The remaining causes of acute scrotal pain are less common in all age groups (**Table 7–1**).

Diagnostic Evaluation

Differentiations Torsion from Infection

Differentiating torsion from infection is an urgent problem. Torsion can lead to infarction of the testis within a few hours, so rapid reduction of the torsion is necessary. The mechanism of infarction is initially venous and lymphatic obstruction, later followed by arterial obstruction. The soft lymphatic and venous structures are prone to obstruction at lower degrees of torsion than are the thicker-walled testicular arteries. The rapidity with which torsion causes infarction varies with the degree of torsion. Infarction may not occur for days if there is only 90 degrees of torsion. On the other hand, 720 degrees of torsion may cause infarction within 2 hours. Intermediate degrees of torsion can lead to infarction in intermediate lengths of time.

An underlying anatomical abnormality, the "bell-clapper deformity," predisposes the patient to torsion in most cases. In the bellclapper deformity, the normal, "low, broad attachment" of the tunica vaginalis to the posterior surface of the testis is absent. Instead, the tunica vaginalis attaches in an abnormally high position to the spermatic cord, and the mesorchium is abnormally long. The lack of attachment of the testis to the tunica vaginalis predisposes the testis to torsion around the high point of attachment to the spermatic cord. Thus, testicular torsion should more properly be termed spermatic cord torsion. The bell-clapper deformity is usually bilateral, predisposing both sides to torsion.

The urgent reduction of torsion can be performed surgically or nonsurgically under local anesthetic. Regardless of whether reduction of torsion is surgical or nonsurgical, orchiopexy is required to prevent repeat torsion at a later date. Orchiopexy is almost always performed bilaterally because the bell-clapper deformity, which is the underlying predisposition to torsion, is usually present bilaterally.

The patient's clinical history can be helpful, but is sometimes quite atypical. The precipitating factor is thought to be an unusually strong contraction of the cremasteric muscle, which can be caused by trauma, strenuous exercise, or sexual activity. However, in many patients the onset of pain occurs during sleep, without any apparent cause for forceful contraction of the cremasteric muscle. The onset of pain in spermatic cord torsion is usually acute. Gradual onset of pain is more typical of infection, but up to 25% of torsion patients also have gradual onset of pain. Spontaneous detorsion does occur, and careful questioning sometimes reveals a past history of repeated episodes of scrotal pain due to intermittent spontaneously resolving episodes of torsion. Urinary symptoms such as dysuria are relatively rare in torsion in comparison with epididymitis.

Table 7–1 Differential Diagnosis of Acute Scrotal Pain

Children
    Torsion
    Infection
    Appendage torsion
    Tumor
    Trauma
    Hernia
    Spermatic versus occlusion
    Vasculitis
Adults
    Infection
    Torsion
    Appendage torsion
    Tumor
    Trauma
    Hernia
    Spermatic versus occlusion
    Vasculitis

Like the clinical history, the patient's physical examination may not reveal the classical signs of torsion. The torsed testis is usually swollen, painful, and tender, but may be nontender. Swelling of the testes and scrotal skin is usually present in both torsion and infection. The torsed testis is usually in an abnormally high, transverse position, with the epididymis rotated anteriorly, but in some cases it is not. The high, transverse testicular position is related to the degree of torsion. It is said that the pain from infection improves if the testis is elevated and supported, but the pain due to torsion does not. However, this is not always the case. The physical examination can be limited and difficult because of pain and tenderness, but injection of the spermatic cord in the inguinal canal with lidocaine may facilitate both a more thorough and accurate physical examination and nonsurgical external reduction of the torsion.

In patients in whom the history and physical examination are not classical for torsion, ultrasound with Doppler can be used to help differentiate torsion from infection. Our ability to demonstrate specific gray-scale patterns of edema within the testes, epididymis, and spermatic cord has improved. The sensitivity of color duplex sonography and power Doppler sonography for demonstrating the relatively slow and sparse flow within the testes has also improved markedly over the years. The combination of improved gray-scale imaging and Doppler capabilities now make ultrasound and Doppler the imaging procedures of choice for evaluation of acute scrotal pain.

Ultrasound Imaging

Ultrasound Equipment and Machine Setup

Scrotal sonography requires both high-frequency, high-resolution, near-field, real-time, gray-scale imaging and superb color and/or power Doppler sensitivity. These are best accomplished with high-frequency electronically focused transducers in the 10 to 12 MHz range. In children, frequencies as high as 17 MHz can be used. Lower frequency transducers, such as 5 MHz linear array transducers, are designed for peripheral vascular Doppler, not small parts imaging, and will less frequently show normal intratesticular flow than will higher-frequency transducers. Failure to show normal flow on the contralateral asymptomatic side reduces the value of Doppler in assessment of acute scrotal pain caused by torsion. In addition to Doppler sensitivity limitations, most 5 MHz transducers also have short-axis fixed focal lengths that are too deep for optimal scanning of the scrotal contents, especially in children. However, in patients with large hydroceles or hematoceles, severe testicular enlargement, a large testicular mass, or severe skin swelling, the greater focal length of the 5 MHz linear probe may be an advantage.

Power Doppler imaging is more sensitive than color Doppler flow imaging for showing relatively slow flow in small vessels, such as those within the substance of the normal testes. This is especially true in young boys and very old men, who tend to have less flow within the testes. Power Doppler is also less angle dependent than color Doppler, showing small vessels that course near 90 degrees to the Doppler beam better than does color Doppler. Being able to demonstrate flow within the normal contralateral asymptomatic testis is critical to the diagnosis of torsion because failure to do so makes lack of demonstrable flow in the symptomatic testis meaningless, and in a few cases power Doppler can show normal flow better than color Doppler does.

Some ultrasound equipment enables the user to downshift the Doppler frequency to a lower frequency than is normally used for imaging (i.e., the Doppler frequency on a 10 MHz linear transducer might be 7 MHz rather than 10 MHz). This downshift allows better penetration for peripheral vascular applications and also allows a greater degree of beam steering to optimize angles of incidence in peripheral vessels, such as the carotid and femoral arteries. However, downshifted Doppler frequencies and beam steering both reduce Doppler sensitivity and generally should not be used for evaluating intratesticular blood flow except in rare cases where large masses or marked scrotal enlargement makes penetration with higher frequencies suboptimal. If the vessels of interest within the scrotum are coursing at an obtuse angle of incidence, it is easy to move the probe along the surface of the scrotum to a position in which the angle of incidence is more acute. Angles as close to 0 degrees as possible should be sought and are usually possible. Sliding the transducer parallel to its long axis to a different location on the surface of the scrotum is a better way to improve angles of incidence than is beam steering.

Doppler sensitivity settings should be maximized. This is especially important in young children and old men, who have less flow and slower flow than young adult and middle-aged men. Full color and pulsed Doppler power, low-velocity scales, low wall filters, and high gray-scale-write-priorities maximize sensitivity. Many units, due to U.S. Food and Drug Administration requirements, boot up at low-power settings for safety purposes. These low-power settings can adversely affect Doppler sensitivity for the detection of normal intratesticular blood flow, especially in children and elderly men. The risk:benefit ratio of Doppler imaging in these patients demands full power, if flow within the asymptomatic testis cannot be demonstrated at the default low-power setting. Low-velocity scales (pulse-repetition frequency) and low wall-filter settings also maximize our chances of demonstrating flow. The ultrasound unit can usually only write either color or gray scale to each pixel, but not both. The write-priority tells the unit how white a gray-scale pixel can be overwritten with color. Peripheral vascular applications, with large lucent vessels, require low write-priority settings (that is, toward the black end of the gray scale). In such cases, high write-priorities (toward the white end of the gray-scale spectrum) would result in too much artifactual color being written into echogenic tissues outside of the vessels. In contrast to large peripheral vessels, the testes and epididymis are relatively echogenic. Many of the vessels within them that are being interrogated are too small to resolve on the B-mode image. Therefore, color flow must be displayed on a relatively white background by using a high write-priority. If the B-write-priority settings are too low (like those used for peripheral vascular imaging), color may not be written onto the image of the testis, even when the unit has correctly detected it. Some ultrasound units do not have a separate control for write-priority and have combined control of this parameter with other parameters (i.e., threshold control).

In most cases, color Doppler or power Doppler imaging alone is sufficient to distinguish between infection and torsion by showing markedly increased or decreased flow within either or both the symptomatic testis and epididymis. However, occasionally, obvious color or power Doppler asymmetry may not be demonstrable. In such cases, pulsed Doppler spectral analysis can be helpful. As is the case for color and power Doppler imaging, electronic beam steering reduces the sensitivity of pulsed Doppler spectral analysis and should not be used. In our experience, it is possible to maneuver the transducer on the surface of the scrotal skin to create an angle of incidence of the pulsed Doppler beam that is near 0 degrees without steering in virtually all cases. We have also found that using a wider sample volume improves the quality of the spectral tracing when the vessel being interrogated is small and the angle of incidence is near 0 degrees.

Occasionally, the testis is too long to measure with a standard 38 mm long 10 or 12 MHz linear array transducer. Five centimeter long transducers, trapezoidal beam shapes, extended field of view, or 5 MHz curved linear array transducers all offer workarounds to this problem.

Sonographic and Duplex Technique

Ultrasound examination of the scrotum in patients with acute scrotal pain should always include Doppler studies in addition to gray-scale imaging. On the other hand, Doppler evaluation is usually not necessary when the patient has a nonpainful, nontender, palpable nodule or mass. In patients in whom the clinical index of suspicion of torsion is high and in those who have gross enlargement of the testis, color Doppler flow imaging should be used early in the examination to make as prompt a diagnosis of torsion as possible. A color or power Doppler examination of the symptomatic testis can usually be performed very quickly. If there is no demonstrable flow within the symptomatic testis, one should quickly make sure that flow is demonstrable in the contralateral asymptomatic testis. This will be discussed in greater detail later.

After the quick color or power Doppler survey, the entire symptomatic testis and epididymis should be scanned in real time gray scale to get an overall picture of the scrotal contents and alignment of the testis and epididymis. The contralateral asymptomatic side should also be quickly surveyed to get an idea about symmetry in size and echogenicity between the two sides and also to assess the position and alignment of the contralateral testis and epididymis. The spermatic cord should be inspected from several centimeters superior to the epididymal head to the tail of the epididymis. The presence of a complex hydrocele and debris or adhesions within it should be noted. Intratesticular nodules or masses should be excluded, and the testes measured. The presence of a solid mass or nodule within the testis suggests the presence of a neoplasm. A complex cystic lesion within the testis may represent an abscess resulting from orchitis or necrosis resulting from infarction or tumor.

One advantage of scrotal–testicular color duplex sonography is that there is almost always a mirror-image contralateral normal structure with which the painful side can be compared. This advantage should be utilized to its fullest extent. When the color Doppler findings do not indicate torsion and the need for immediate surgery, we make this comparison by obtaining split-screen images of corresponding right and left intrascrotal contents in both transverse and longitudinal planes. Split-screen long-axis images of the epididymal heads (**Fig. 7–1**) and long- and short-axis split-screen images of both testes are recorded (**Fig. 7–2**). The epididymal tails are usually best shown on coronal views that are angled from anterosuperior to posteroinferior. Obtaining such a view often requires the patient to temporarily assume a frogleg position. The shape of the epididymis varies from straight (**Fig. 7–3A**) to C-shaped (**Fig. 7–3B**). Imaging the epididymal tails is very important because infection is often most apparent and

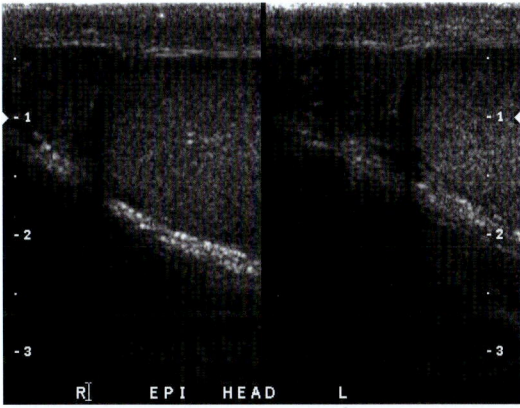

Figure 7–1 Long-axis split-screen images of bilaterally normal epididymal heads. The heads are triangular and symmetrical in size and shape. The transducer position needed to obtain these views varies not only from one patient to another, but from right side to left.

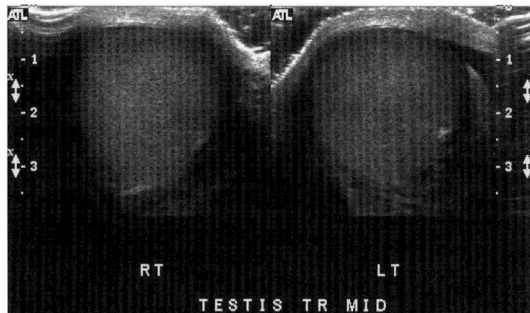

Figure 7–2 Split-screen transverse images through the normal right and left testes—size and echogenicity are symmetrical from right to left.

manifests itself most definitively there. Transverse split-screen images of the spermatic cords just superior to the epididymal heads are also obtained (**Fig. 7–4**). Occasionally, scanning the spermatic cords within the inguinal canals can be helpful. We also obtain an oblique short-axis view through the median raphe of the scrotum to compare the size and echogenicity of the testes on a single image. It is important that the angle of incidence of the beam into the testes be bilaterally symmetrical on this view to minimize the chance that critical angle shadowing will make a testis artifactually look hypoechoic. Usually the left end of the probe must be angled inferiorly because the left testis usually lies lower than the right, but this relationship may be altered in torsion. It is important to make sure that all of the split-screen images are obtained symmetrically through the widest part of the structures being imaged and that the angles of incidence be as close to 90 degrees as possible to minimize artifactual shadowing and errant assessment of relative echogenicities and thicknesses (**Fig. 7–5**). The right and left testes, epididymi, and spermatic cords should be symmetrical in size and echogenicity.

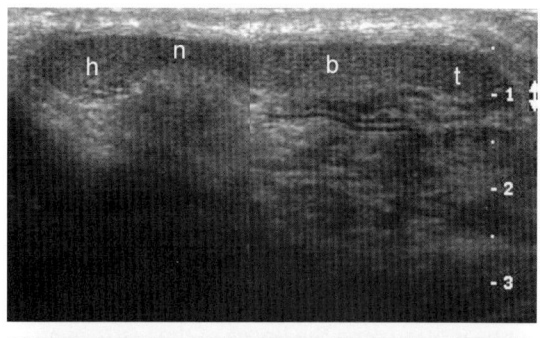

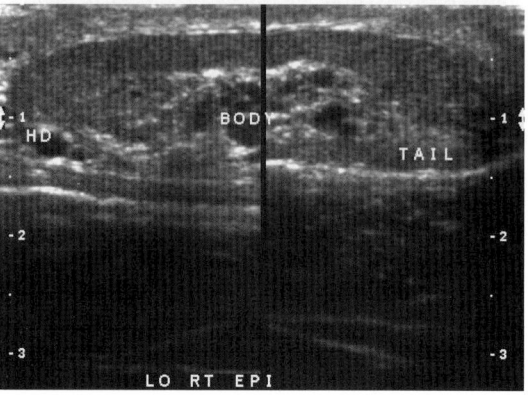

Figure 7–3 (A) Coronal or C view of normal straight epididymis. Combined view of entire length of normal epididymis shows the head (h), neck (n), body (b), and tail (t). **(B)** Coronal or C view of normal curved epididymis.

Demonstrating symmetrical sections through right and left sides may require grossly different probe orientations on the right and left sides because the position of the testes within the scrotal sac in normal individuals is often asymmetrical. In torsion, this asymmetry of position is even more pronounced. The relative position of the right and left sides is ascertained at the time of the initial survey.

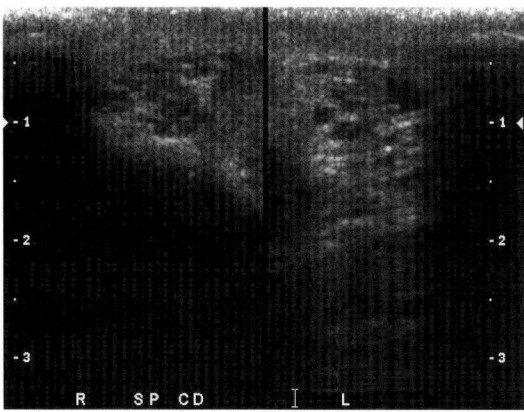

Figure 7–4 Short-axis split-screen images of spermatic cords. These short-axis views were obtained through the spermatic cords just superior to the epididymal heads. The cords are symmetrical in size and echogenicity. Because of tortuosity of the cord, obtaining such views in nonredundant segments of cord can be difficult.

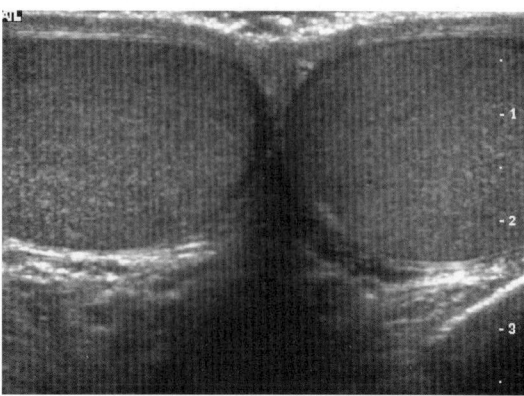

Figure 7–5 Oblique median raphe view through the medial half of each testis. This median raphe view shows the testes to be equal in size and echogenicity. Because the left testis is usually lower than the right, this view cannot be obtained in a true transverse plane and usually requires an oblique view with the left side lower.

Because the testes are freely mobile within the scrotal sac, the alignment of the testis may change during the examination. The goal of this systematic imaging approach is to detect a pattern of swelling or abnormal echogenicity that favors a diagnosis of either infection or torsion. For example, swelling of the epididymal tail and spermatic cord out of proportion to swelling within the epididymal head and testis strongly suggests epididymitis. Furthermore, systematic scanning minimizes the chances of missing the key findings of infection. For example, mild or early epididymitis, or partially treated epididymitis, can affect only the spermatic cord and epididymal tail, sparing the epididymal head and testis. Failure to evaluate the spermatic cords and epididymal tails will cause these findings to be missed.

We are not in favor of using a rolled-up towel to support the testis. Although this may offer symptomatic relief to a patient with epididymitis, it blocks inferior and coronal approaches to the testis and also pushes the scrotal contents superiorly, interfering with the evaluation of the epididymal heads, appendices, and spermatic cords above the testes. Additionally, the rolled-up towel redistributes physiological amounts of fluid within the scrotal sac posteriorly, where it cannot be used to outline small structures such as the appendix testis. Scanning without a rolled-up towel allows the scrotal contents to fall inferiorly and posteriorly and redistributes physiological hydroceles to the upper pole, nicely outlining appendices, epididymal heads, and spermatic cords. It also stretches out the epididymis, facilitating demonstration of the entire epididymis on a single coronal view.

The Doppler examination begins with color or power Doppler interrogation of the testes. We usually quickly evaluate the asymptomatic testis first to make sure that flow is detectable on the side on which torsion is not suspected. If no flow exists in the asymptomatic side, decreased or absent flow in the symptomatic side will have no meaning. If flow cannot be detected within the asymptomatic contralateral testis, velocity scale, wall filter, B-write priority, and Doppler power can be adjusted as needed to demonstrate flow. Increased flow in the symptomatic testis is always important, regardless of the contralateral findings. It indicates inflammatory hyperemia, which is almost always due to infection; in rare cases, it can be a manifestation of reactive hyperemia after spontaneous detorsion.

If flow is present in the asymptomatic testis, but absent or decreased in the symptomatic testis, then torsion is likely. Duplex sonographic interrogation with spectral tracings and complete color Doppler and duplex sonographic studies of the remainder of the intrascrotal contents are usually not performed because it is important for the patient to undergo surgery as soon as possible. Additional examinations in such patients may waste valuable time in which the patient could be prepared for surgery. It should be kept in mind, however, that severe infection, trauma, and inguinal hernia surgery can lead to ischemia of a testis, which appears similar to torsion on color Doppler flow imaging or power Doppler imaging. The pattern of oligemia can be helpful. Spermatic cord torsion tends to cause global absence or decrease in flow within the testis, whereas in ischemia caused by conditions other than torsion, the ischemic changes often appear focal or patchy rather than diffuse.

If flow is present in both testes but increased in the symptomatic testis, or if there appears to be normal and symmetrical flow in both testes, torsion is unlikely. Complete gray-scale imaging with split-screen images and color duplex sonographic examination of intrascrotal contents can then be performed. In some cases, spectral Doppler analysis will show asymmetries in velocities and resistivity indexes, even when color Doppler appears symmetrical. The goal of complete gray-scale and Doppler in assessing testes, epididymi, and spermatic cords is to detect a pattern of hyperemia that suggests a specific diagnosis. For example, abnormally high velocities and low resistivity indexes in the epididymis, but normal velocities in the testes, strongly favor a diagnosis of epididymitis over other causes.

It is very important to assess the intratesticular vessels (centripetal) as well as the more easily seen capsular arteries. In cases of missed torsion, the tunica vaginalis, the lining of the scrotal sac, can be markedly hyperemic. Because the inflamed tunica vaginalis may become adherent to the immediately adjacent tunica albuginea, reactive hyperemia within the tunica vaginalis can be mistaken for flow within a capsular testicular artery, resulting in a missed diagnosis of torsion. By assessing intratesticular arteries rather than capsular arteries, this potential mistake can usually be avoided. As mentioned earlier, it is possible to create an optimal angle of incidence of near 0 degrees without electronically steering the ultrasound beam to maximize Doppler sensitivity.

In most cases the combined pattern of swelling, altered echogenicity, and increased or decreased flow on Doppler ultrasound examination suggest the exact cause of scrotal pain.

Normal Imaging and Doppler Findings

Normal testes, epididymi, and spermatic cords are bilaterally symmetrical in size and texture. The epididymi and testes are normally relatively homogeneous and have mid-level echogenicity. The spermatic cords have heterogeneous texture due to the venous plexus and abundant loose connective tissues they contain. The tortuosity of the spermatic cord makes it difficult to obtain precisely symmetrical images and to precisely measure the spermatic cord, but an eyeball estimate of size and echogenicity is usually possible. Marked asymmetries in size, shape, homogeneity, and echogenicity between right and left sides are abnormal.

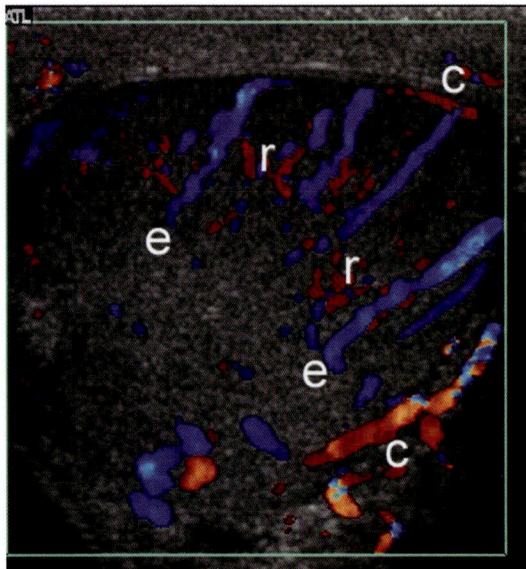

Figure 7–6 Color Doppler image through equator of testis. Capsular arteries (c) course on the outer surface of the testis, centripetal arteries (e) penetrate into the substance of the testis from peripheral to central, and recurrent rami (r) double back toward the surface of the testis. Demonstrating flow in centripetal arteries is important in excluding torsion because vessels within adherent tunica vaginalis can simulate capsular arteries in patients with "missed" torsion.

With current equipment, flow is demonstrable within the capsular arteries, the intratesticular vessels (centripetal and, sometimes, recurrent rami), in almost all adults within the reproductive age groups (**Fig. 7–6**). Demonstrable color Doppler flow should be roughly symmetrical in the right and left testes, with only minimal asymmetry in the number of vessels in right and left testes

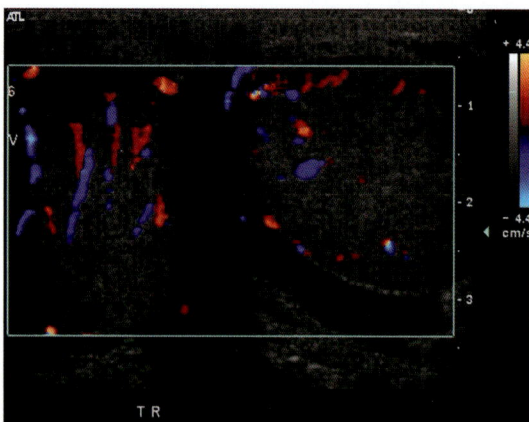

Figure 7–7 Oblique median raphe color Doppler view can be helpful in comparing blood flow in the right and left testes on a single view. In normal individuals, flow should be roughly symmetrical on right and left sides.

shown on oblique transverse median raphe views (**Fig. 7–7**). However, normal intratesticular flow can be more difficult to demonstrate in children, particularly very young children and newborns, and in very elderly men. Additionally, the intratesticular vessels pass through the testis in a few discrete vascular planes. If the ultrasound probe is parallel to the vascular plane on one side, but out of the vascular plane in the contralateral testis, the flow may appear falsely asymmetrical. Every effort should be made to compare comparable tissue planes within the two testes. The vascular planes of the testis are oriented in the long axis of the testis. Therefore, errors in assessment of vascularity are more likely to occur in the longitudinal planes than in transverse plans. The capsular arteries are

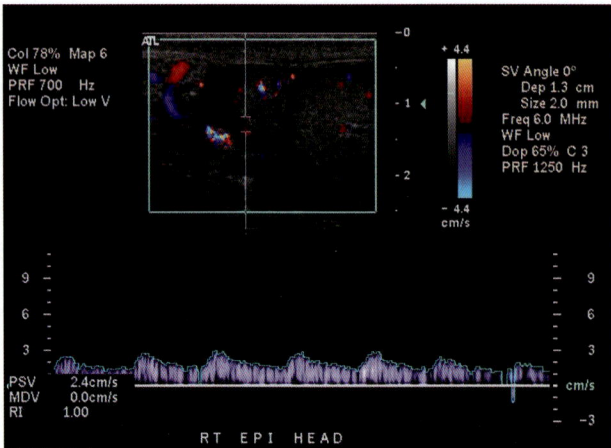

Figure 7–8 Spectral waveforms obtained from a normal epididymal head. Epididymal head waveforms can be obtained in most normal adult patients with current equipment, are low resistance type, and demonstrate rounded systolic peaks. Normal epididymal head peak systolic velocities are ≤5 cm/s and normal end-diastolic velocities are ≤3 cm/s.

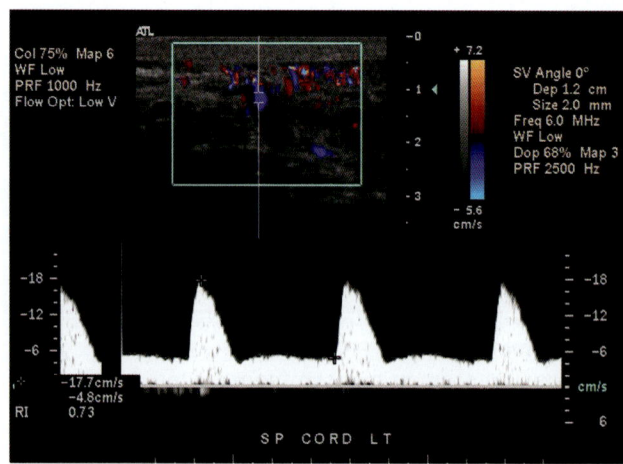

Figure 7–9 Spectral waveform from a normal testicular artery within the spermatic cord superior to the epididymal head. Testicular artery waveforms can be obtained in all normal patients, have a higher resistance pattern than do normal testicular and epididymal waveforms, and have sharp systolic peaks. Peak systolic velocities vary greatly but should be within 50% of contralateral testicular artery peak systolic velocities.

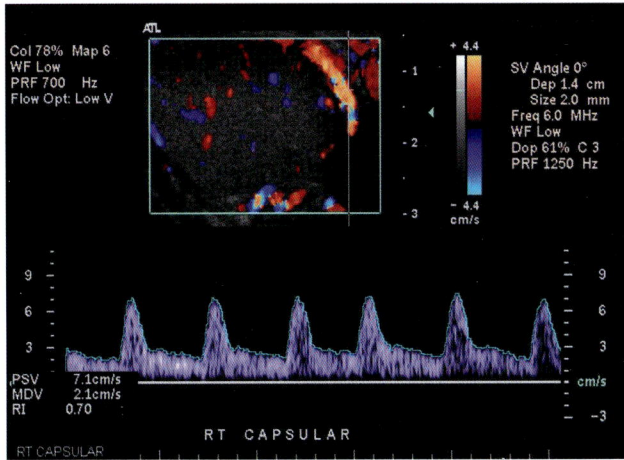

Figure 7–10 Spectral waveform obtained from a capsular artery. These should be obtainable in virtually all normal patients. The waveform resistance index is intermediate between that of the testicular artery within the spermatic cord and those obtained from the epididymis or centripetal arteries within the substance of the testis. Normal peak systolic velocities within capsular arteries are ≤15 cm/s and normal end-diastolic velocities are ≤7 cm/s. Capsular artery velocities are higher than those of the centripetal arteries in most, but not all, patients. Velocities from capsular arteries on one side should not be compared with centripetal arteries on the other side.

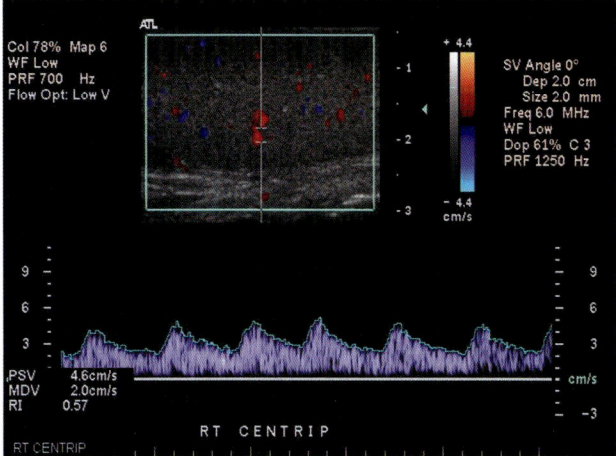

Figure 7–11 Spectral waveform obtained from a centripetal artery. These should be obtainable in almost all adult patients but can be difficult to obtain in infants and young children. Like those from within the epididymal head, waveforms from centripetal arteries are low-resistance type and the systolic peaks are rounded. Normal peak systolic velocities within centripetal arteries vary too greatly to use a fixed number as a cutoff. Comparison should be made with similar contralateral centripetal arteries. There should be less than 50% difference between sides. Centripetal artery velocities are lower than those of the capsular arteries in most, but not all, patients. Velocities from centripetal arteries on one side should not be compared with capsular arteries on the contralateral side.

usually best seen in segments that course at nearly a 0 degree angle of incidence to the beam. This most commonly occurs on the inferomedial surface of the testes. Multiple intratesticular vessels are visible in most adult testes, but may be more or less evident, depending upon the angle of incidence and scan plane.

With current equipment, some flow is demonstrable within the epididymal head in a majority of adult patients. Flow is not demonstrable within the epididymal head in a small percentage of adults and in most children. Flow within the epididymal tail is demonstrable in a larger percentage of adult patients than within the epididymal head but, once again, not always demonstrable in children. On color or power Doppler assessment it can be difficult to determine whether flow that is being detected is within the epididymal head or the adjacent spermatic cord. However, the spectral waveforms obtained from the epididymal head and spermatic cord differ greatly from each other. Waveforms obtained from vessels within the epididymal head have a low impedance pattern, low velocities (peak systolic velocity of ≤ 5 cm/s and end diastolic velocities of ≤ 3 cm/s), and a rounded systolic peak, and they lack an early diastolic notch (**Fig. 7–8**). On the other hand, waveforms obtained from within the spermatic cord (testicular artery or supratesticular artery) have much higher impedance, higher systolic velocities, sharp systolic peaks, and early diastolic notches (**Fig. 7–9**).

Normal spectral waveforms obtained from within the testicular substance should be symmetrical on the right and left sides in most patients, as long as they are obtained from vessels that appear to be similar in size, angle of incidence, and depth on both sides. One should not compare a capsular artery waveform on one side to a centripetal artery waveform on the other side. The velocities in centripetal and capsular arteries differ from each other in most cases. Velocities are usually, but not always, higher within the capsular than within the intratesticular arteries. Peak systolic velocities in capsular arteries usually range from 5 to 14 cm/s (**Fig. 7–10**). Peak end-diastolic velocities vary from 2 to 6 cm/s (**Fig. 7–11**). Peak systolic velocities obtained from centripetal arteries are far more variable and need to be compared with similar arteries on the contralateral side.

The appearance of pulsed Doppler spectral waveforms obtained from the epididymal tails varies greatly, depending upon the location within the epididymal tail from which the waveforms are obtained. Waveforms obtained farthest from the reflection with the distal spermatic cord have velocities and appearances similar to those obtained from the epididymal head (**Fig. 7–8**). On the other hand, waveforms obtained closer to the reflection with the distal spermatic cord have an appearance more similar to that of the spermatic cord (**Fig. 7–9**).

In normal individuals, peak systolic velocities are much lower in the epididymal head than within the spermatic cord, testes, or epididymal tail, but in cases of severe epididymitis, the velocities in the epididymal head can exceed those within the testes.

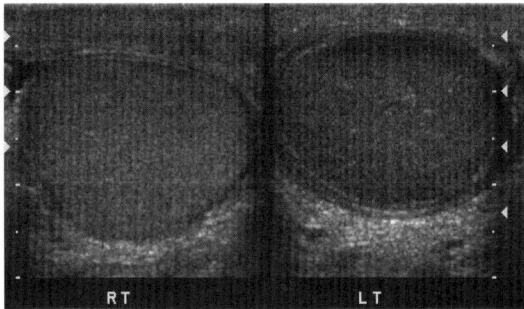

Figure 7–12 Split-screen images in long axis through the midtestes in a patient with acute left spermatic cord torsion show decreased echogenicity in the torsed left testis. In bland infarction, the testicular substance is usually hypoechoic, but in areas that have undergone hemorrhagic infarction, the affected areas usually become hyperechoic.

The velocities within similar vessels on the right and left sides should be symmetrical, but there is enough variability and difficulty in obtaining and measuring spectral waveforms that a 50% or greater difference in velocities between the right and left sides is usually necessary to document a significant difference.

Findings in Testicular Torsion

Imaging Findings

The spermatic cord below the point of spermatic cord torsion, the epididymis, and testis are all abnormally enlarged. The enlargement increases over time, so patients who are very early in the course of torsion may have only minimal enlargement, whereas patients with more severe or longstanding torsion have more severe enlarge-

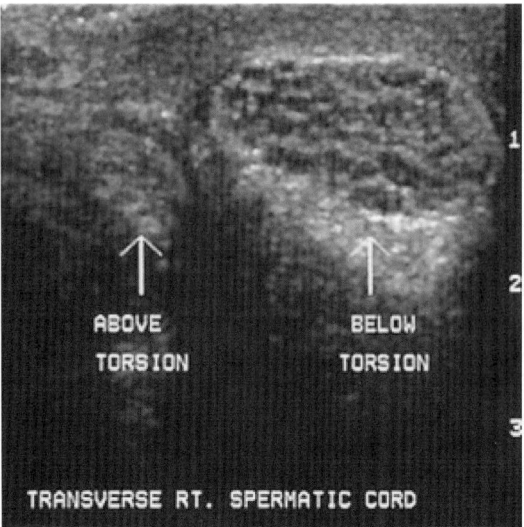

Figure 7–14 Long-axis view of a torsed spermatic cord shows the normal-sized cord above the torsion and the enlarged cord below the torsion. The cord below the torsion contains many distended hypoechoic veins due to either or both venous stasis and thrombosis.

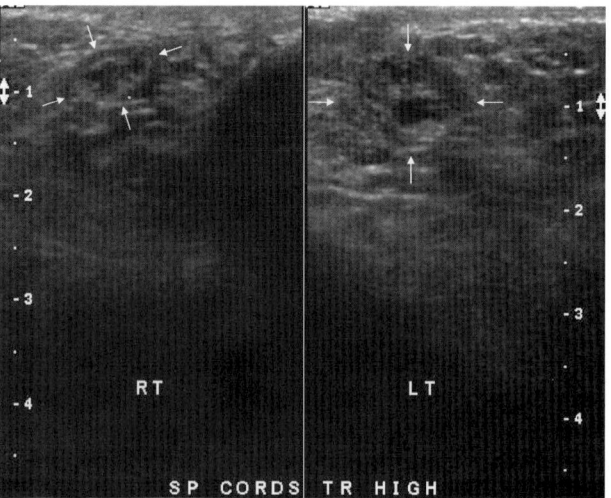

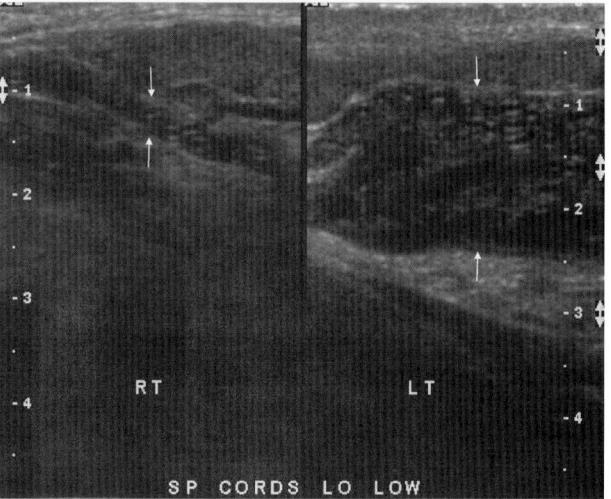

Figure 7–13 (A) Split-screen images of the spermatic cords above the epididymal heads, but below the torsion, in a patient with acute left spermatic cord torsion. Note the left spermatic cord (*arrows*) is larger than the right and that there is a distended pampiniform plexus vein. The distension can be due to stasis early or due to thrombosis late. **(B)** Split-screen long-axis images of the distal spermatic cords and cremasteric plexes (*arrows*) on the right and left side show the cord to be markedly swollen on the left side.

ment. The echogenicity of the testis is usually decreased (**Fig. 7–12**), although very early in the process the echogenicity may be normal, and very late in the process, after infarction has occurred, hemorrhage into the testis may cause heterogeneously increased echogenicity. The echogenicity of the epididymis and spermatic cord also varies, depending on whether hemorrhage has occurred. Enlarged acutely thrombosed pampiniform plexus veins within the spermatic cord can also be demonstrable in some cases and are what make the spermatic cord appear abnormally hypoechoic (**Fig. 7–13**). If the spermatic cord is carefully examined, an abrupt increase in the size and alteration of the spermatic cord may be noted below the point of torsion (**Fig. 7–14**). In other cases, actual twisting

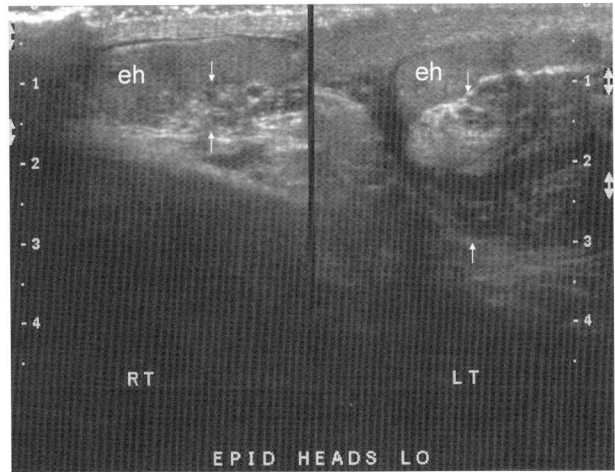

Figure 7–15 (A) Long-axis, split-screen images of the epididymal heads in a patient with acute left spermatic cord torsion. Note that the spermatic cord and loose areolar tissues (between arrows) that lie posterior to the epididymal head are greatly swollen, but that the

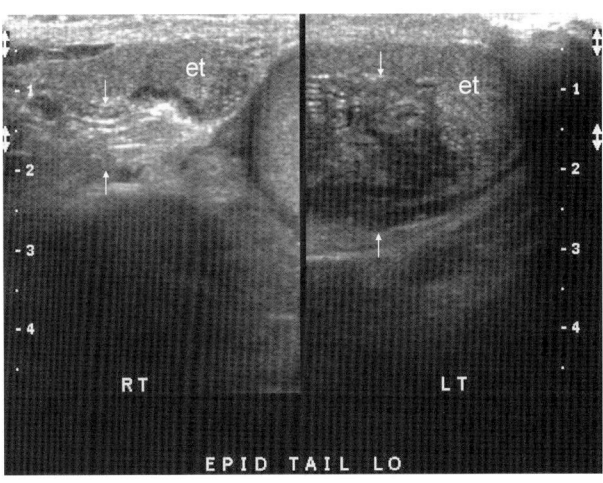

left epididymal head (eh) is only minimally enlarged. **(B)** Long-axis split-screen images of the epididymal tail–spermatic cord junction shows marked enlargement of the left spermatic cord (between arrows), but little swelling in the adjacent epididymal tail (et).

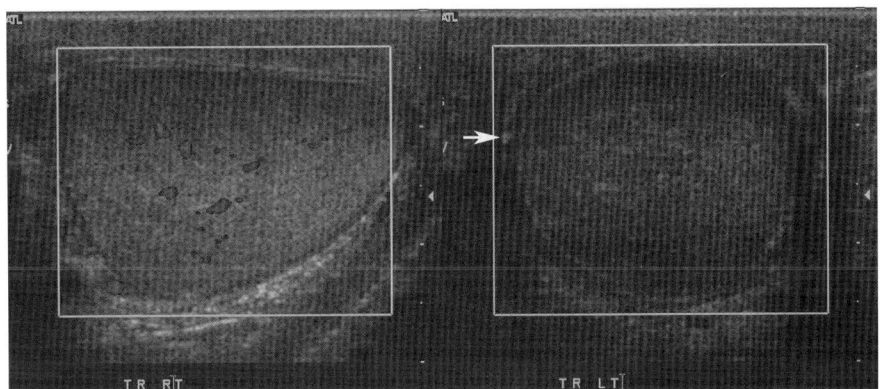

Figure 7–16 Short-axis color Doppler images of the right and left testes in a patient with acute left spermatic cord torsion. There is no demonstrable flow within the torsed left testis, but normal flow within the right testis. Note that a vessel in the medial tunica vaginalis (*white arrow*) could be mistaken for a capsular artery.

of the cord can be seen. The literature mentions enlargement and increased echogenicity within the epididymal head in torsion. However, in our experience, in most cases of torsion the epididymisa head is only minimally enlarged, but the spermatic cord, which passes just superiorly and posteriorly to the epididymal head is grossly enlarged and mistaken for enlargement of the epididymal head. (**Fig. 7–15**).

Doppler Findings

In most cases, flow within the substance of the torsed testis is absent, but there is flow within the contralateral asymptomatic testis demonstrable on split-screen imaging (**Fig. 7–16**) or on the transverse oblique median raphe view (**Fig. 7–17**). However, in cases with lesser degrees of torsion (180 degrees or less), some flow may still be present within the torsed testis (**Fig. 7–18**). In such cases the peak systolic velocities will be abnormally low compared with the contralateral asymptomatic testis. These abnormally low velocities can be associated with resistivity indices that are normal, increased, or decreased. Because of such cases, simply showing some flow

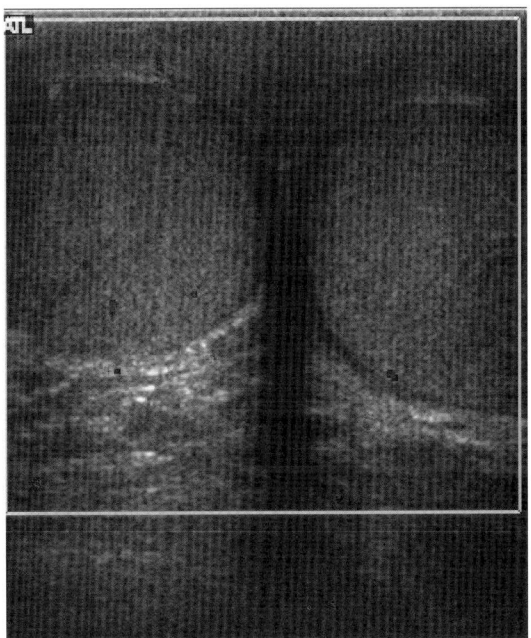

Figure 7–17 Oblique median raphe color Doppler view of both testes in a patient with acute left torsion shows normal flow in the normal right testis, but no demonstrable flow within the torsed left testis.

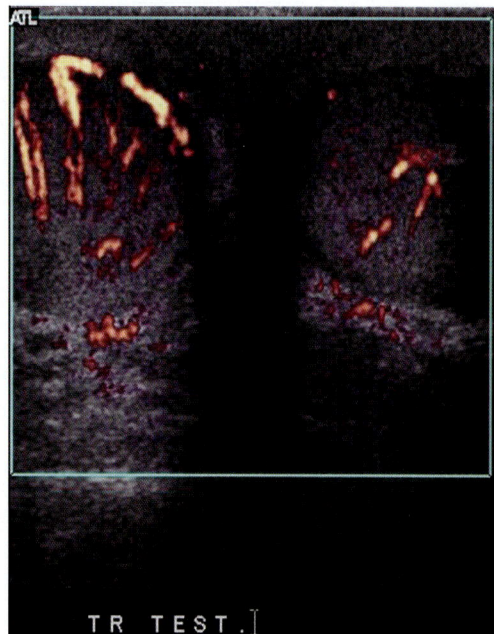

Figure 7–18 Oblique median raphe power Doppler view of both testes in a patient with acute left torsion shows normal flow in the normal right testis and reduced rather than absent flow on the torsed left side. The torsion was less than 360 degrees, allowing some flow past the torsion.

within a torsed testis does not completely exclude a diagnosis of torsion. It is still necessary to compare the flow to that in the contralateral side. Flow that appears to be only on the surface of the testis also does not exclude a diagnosis of torsion. Flow must be shown within the intratesticular branches of the testicular artery, the centripetal arteries, and recurrent rami. Demonstrating intratesticular flow is necessary because, in patients with torsion, the tunica vaginalis can adhere to the surface of the testis, and reactive hyperemia within the adherent tunica vaginalis can be mistaken for testicular capsular artery flow, potentially causing the diagnosis of torsion to be missed (**Fig. 7–16**).

Obviously, no significance can be attributed to a lack of demonstrable flow in the painful testis if flow is not demonstrable in the contralateral asymptomatic testis.

Spermatic cord torsion also results in reduced or absent flow within the swollen spermatic cord and epididymis (**Fig. 7–19**). On the other hand, any evidence of hyperemia within the epididymis and spermatic cord strongly favors a diagnosis of infection over one of torsion.

Occasionally, spontaneous detorsion may occur before the color duplex sonographic examination can be performed. If infarction has already occurred, the findings will be the same as if torsion still exists. However, in patients in whom spontaneous detorsion occurs before infarction, the ultrasound scan and Doppler findings may return to normal or may show residual swelling with reactive hyperemia, findings identical to those seen in patients with epididymo-orchitis. In such patients, the history may be the only way to distinguish infection from spontaneous detorsion. A history of pain rapidly decreasing prior to sonography favors spontaneous detorsion. A history of previous episodes of spontaneously resolving pain might also be elicited from such patients. Most untreated patients with epididymo-orchitis, on the other hand, will not have any abatement of pain before sonography.

Findings in Epididymitis, Orchitis, and Epididymo-orchitis

Imaging Findings

Most cases of infection are sexually transmitted or ascend from the prostate or urinary tract. The infection ascends, in order, through the vas deferens and the spermatic cord, to the epididymal tail, the epididymal body, the epididymal head, and finally the testis. The patient may undergo a

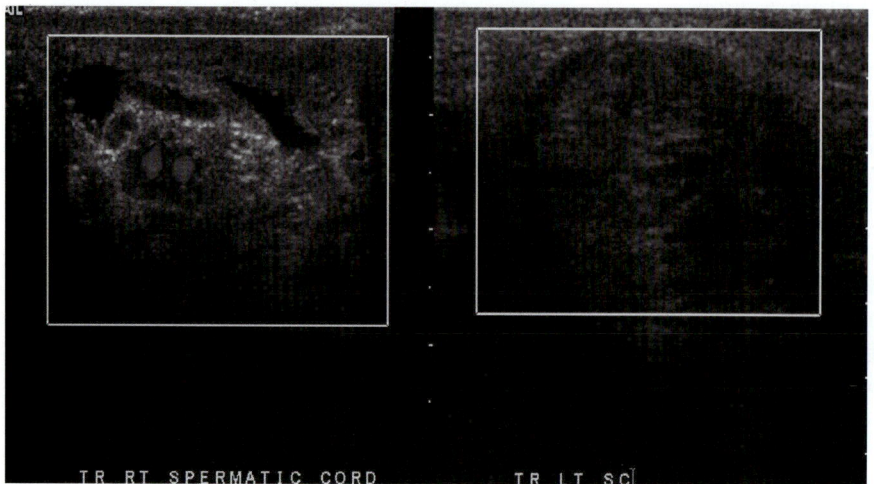

Figure 7–19 Short-axis color Doppler views of the spermatic cords in a patient with acute left torsion shows normal flow within the nontorsed right spermatic cord, but no demonstrable flow within the swollen left spermatic cord below the level of torsion.

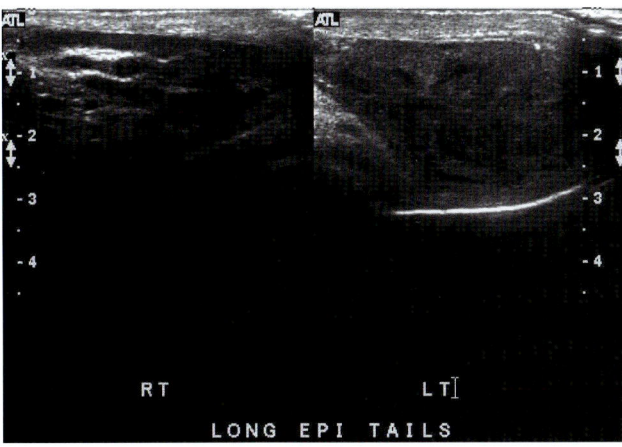

Figure 7–20 Long-axis split-screen images of the epididymal tails in a patient with early acute epididymitis on the left shows focal swelling of the left epididymal tail that is most easily assessed when compared with the contralateral side. Isolated swelling of the epididymal tail is the most common finding in early epididymitis.

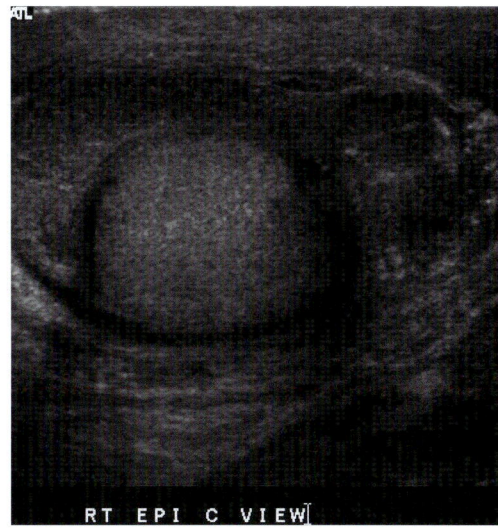

Figure 7–21 Coronal or C view of the epididymis in a patient with later or more severe epididymitis. The entire epididymis is severely swollen.

sonographic examination at any point in this progression. The pattern of swelling and altered echogenicity will reflect the pattern of infectious involvement at the time that the scan is performed.

With isolated vasitis or funiculitis, which occurs very early in the course of ascending infection, only the spermatic cord will be infected and swollen. Later in the process the epididymal tail becomes involved. The pattern of edema and hyperemia isolated to the epididymal tail is actually quite common in patients with epididymitis who present for sonography, making it essential that the epididymal tails be evaluated in all patients with acute scrotal pain who do not show immediate evidence of torsion. The swelling is much more obvious when compared with the contralateral side on split-screen images (**Fig. 7–20**). Finally, the head and tail become involved and the entire epididymis is swollen and hyperemic. This is best shown on coronal or "C" views (**Fig. 7–21**). In some cases, the swelling of the epididymal tail may be so massive that the tail indents and distorts the testis and simulates an epididymal neoplasm (**Fig. 7–22A**). In such cases, liquefactive necrosis and early abscess formation can occur within the epididymal tail (**Fig. 7–22B**). In cases of very severe epididymitis, the venous outflow from the testis can become obstructed, leading to a venous infarction of the testis similar to that caused by torsion.

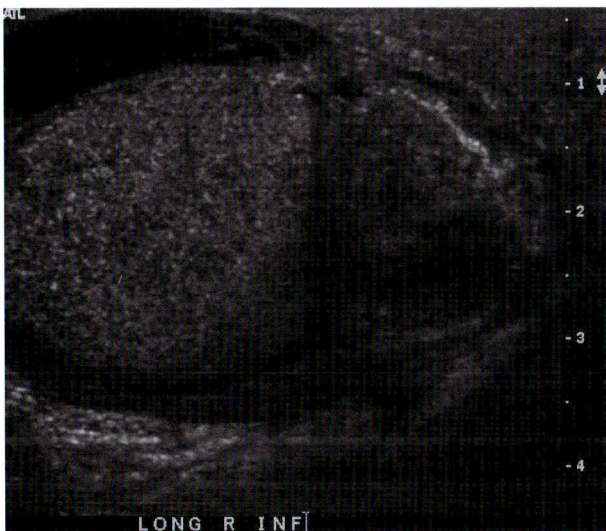

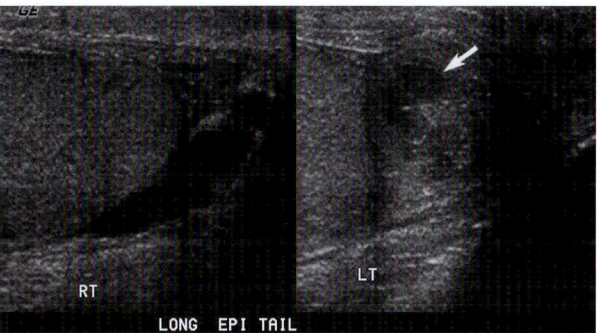

Figure 7–22 (A) Long-axis view of the right epididymal tail in a patient with severe right epididymitis affecting primarily the tail. The tail is so swollen that it appears masslike and flattens and indents the lower pole of the testis. **(B)** Long-axis split-screen images of the epididymal tails shows severe swelling of the left epididymal tail, which is undergoing cystic or hemorrhagic necrosis and early abscess formation (*white arrow*).

Occasional cases of epididymitis will more severely affect the head than the tail. We believe this most commonly occurs in partially, but incompletely, treated cases of epididymitis. It occurs in patients who are treated for epididymitis based upon characteristic clinical findings alone, but who do not respond to antibiotics as quickly as expected. It is our experience that patients with epididymitis are frequently treated with an antibiotic course that is too short—often only 7 days. In many cases this is insufficient to eradicate the infection. It appears that the tail is better vascularized than is the head, and, therefore, it heals more quickly than does the head on antibiotic treatment. Patients who respond completely to short courses of antibiotic treatment are never referred for sonography. We tend to see the highly selected subset of patients who respond suboptimally to treatment, and thus, the subgroup that is more likely to have disproportionate residual swelling of the epididymal head after the swelling in the tail has already cleared.

In cases of epididymitis without associated orchitis, the degree of swelling and hyperemia within the affected part of the epididymis will exceed the swelling and textural abnormality and hyperemia within the ipsilateral testis. This pattern of isolated edema of the epididymis on gray-scale imaging is so typical of epididymitis that it virtually excludes a diagnosis of torsion, even before Doppler ultrasound examination is performed.

Untreated cases of epididymitis may eventually lead to orchitis, resulting in epididymo-orchitis. In such cases, in addition to the spermatic cord and epididymis, the testis will be affected. The ipsilateral testis will be larger and usually more hypoechoic, although the echogenicity can vary (**Fig. 7–23**). This pattern of involvement is so similar to that caused by torsion that Doppler is necessary to distinguish epididymo-orchitis from torsion with certainty.

Hemorrhagic or ischemic necrosis secondary to severe epididymo-orchitis can lead to testicular abscess, which presents as a complex cystic lesion within the testicular

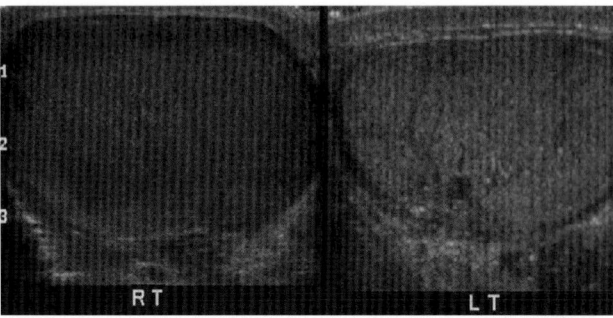

Figure 7–23 Short-axis split-screen images of testes in a patient with acute orchitis shows the infected right testis to be larger and more hypoechoic than the normal contralateral testis. Echotexture of infected testes is usually hypoechoic but can be isoechoic very early, or can demonstrate mixed echogenicity in cases where hemorrhagic necrosis has occurred.

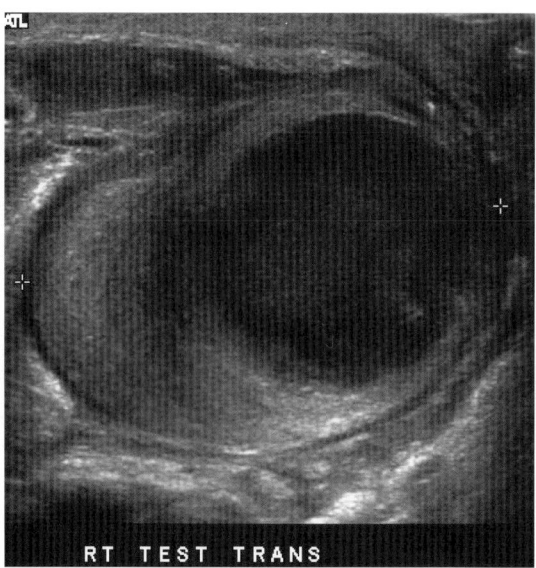

Figure 7–24 Long-axis view of a testicular abscess in a patient with severe epididymo-orchitis who responded poorly to antibiotic treatment.

substance (**Fig. 7–24**). Testicular abscesses can, in turn, rupture through the tunica albuginea into the scrotal sac, leading to a scrotal abscess. Poor or delayed improvement to a priori antibiotic treatment may be the first indication of a developing testicular abscess, so patients who present with a history of many days of pain that is not improving represent a subgroup of scrotal pain patients more likely to have developed a testicular abscess. Treatment of testicular abscess is surgical.

In cases of viral orchitis, the infection spreads to the testis hematogenously and does not ascend through the spermatic cord and epididymis. As would be expected, this causes disproportional swelling and altered echogenicity in the testis, with relative sparing of the spermatic cord and epididymis.

Any infective process can lead to hydrocele, complex hydrocele, or pyocele. Diffuse low-level echoes and fibrinous adhesions within the hydrocele suggest an exudative or inflammatory etiology (**Fig. 7–25**).

Some cases of acute scrotal pain and swelling are the result of scrotal cellulitis. In such cases the scrotal skin and subcutaneous tissues are infected, but the contents of the scrotum inside the tunica vaginalis are spared. This process is usually bilateral. The swelling and tenderness may prevent adequate clinical examination of such cases, making sonography valuable for assessment of intrascrotal contents. Fournier's gangrene is a more serious and potentially life-threatening form of necrotizing scrotal cellulitis. It can involve the tissues of the perineum and the base of the penis as well as the scrotal tissues. It is a necrotizing infection that can be caused by a variety of aerobic and anaerobic bacteria that produce enzymes which allow the infection to break down tissues and spread, cause

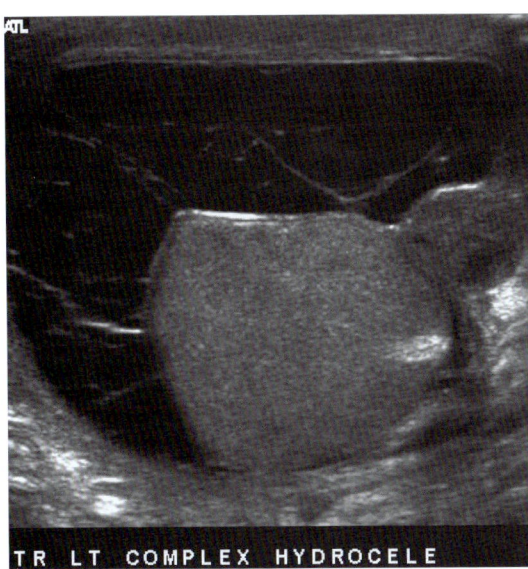

Figure 7–25 Short-axis view of a patient with severe epididymitis and a large complex hydrocele. Fibrinous adhesions bridge the hydrocele, indicating an exudative rather than transudative etiology.

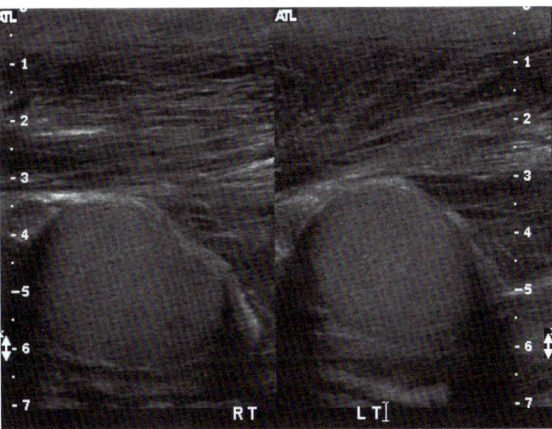

Figure 7–26 Short-axis split-screen images of the midtestes in a quadriplegic patient with acute scrotal cellulitis. Note the marked thickening of the scrotal skin and subcutaneous tissues bilaterally without associated testicular abnormalities. The thickened skin was also markedly hyperemic.

endarteritis and infarction of tissues, and produce gas within the infected tissues. If Fournier's gangrene results in bacteremia, it can be fatal. It is more common in men than in women. Predisposing factors are alcoholism, diabetes, morbid obesity, and immunologic deficiencies. The unusual cases that occur in women are generally related to obstetric trauma or obstetric and gynecologic surgical procedures. We have also found scrotal cellulitis and Fournier's gangrene to be more common in spinal cord injury patients, where a combination of indwelling Foley or suprapubic catheters and decubitus ulcers near the perineum predispose the patient to scrotal cellulitis.

In scrotal cellulitis, sonography shows severe edema and hyperemia within the skin and subcutaneous tissues of the scrotal sac. The testis, epididymis, and spermatic cord are spared (**Fig. 7–26**), but there may be reactive hydrocele. The gray-scale sonographic findings in Fournier's gangrene are similar to those of scrotal cellulitis, but bright echoes with "dirty shadowing" suggestive of air occur within the thickened scrotal tissues (**Fig. 7–27**). The swollen tissues in Fournier's gangrene are typically ischemic, so, unlike inflamed tissues in simple scrotal cellulitis, they will not have demonstrable inflammatory hyperemia.

In summary, the pattern of edema on gray-scale imaging parallels the pattern of inflammation. In epididymo-orchitis the testes, epididymal heads and tails, and spermatic cords are all swollen. However, in epididymitis without associated orchitis, the spermatic cord and all or part of the epididymis is swollen. In vasitis or funiculitis, only the spermatic cord is swollen.

Doppler Findings

Acute inflammation leads to arteriolar, venular, and capillary dilatation. This dilatation, in turn, increases blood flow within vessels supplying the inflamed organ. The inflammatory hyperemia of vasitis, funiculitis, epididymitis, and orchitis is readily demonstrable by color or power Doppler sonography. Compared with the contralateral uninfected

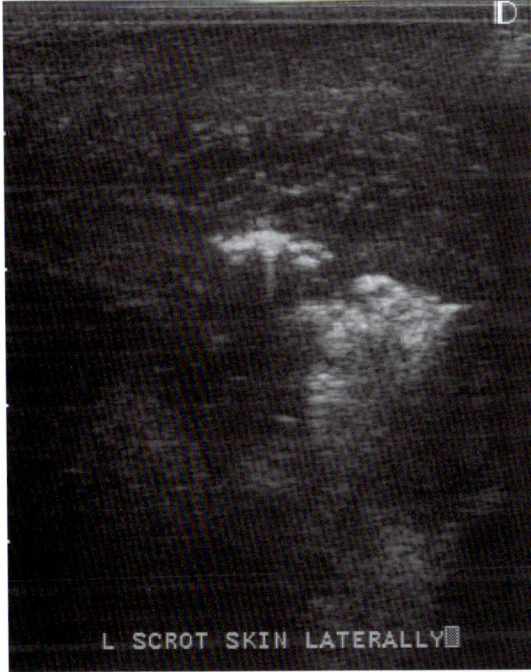

Figure 7–27 Transverse view through the scrotal skin lateral to the left testis in an elderly diabetic male patient with Fournier's gangrene. There is severe edema of the scrotal skin and subcutaneous tissues, and there are bright echoes caused by air within the soft tissues. The bright echo on the right has "dirty shadowing," whereas the bright echo on the left side of the image has ringdown or comet tail artifact.

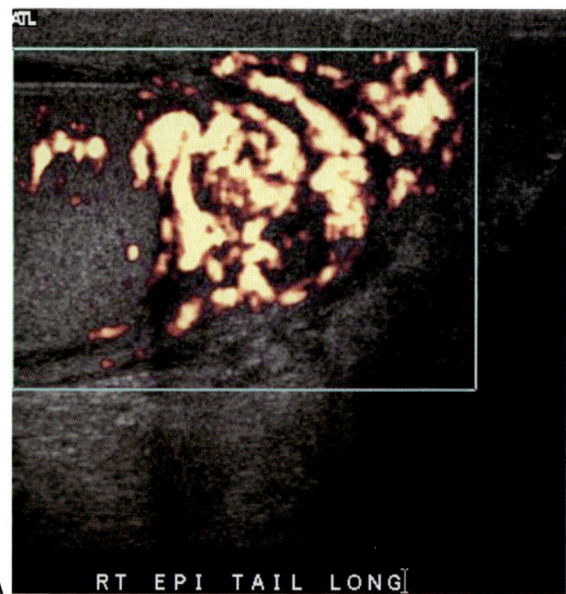

Figure 7–28 (A) Long-axis power Doppler view of the epididymal tail. In early epididymitis there is hyperemia as well as swelling in the epididymal tail. **(B)** Coronal power Doppler view of epididymitis. In severe or later epididymitis, the entire epididymis becomes hyperemic as well as swollen.

side, the inflamed organ shows more numerous and larger vessels on color or power Doppler imaging and more saturation of color, indicating higher mean velocities.

As is the case for gray-scale evidence of edema, the pattern of hyperemia parallels the pattern of inflammation. When epididymitis primarily affects the epididymal tail, the greatest and most obvious degree of hyperemia will occur within the swollen epididymal tail (**Fig. 7–28A**). When the entire epididymis is infected, the entire epididymis will be hyperemic (**Fig. 7–28B**). In epididymo-orchitis, the ipsilateral testis will be hyperemic in addition to the epididymis (**Fig. 7–29**). In occasional cases, the development of inflammatory hyperemia can precede any demonstrable enlargement (**Fig. 7–30**).

In most cases of infection, the increased flow within the inflamed organ will be so obvious with color or power Doppler alone that duplex sonographic spectral analysis will not be necessary. However, in a few cases, color or power Doppler alone may fail to demonstrate hyperemia.

In such cases, pulsed Doppler spectral analysis can help. A peak systolic velocity within the capsular testicular arteries in an adult reproductive-aged male over 15 cm/s suggests hyperemia, as does peak systolic velocity on the ipsilateral symptomatic side that is 5 cm higher than the velocity on the contralateral side. In infants, young children, and elderly adults, velocities are so low that absolute velocities and velocity differences may be difficult to use. In these patients, ratio peak systolic velocities from mirror image vessels within the symptomatic ipsilateral and asymptomatic contralateral testes of 1.7 or greater suggest the presence of hyperemia on the symptomatic side (**Fig. 7–31**).

Peak systolic velocities in the epididymal head over 5 cm/s and end-diastolic velocities over 3 cm/s usually indicate epididymitis. The peak systolic velocity of the epididymal tail and spermatic cord is more variable, and comparison with contralateral asymptomatic side is more important than the absolute value of the velocity. A ratio of the peak systolic velocity of 1.5 or greater between the

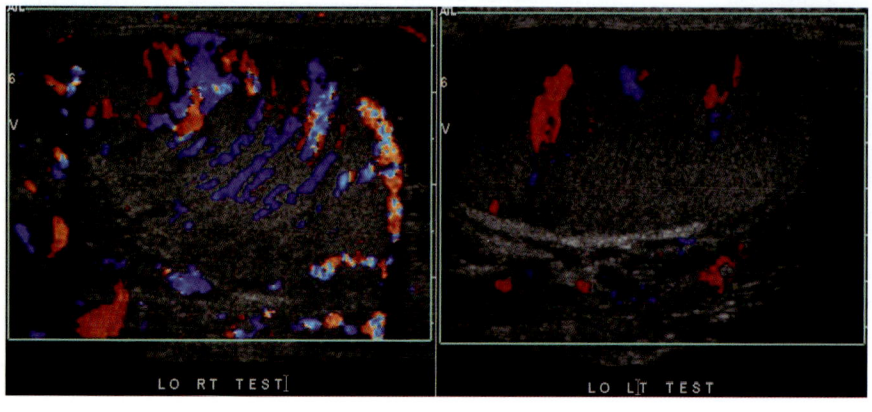

Figure 7–29 Long-axis color Doppler images of the right and left testes in a patient with acute orchitis on the right. The infected right testis is hyperemic compared with the normal left side.

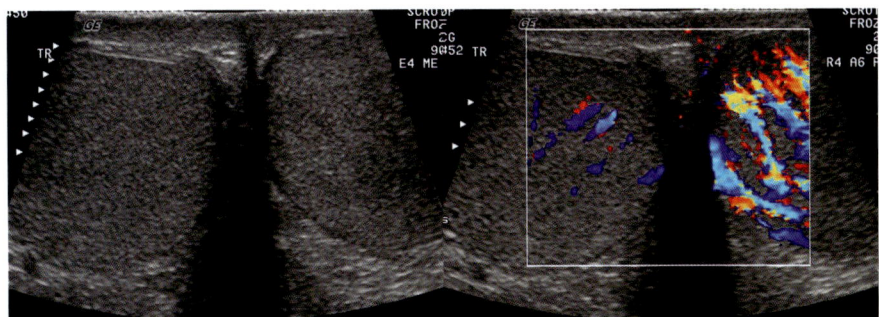

Figure 7–30 Medial raphe gray-scale and color Doppler images of both testes in a patient with acute left orchitis. In a few cases Doppler may become abnormal before the testis enlarges and changes echogenicity. The gray-scale (left image) median raphe image shows symmetrical testicular size and echogenicity on the right and left. The median raphe color image (right image), however, shows obvious hyperemia within the left testis.

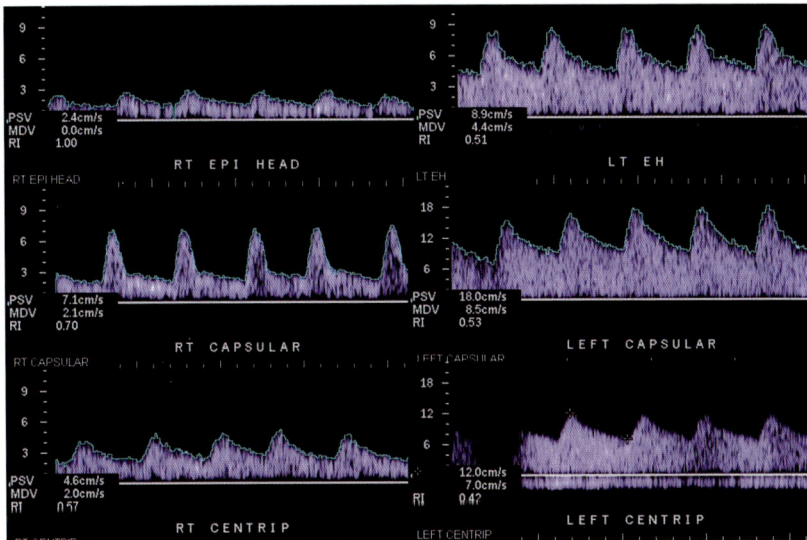

Figure 7–31 Spectral waveforms from the epididymal head, capsular arteries, and centripetal arteries on the right and left sides in a patient with acute left epididymo-orchitis show higher velocities and generally lower resistance on the infected left side. The infected left epididymal head has peak systolic velocity > 5 cm/s and an end-diastolic velocity > 3 cm/s. The capsular artery from the infected left side has a peak systolic velocity > 15 cm/s and an end-diastolic velocity > 7 cm/s. The absolute velocities of the centripetal arteries are more variable and usually require comparison with the opposite side. All the peak systolic velocities on the infected left side are more than 1.7 times greater than the velocities of the corresponding artery on the normal side.

symptomatic and the asymptomatic epididymitis suggests hyperemia on the symptomatic side (**Fig. 7–31**).

Most adults with acute scrotal pain have infection rather than torsion and will show obviously increased color flow. Inflammatory hyperemia is a positive finding, as opposed to torsion-induced oligemia, which is a negative finding. Positive findings are inherently more believable and reliable than negative findings. The presence of hyperemia is, therefore, strongly predictive that the testis is not torsed.

Findings in Torsion of the Appendix Testis

Imaging Findings

In children, torsion of the appendix testis or appendix epididymis is more common than epididymitis and can present with clinical findings indistinguishable from spermatic cord torsion or epididymo-orchitis. The torsed appendix testis will be visible as a small hyperechoic or mixed hyperechoic and hypoechoic nodule medial to the epididymal head. The enlargement and alteration in echotexture of the torsed appendix testis is due to infarction with or without hemorrhage. The epididymal head and spermatic cord immediately adjacent to the torsed appendix testis are usually sympathetically swollen and inflamed (**Fig. 7–32**). The

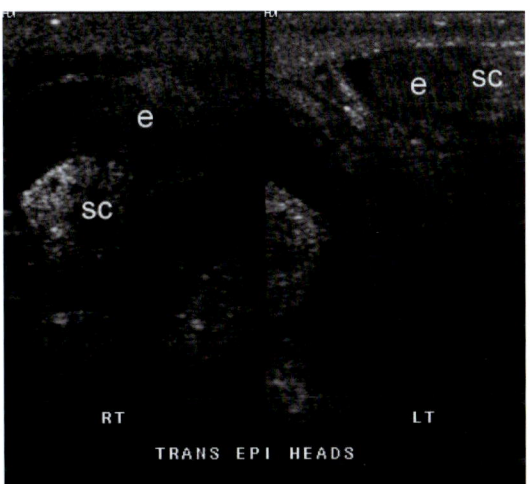

Figure 7–32 Short-axis split-screen images through the epididymal heads in a young boy with acute torsion of the appendix testis on the right. Note that the right epididymal head (e) and spermatic cord (sc) are swollen compared with the left. The reactive inflammation within the epididymal head and spermatic cord are indistinguishable from the primary inflammation caused by acute epididymitis involving the epididymal head unless the appendix testis is specifically evaluated.

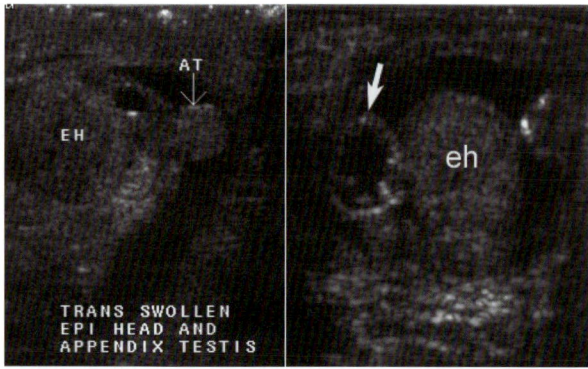

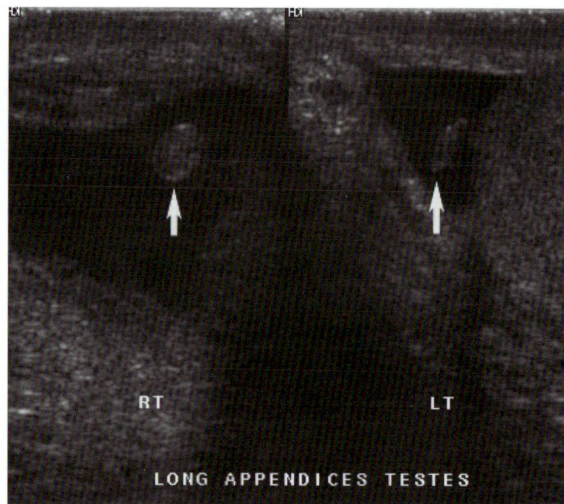

Figure 7–33 The left image shows an enlarged echogenic appendix testis (AT) (*arrow*) that has torsed and undergone bland infarction. Most torsed appendices have this appearance. The right image shows an enlarged complex cystic appendix testis (*arrow*) that has torsed and undergone secondary hemorrhagic infarction. The hemorrhage into the torsed appendix creates the cystic appearance. Only a minority of torsed appendices have this appearance.

Figure 7–34 Long-axis split-screen images of the right and left appendix testes in a patient with an acutely torsed appendix testis. Note that the normal left appendix has a thin, elongated vermiform shape, like that of a grain of rice. The swollen torsed appendix is plumper and rounder, more like the shape of a snow pea.

testis is usually sonographically normal. A small, associated reactive hydrocele often exists. If no specific attempts are made to image the appendix testis, then the diagnosis of torsed appendix will likely be missed and the reactive swelling within the adjacent epididymal head and spermatic cord will be misinterpreted as epididymitis that involves primarily the epididymal head. The sonographic appearance of the torsed appendix depends upon whether infarction is bland or hemorrhagic. Bland infarction results in hyperechoic echotexture, whereas superimposed hemorrhage gives the enlarged appendix a complex cystic appearance (**Fig. 7–33**). Longitudinal split-screen imaging of the appendices testes is definitive, but not always possible (**Fig. 7–34**). As a practical matter, the misdiagnosis of a torsed appendix testis as epididymitis is relatively unimportant—as long as the patient is not taken to surgery for suspected testicular torsion—because both epididymitis and torsion of the appendix testis are managed medically, not surgically. The pain eventually (in a few days) spontaneously abates and the hemorrhagic infarcted appendix testis may slough into the scrotal sac, calcify, and form a "scrotal pearl."

Doppler Findings

No demonstrable flow exists within the enlarged, infarcted, and hemorrhagic torsed appendix testis. Unfortunately, we are so rarely able to demonstrate flow within a normal appendix testis that no importance can be attached to a lack of flow within the enlarged ipsilateral appendix. However, sympathetic or reactive hyperemia will usually be found in the enlarged epididymal head and spermatic cord, immediately adjacent to the torsed appendix testis (**Fig. 7–35**). As is the case for imaging findings, the pattern of inflammatory hyperemia may mimic that of epididymitis that predominantly involves the head. Thus one must have a clinical index of suspicion for torsion of an appendix to make the diagnosis and to distinguish it from epididymitis involving primarily the epididymal head.

Findings in Testicular Tumors

Imaging Findings

Occasionally, necrosis of or hemorrhage into a testicular tumor causes acute scrotal pain. In fact, ~10% of testicular

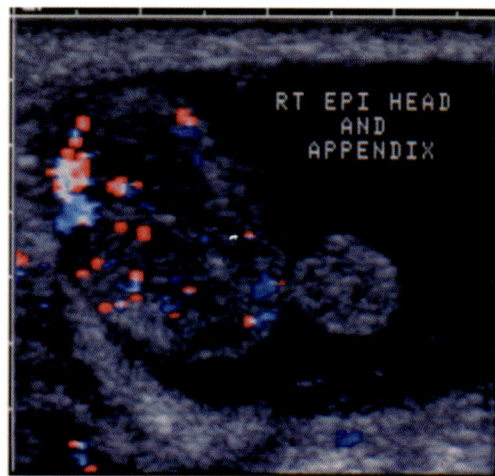

Figure 7–35 Short-axis color Doppler view of torsed appendix testis and adjacent torsed appendix shows no flow in torsed appendix and reactive hyperemia in the adjacent epididymal head. The problem is that we can almost never demonstrate flow in a normal appendix testis. Thus absence of flow in a suspect appendix testis has little value. The diagnosis rests upon clinical suspicion and the gray-scale images.

7 Acute Scrotal Pain   97

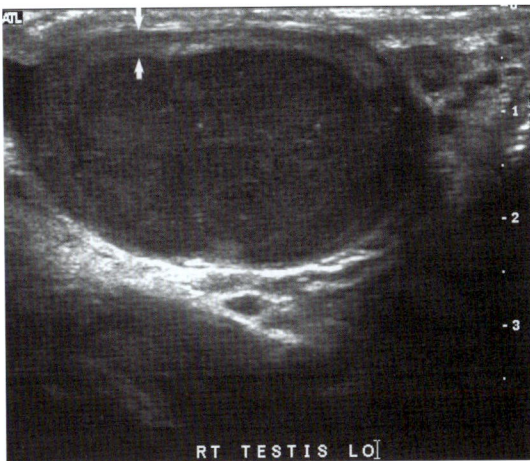

Figure 7–36 Long-axis gray-scale view of a large testicular tumor that presented with acute pain. A small percentage of testicular tumors present with acute pain. In a few cases the tumor may almost completely replace normal tissue, leaving only a thin peripheral rim of normal tissue (between arrows). If the thin rim of normal tissue is not appreciated, there is a risk of misdiagnosing the cause of pain as orchitis.

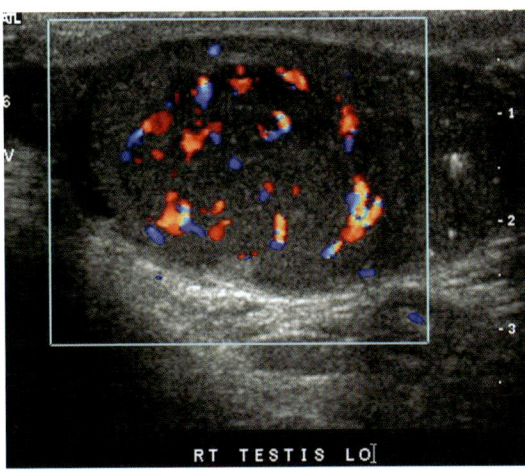

Figure 7–37 Long-axis color Doppler image of a large testicular tumor that replaces nearly all of the substance of the testis. Such large testicular tumors usually have increased vascularity that is more disorganized than hyperemia that occurs within an inflamed testis.

tumors present with pain and swelling that simulate those of infection or torsion. Smaller masses or nodules within the testis are usually easily recognized, but very large tumors that almost completely replace the testicular substance can be mistaken for an edematous testis due to orchitis or torsion. However, careful inspection will usually show a thin rim of compressed testicular tissue on one side of the mass (**Fig. 7–36**). Care must also be taken not to mistake a hugely swollen epididymal tail caused by epididymitis for a primary testicular tumor. In some cases, the tail may be so swollen that it compresses and indents the lower pole of the testis sufficiently that it appears to arise from the testis. With a coronal approach, ultrasound imaging can show that the tail is connected to the epididymal body. Additionally, the borders of the indented testis are rounded rather than pointed and claw shaped, as they are when the mass arises from within the testis.

Doppler Findings

Whether abnormally increased flow exists within neoplastic testicular masses depends almost entirely on their size rather than their cell type. Small testicular nodules (< 1.5 cm in maximum diameter) generally do not have any demonstrable flow, and masses larger than 1.5 cm are more likely to have demonstrable tumor flow, regardless of whether the nodules are benign or malignant (**Fig. 7–37**). In general, color Doppler imaging is not as useful in assessing intratesticular masses as it is for evaluating pain.

Findings in Testicular Trauma

Imaging Findings

Trauma can increase the risk of torsion, lead to epididymo-orchitis, and result in fracture of the testis, with or without a large hematocele. Because the differential diagnosis for trauma is essentially the same as for acute scrotal pain in the absence of trauma, the standard workup for scrotal pain should be used. The only difference is that a specific attempt should be made to identify testicular fracture. Large hematoceles can make it difficult to determine whether testicular fracture exists. Foci of abnormal echotexture within the substance of the testis can be manifestations of either contusion or occult fracture. Textural abnormalities that extend to the tunica albuginea are more suspicious for occult laceration than are centrally located foci of abnormal echotexture. Macroscopic lacerations can contain liquid blood or echogenic clot (**Fig. 7–38**). One should err on the

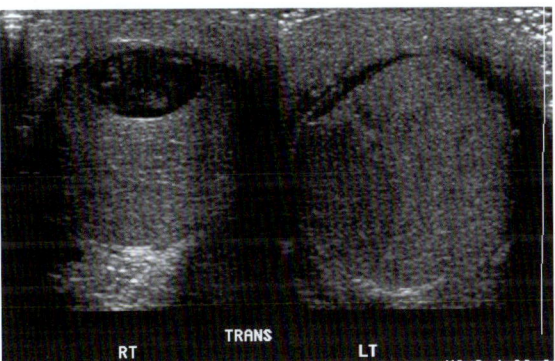

Figure 7–38 Short-axis split-screen images of bilaterally lacerated testes due to blunt trauma. The laceration in the right testis contains liquid blood and appears complex cystic. The laceration in the left testis contains echogenic clot.

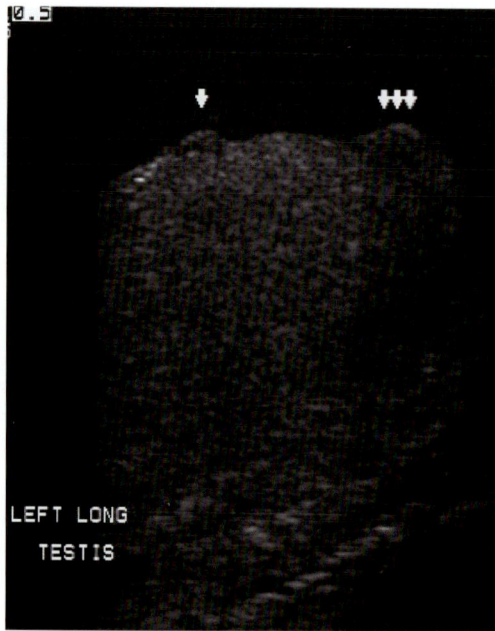

Figure 7-39 Long-axis view of a lacerated testis. The lacerations are not seen. Only mild irregularity of the tunica albuginea gives evidence of underlying lacerations (arrows).

side of aggressiveness when assessing the testis for fracture because early surgical repair improves salvage rate and recovery time. Any irregularity or flap of the tunica albuginea should be viewed as suspicious for a rent in the tunica albuginea with herniation of testicular tissue through the rent or adherent clot (**Fig. 7-39**).

Doppler Findings

The Doppler findings, like the imaging findings of trauma, include the entire gamut of causes of scrotal pain. The

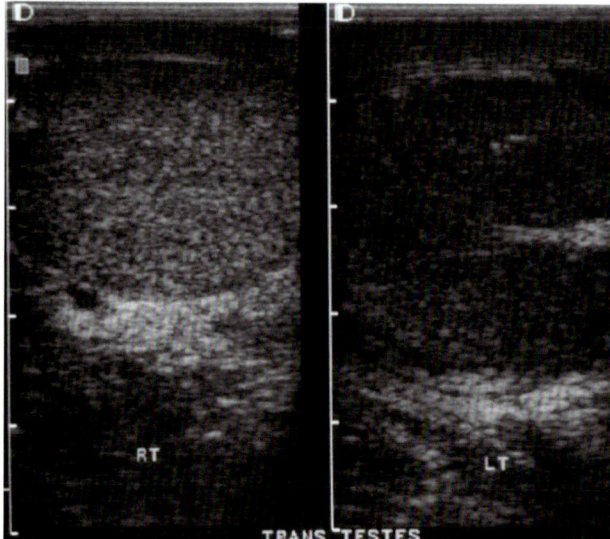

Figure 7-41 Short-axis split-screen images in a patient with an infarcted left testis that is the result of acute spermatic cord compression caused by a posthemiorrhaphy hematoma.

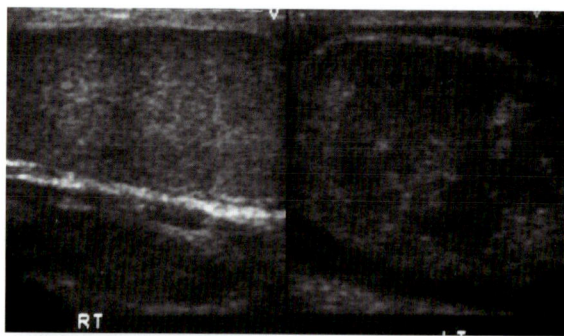

Figure 7-40 Long-axis view of right and left testes in a patient who has undergone ischemic infarction because of venous occlusion caused by severe epididymitis. Notice that the alteration in echogenicity due to venous occlusion is not homogeneous.

Doppler workup should be the same as for any other patient with acute scrotal pain. Doppler can demonstrate inflammatory hyperemia in the days or weeks after trauma in patients who develop posttraumatic orchitis or epididymitis.

Findings in Spermatic Cord Thrombosis from Causes Other than Torsion

Imaging Findings

The imaging findings of spermatic cord compression or thrombosis, whether due to severe epididymitis (**Fig. 7-40**), inguinal hernia surgery (**Fig. 7-41**), trauma, or spontaneous thrombosis (in patients who are hypercoagulable), are similar to those of testicular torsion at a similar temporal stage. The findings are manifestations of venous and lymphatic occlusion. The ultimate result, if not treated promptly, is hemorrhagic venous infarction, the same pathological condition caused by torsion. The testicular and epididymal findings are indistinguishable from those of torsion. The only imaging difference between spermatic cord thrombosis resulting from inguinal herniorrhaphy and torsion is the level at which the spermatic cord

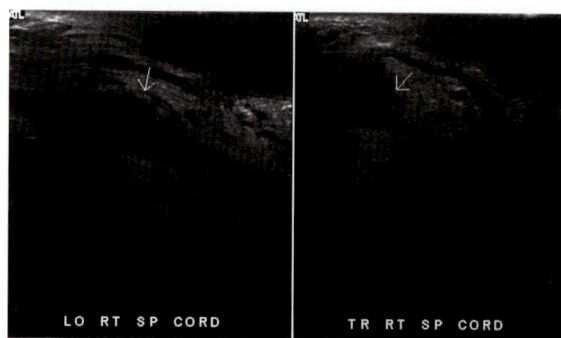

Figure 7-42 Long-axis (left) and short-axis (right) images of the spermatic cord in a patient with acute right-sided pain immediately postvasectomy. There is a small acute hematoma within the spermatic cord just deep to the cremasteric muscle.

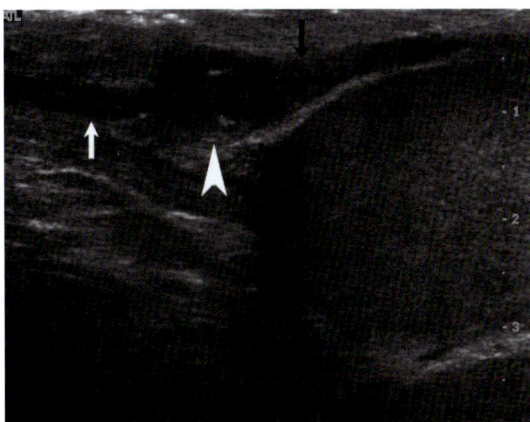

Figure 7–43 Long-axis view of the vas deferens postvasectomy in a patient who developed acute pain postvasectomy. The vas deferens is dilated below the vasectomy site (*white arrow*) There is an acute spermatic cord granuloma (*white arrowhead*). The vas deferens below the sperm granuloma is quite disorganized (*black arrow*).

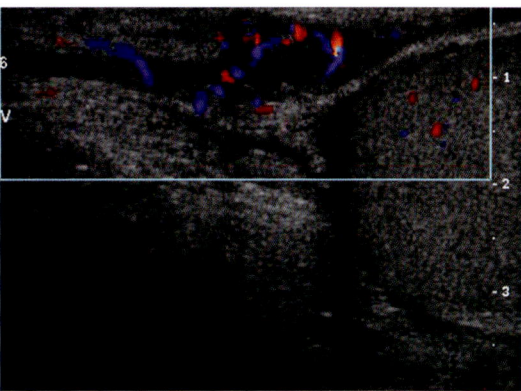

Figure 7–44 Long-axis color Doppler view of the acute sperm granuloma shown in the previous image shows inflammatory hyperemia in the walls of the granuloma. Some degree of inflammation is commonly associated with sperm granulomas, but whether it is due to a chemical inflammation or low-grade infection is difficult to determine.

swelling and hemorrhage arise. In most adult cases of torsion, the level of torsion is in the spermatic cord slightly above the testis, whereas in cases of spermatic cord occlusion due to inguinal hernia repair, the level of obstruction is at the internal inguinal ring or within the inguinal canal. The spermatic cord within the inguinal canal lateral to the penis will, therefore, be normal in size in most cases of spermatic cord torsion but abnormal in cases of testicular venous thrombosis resulting from inguinal hernia surgery. This is because compression of the spermatic cord in such cases occurs either within the inguinal ring or within the inguinal canal. Severe epididymitis may impede venous outflow from the testis, leading to venous infarction. This infarction is usually patchy and inhomogeneous but may be global and uniform. Global, uniform changes are more difficult to distinguish from changes caused by torsion than are patchy inhomogeneous changes. Evaluation of the spermatic cord for flow, twist, or the level of abrupt change in size, and the presence or absence of loose connective tissue edema provide additional clues that help make the distinction.

Doppler Findings

Doppler findings of testicular vein occlusion are identical to those of torsion.

Findings in Postvasectomy Pain

Pain occurring immediately after vasectomy is usually related to spermatic cord hematoma (**Fig. 7–42**) or an immediately developing sperm granuloma. These occur directly in and around the vasectomy site superior to the epididymal head (**Fig. 7–43**). There is usually some hyperemia associated with acute or subacute sperm granulomas (**Fig. 7–44**).

Delayed postvasectomy pain is usually related to chronic ectasia of the vas deferens, chronic epididymitis, and chronic sperm granuloma, which is most likely to occur in the distal spermatic cord near the epididymal tail. Chronic sperm granulomas can be single or multiple, and the echotexture can vary greatly from complex cystic appearance, with and without an echogenic outer rim, to solid and hyperechoic (**Fig. 7–45**). As is the case with acute

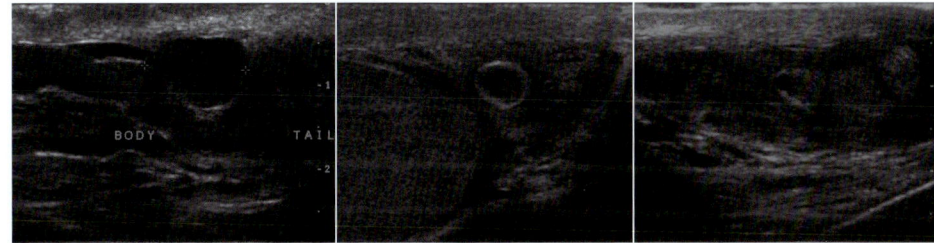

A–C

Figure 7–45 **(A)** The left image shows a sperm granuloma at the junction of the epididymal tail with the spermatic cord that has the appearance of a complicated cyst. **(B)** The middle image shows a sperm granuloma in a similar location with similar internal texture, but with a bright echogenic rim. **(C)** The image on the right shows multiple sperm granulomas with variable appearances, including that of a solid hyperechoic nodule. These three patients all presented with low-grade pain years after vasectomy. For unknown reasons, acute sperm granulomas tend to occur superiorly, near the vasectomy site, but chronic sperm granulomas tend to occur within the distal spermatic cord or epididymal tail.

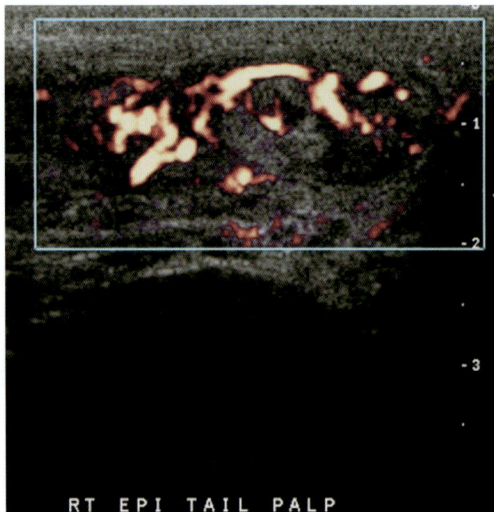

Figure 7–46 Long-axis power Doppler view of the three sperm granulomas shown in the right image of **Fig. 7–42** shows moderate hyperemia, indicating secondary inflammation or infection, just as there is in acute sperm granulomas.

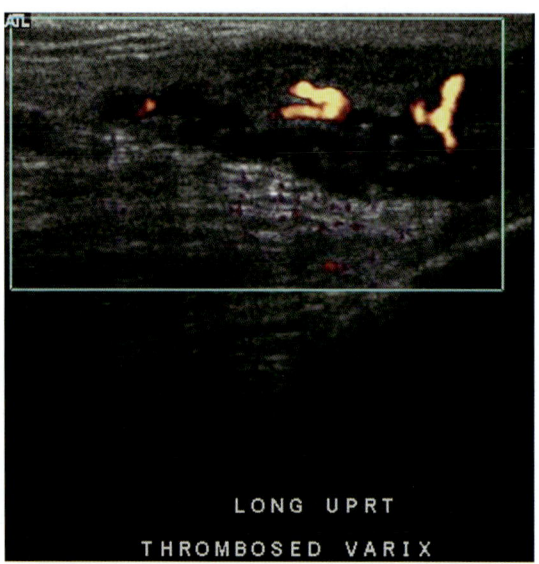

Figure 7–47 Long-axis power Doppler view of the spermatic cord in a patient who has acute thrombosis of a vein within a varicose pampiniform plexus.

sperm granulomas, there is an associated low-grade epididymitis in most cases (**Fig. 7–46**).

Findings in Thrombosis of Varicocele

Varicocele is generally not a cause of acute pain. It can cause infertility, testicular atrophy, and chronic aching, heaviness, or tugging, but usually not acute pain. However, occasionally, because of slow flow, a varicose vein within either the pampiniform plexus or the cremasteric plexus thromboses, causing acute pain. Typically only a single vein thromboses, not the entire plexus.

Gray-scale imaging findings can be helpful if echogenic flow is visible in nonthrombosed veins. Harmonics and "B-flow" can make flow more apparent. Such techniques have an advantage over Doppler in that they are not limited by "slow flow," the typical pattern of flow within varicoceles.

Doppler can be definitive in diagnosing thrombosis within a varicocele. Color Doppler is less sensitive for slow flow and more angle dependent than is power Doppler and thus is more likely than power Doppler to be unable to demonstrate slow flow within a nonthrombosed varicocele, resulting in the false impression of thrombosis where none exists. Thus power Doppler will generally be more effective than color Doppler in evaluating for thrombosis of a varicocele. Additionally, in most patients, especially on the left side, the velocity of flow within a varicocele will increase markedly when the patient is standing rather than lying down. Thus we recommend examining veins within a varicocele for thrombosis while the patient is standing (**Fig. 7–47**). Treatment usually consists only of rest, heat, and antiplatelet therapy, and, perhaps, embolization or ligation of the testicular vein.

Findings in Inguinal Hernia Extending into the Scrotum

Some patients who have large, indirect inguinal herniasm that extend into the scrotum present with pain and swelling in the ipsilateral hemi scrotum. The hernia can contain bowel loops, but most contain only mesenteric and/or omental fat (**Fig. 7–48**). Hernias this large can almost never be reduced completely.

The hernia can cause pain simply by its size and weight, by traction on the omentum or mesentery, or by incarceration or strangulation. Signs of strangulation include abnormally echogenic fat, isoechoic thickening of the hernia sac wall, and abnormal thickening and hypoperistalsis of bowel loops that might be present in the hernia.

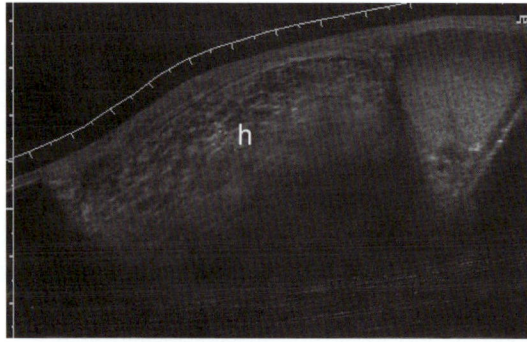

Figure 7–48 Extended field of view of left scrotum and distal left inguinal canal shows large fat-containing indirect inguinal hernia (h), extending into the scrotum to the upper pole of the left testis.

Summary

Color duplex sonography is the procedure of choice for evaluation of acute scrotal pain. The initial goal is to quickly determine whether torsion is the cause of pain. If torsion is present, then the patient immediately undergoes surgery. Once a diagnosis of torsion has been excluded, complete imaging and Doppler evaluation of the testes, epididymi, and spermatic cords will usually enable a specific diagnosis to be made and the most appropriate treatment to be instituted.

Suggested Readings

Benson CB, Doubilet PM, Richie JP. Sonography of the male genital tract. AJR Am J Roentgenol 1989;153:705–713

Bird K, Rosenfield AT. Testicular infarction secondary to acute inflammatory disease: demonstration by B-scan ultrasound. Radiology 1984;152:785–788

Brown JM, Hammers LW, Barton JW, et al. Quantitative Doppler assessment of acute scrotal inflammation. Radiology 1995;197:427–431

Burks DD, Marky BJ, Burkhard TK, et al. Suspected testicular torsion and ischemia: evaluation with color Doppler sonography. Radiology 1990;175:815–821

DeWire DM, Begun FP, Lawson RK, Fitzgerald S, Foley WD. Color Doppler ultrasonography in the evaluation of the acute scrotum. J Urol 1992;147:89–91

Dunn EK, Macchia RJ, Chauhan PS, Laugani GB, Solomon NA. Scintiscan for acute intrascrotal contents. Clin Nucl Med 1986;11:381–388

Fitzgerald SW, Erickson S, DeWire DM, et al. Color Doppler sonography in the evaluation of the adult acute scrotum. J Ultrasound Med 1992;11:543–548

Holder LE, Martire JR, Holmes ER, Wagner HN. Testicular radionuclide angiography and static imaging: anatomy, scintigraphic interpretation and clinical indications. Radiology 1977;125:739–752

Horstman WG, Middleton WD, Melson GL. Scrotal inflammators disease: color Doppler US findings. Radiology 1991;179:55–59

Horstman WG, Middleton WD, Melson GL, Siegel BA. Color Doppler US of the scrotum. Radiographics 1991;11:941–957

Kass EJ, Stone KT, Cacciarelli AA, Mitchel B. Do all children with an acute scrotum require exploration? J Urol 1993;150:667–669

Kissane JM, ed. Anderson's Pathology. 8th ed. Vol 1. St. Louis: CV Mosby; 1985:796–811

Leopold GR, Woo VL, Scheible FW, Nachtsheim D, Gosink BB. High-resolution ultrasonography of scrotal pathology. Radiology 1979;131:719–722

Lerner RM, Mevorach RA, Hulbert WC, Rabinowitz R. Color Doppler US in the evaluation of acute scrotal disease. Radiology 1990;176:355–358

Luker GD, Siegel MJ. Color Doppler sonography of the scrotum in children. AJR Am J Roentgenol 1994;163:649–655

Martin B, Conte J. Ultrasonography of the acute scrotum. J Clin Ultrasound 1987;15:37–44

Mevorach RA, Lerner RM, Greenspan BS, et al. Color Doppler ultrasound compared to a radionuclide scanning of spermatic cord torsion in a canine model. J Urol 1991;145:428–433

Middleton WD, Siegel BA, Melson GL, Yates CK, Andriole GL. Acute scrotal disorders: prospective comparison of color Doppler US and testicular scintigraphy. Radiology 1990;177:177–181

Phillips GN, Schneider M, Goodman JD, Macchia RJ. Ultrasonic evaluation of the scrotum. Urol Radiol 1979–1980;1:157–163

Ralls PW, Jensen MC, Lee KP, et al. Color Doppler sonography in acute epididymitis and orthicitis. J Clin Ultrasound 1990;18:383–386

Rifkin MD, Kurtz AB, Goldberg BB. Epididymitis examined by ultrasound: correlation with pathology. Radiology 1984;151:187–190

See WA, Mack LA, Krieger JN. Scrotal ultrasonography: a predictor of complicated epididymitis requiring orchiectomy. J Urol 1988;139:55–56

Symmers WStC, ed. Systemic Pathology. 2nd ed. Vol 4. London: Churchill Livingstone; 1979

Tumeh SS, Benson CB, Richie JP. Acute diseases of the scrotum. Semin Ultrasound CT MR 1991;12:115–130

Wilbert DM, Schaerfe CW, Stern WD, Strohmaier WL, Bichler KH. Evaluation of the acute scrotum by color-coded Doppler ultrasonography. J Urol 1993;149:1475–1477

8 Acute Pelvic Pain
John S. Pellerito

Acute pelvic pain is a common problem seen in everyday practice. There are multiple possible causes of acute pelvic pain, and a quick, cost-effective evaluation is desirable for timely diagnosis. Because ultrasound can distinguish between many of the diagnostic possibilities noninvasively, it is the preferred initial imaging modality performed to evaluate this condition. This chapter addresses the role of ultrasound in the clinical evaluation of acute pelvic pain. The value of other diagnostic modalities is also discussed.

Differential Diagnosis

Causes of acute pelvic pain can be divided into gynecologic and nongynecologic etiologies. Gynecologic causes of pelvic pain include ovarian cysts, pelvic inflammatory disease, ectopic pregnancy, and ovarian torsion. Less commonly, benign or malignant adnexal masses, such as fibroids or ovarian cancer, and endometriosis, may produce acute pelvic pain. Nongynecologic causes of pelvic pain include appendicitis, urinary calculi, mesenteric adenitis, inflammatory bowel disease, bowel obstruction, metastatic disease, and diverticulitis.

Diagnostic Evaluation

Nonimaging Tests

The evaluation of the patient with acute pelvic pain begins with the clinical history and physical examination. The value of any imaging technique is enhanced by the addition of clinical information. Because multiple disease processes may present with a similar clinical syndrome, the differential diagnosis is constructed from data obtained from the clinical history, including the age of the patient and menopausal status. The duration and recurrence of the problem as well as current medications are important considerations. Significant historical information concerning prior urinary or gynecologic problems also guide the diagnostic evaluation. For example, a prior history of ectopic pregnancy will focus the workup to exclude recurrence of the disease.

This diagnostic evaluation is also supported by the physical examination. The location of pain as well as signs of pelvic mass limit the differential diagnoses. Signs of infection, including fever and rebound tenderness, suggest inflammatory etiologies such as appendicitis or tubo-ovarian abscess (TOA). Sudden decrease in blood pressure or change in mental status portend more serious conditions prompting immediate diagnostic or surgical examinations.

The differential diagnosis is also informed by laboratory information. Hematologic and blood chemistry studies are obviously important tools to determine the origin of pain. An elevated white blood cell count and sedimentation rate support an infectious or inflammatory etiology for pain. Abnormal renal or liver function tests may suggest a specific cause for pain or point to a generalized process such as diffuse metastatic disease. Urine or serum pregnancy tests are essential in premenopausal patients, whereas serum tumor markers may be helpful in postmenopausal women.

Ultrasound Imaging

Ultrasound is the primary imaging modality utilized to distinguish between the different causes of acute pelvic pain. It is a noninvasive examination with no known adverse effects. Other advantages of ultrasound include ready availability, low cost, and high sensitivity for many disease processes.

Endovaginal sonography (EVS) has proven highly accurate for the diagnosis of many gynecologic conditions. EVS offers improved visualization of the pelvic structures compared with the transabdominal approach. EVS demonstrates adnexal masses, collections, free fluid, hydroureter, and other important clues to diagnosis.

Duplex and color flow Doppler techniques demonstrate physiological as well as anatomical information and may provide important diagnostic clues. Detection of tissue vascularity and characterization of specific flow patterns improve diagnostic accuracy and provide specific findings not possible with gray-scale imaging alone. For example, the detection of high-velocity, low-resistance flow signals allows the detection of placental flow in the uterus and adnexa even in the absence of significant gray-scale information. Conversely, the absence of ovarian flow is consistent with ovarian torsion.

Ovarian Cysts

The most common gynecologic cause of acute pelvic pain is the growth of ovarian cysts. The occurrence of pain is closely associated with follicular rupture during the midportion of the menstrual cycle.[1] Mittelschmerz (middle pain) was initially thought to be due to peritoneal irritation

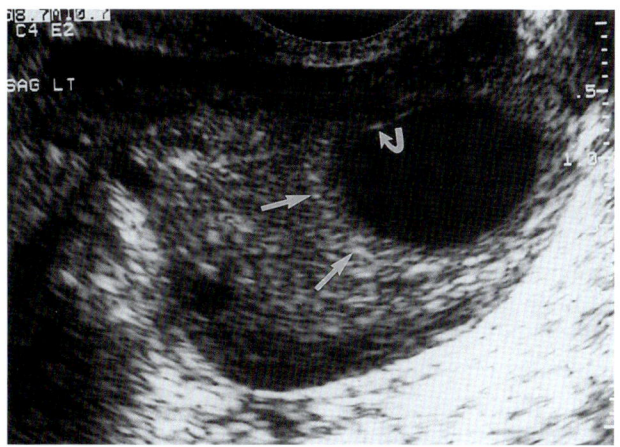

Figure 8–1 Ovarian cyst. A well-circumscribed cyst is identified within the ovary. Note the thickened rim (*arrows*) surrounding the cyst and the echogenic focus (*curved arrow*) consistent with the cumulus oophorus.

from release of blood and follicular contents during ovulation. This coincides with follicle-stimulating hormone/luteinizing hormone (FSH/LH) surge during days 14 through 16 of the menstrual cycle. Sonographic monitoring of midcycle ovaries has shown that the symptoms precede follicular rupture in 97% of cases.[2,3] The pain is usually noted on the side of the dominant follicle and is probably related to follicular enlargement.

Characteristic sonographic findings are associated with the periovulatory period. Prior to ovulation, the mature follicle demonstrates a mean diameter of 20 to 24 mm.[4,5] The cyst will demonstrate an echogenic rim (**Fig. 8–1**). Irregularity of the inner lining of the cyst may be seen when ovulation is imminent.[1] A small echogenic focus or rim may be seen along the wall of the mature follicle. This represents the cumulus oophorus and confirms that the follicle contains the oocyte. Ovulation usually occurs within 36 hours of visualization of the cumulus oophorus.

Following ovulation, the size of the follicular cyst usually decreases. Fluid is commonly seen in the cul-de-sac and surrounding adnexae. This is thought to be due to exudation from the ovary and has been measured to be ~15 to 25 mL at laparoscopy.[6]

Color and pulsed Doppler examination of the mature follicle demonstrates a rim of increased vascularity surrounding the cyst (**Fig. 8–2**). This is best visualized during endovaginal color flow imaging and is helpful in the identification of the corpus luteum.[7] The ring of vascularity ("ring of fire") is initially seen during day 8 of the menstrual cycle and continues through day 24. Although the ring of fire sign was originally described for the peripheral vascularity associated with an extrauterine gestational sac,

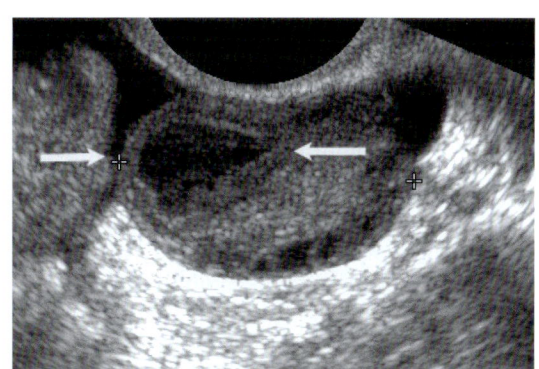

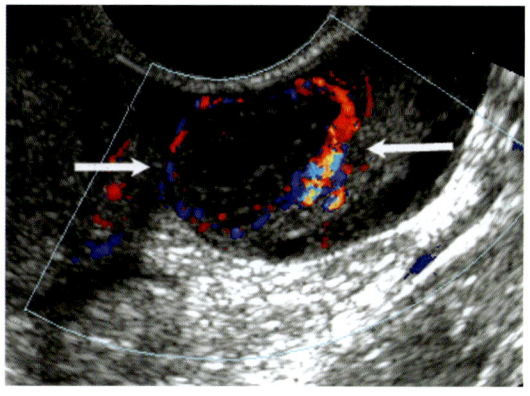

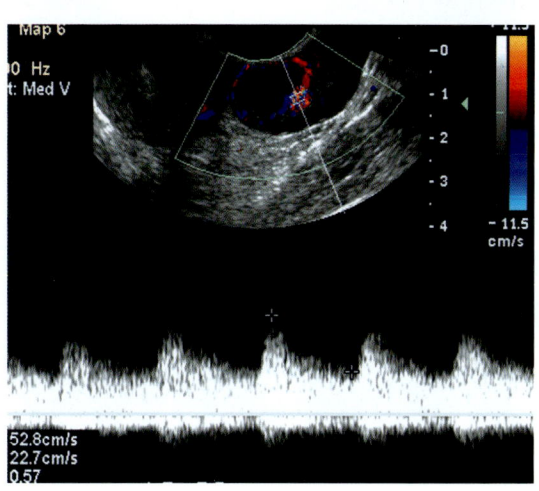

Figure 8–2 Corpus luteum. **(A)** A complex cyst (*arrows*) is seen with internal echoes consistent with hemorrhage. **(B)** Color Doppler demonstrates peripheral vascularity (*arrows*) in a "ring of fire" pattern, consistent with a corpus luteal cyst. **(C)** Pulsed Doppler reveals high velocity, low impedance flow during sampling of the corpus luteum.

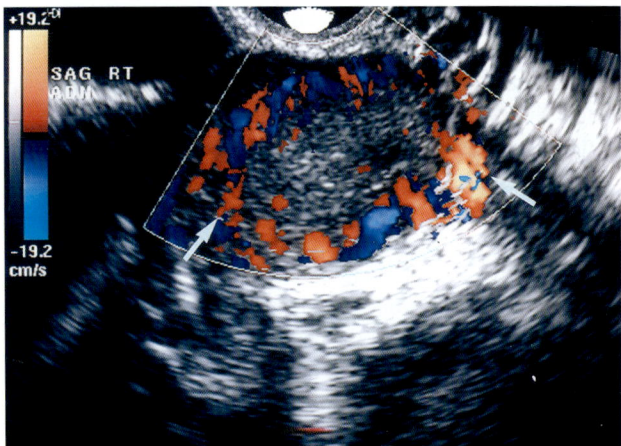

Figure 8–3 Hemorrhagic luteal cyst. A ring of vascularity (*arrows*) surrounds the hemorrhagic corpus luteum, which is isoechoic to the ovarian parenchyma.

the appearance is routinely identified in corpus luteal cysts. Peripheral vascularization of the corpus luteum may persist through the first trimester.

Color Doppler aids in the identification of the hemorrhagic corpus luteum. The cystic component may not be visualized if the hemorrhage within the cyst is isoechoic to the adjacent ovarian parenchyma. Increased vascularity is identified around the periphery of the isoechoic ovarian mass (**Fig. 8–3**). The detection of vascularity in the rim of the cyst, and not in the hemorrhagic component, is an important discriminator between a complex cyst and a solid ovarian mass. The finding of peripheral vascularity in a complex midcycle cyst warrants interval follow-up in 4 to 6 weeks, during the first week of a subsequent menstrual cycle, to confirm interval resolution of the cyst.

Pulsed Doppler sampling of the corpus luteum reveals higher-velocity, low-impedance flow from the vascular ring.[8] Dillon et al demonstrated a peak systolic velocity of 27 ± 10 cm/s and resistive index (RI) = 0.44 ± 0.09 for corpus luteal flow.[9] This low-impedance flow pattern should not be confused with low-resistance flow associated with ovarian cancer. The pain associated with formation of the dominant follicle and ovulation is self-limited, not requiring treatment in most cases.

Ectopic Pregnancy

Ectopic pregnancy is one of the most common indications for pelvic sonography in patients with acute pelvic pain. Ectopic pregnancy represents approximately[1] 4% of all reported pregnancies, with 75,000 cases occurring in the United States each year.[10] The risk of maternal death from ectopic pregnancy is 10 times greater than that from natural childbirth.

Important risk factors include pelvic inflammatory disease, endometriosis, prior tubal surgery and prior ectopic pregnancy. This is probably related to mechanical obstruction of the fallopian tube. Other risk factors include in vitro fertilization and embryo transfer as well as ovulation induction with gonadotropins.

Less than 50% of patients present with the classic clinical presentation of adnexal pain, pelvic mass, and vaginal bleeding.[11,12] Patients typically present with one or more of these nonspecific signs or symptoms. The menstrual history and pregnancy test are essential in the evaluation for ectopic pregnancy. A positive pregnancy test increases the suspicion for ectopic pregnancy. The differential diagnosis includes threatened abortion and gestational trophoblastic neoplasia.

Prompt sonographic examination is indicated to diagnose ectopic pregnancy because delayed diagnosis may result in life-threatening hemorrhage from tubal rupture. Endovaginal sonography is the preferred initial examination because it can diagnose intrauterine and ectopic pregnancy earlier than the transabdominal approach.[13-15] Culdocentesis is no longer considered a first-line diagnostic examination because a negative test does not exclude ectopic pregnancy. Uterine curettage and laparoscopy are useful but should be delayed pending the sonographic results.

The definitive diagnosis of ectopic pregnancy is made based on the observation of an extrauterine embryo or fetal cardiac pulsations (**Fig. 8–4**). If these findings are not identified, then a thorough evaluation of the uterus, adnexae, and cul-de-sac is performed to look for other evidence of pregnancy.

The uterus is evaluated first for evidence of an intrauterine pregnancy. If an intrauterine pregnancy is identified, then the likelihood of a concomitant or heterotopic ectopic pregnancy is low, occurring in one of 30,000 spontaneous pregnancies. The frequency of heterotopic pregnancy increases if the patient has undergone ovulation induction. If the uterus fails to demonstrate evidence of pregnancy, the adnexae are carefully surveyed for signs of ectopic pregnancy. Other possibilities include a complete

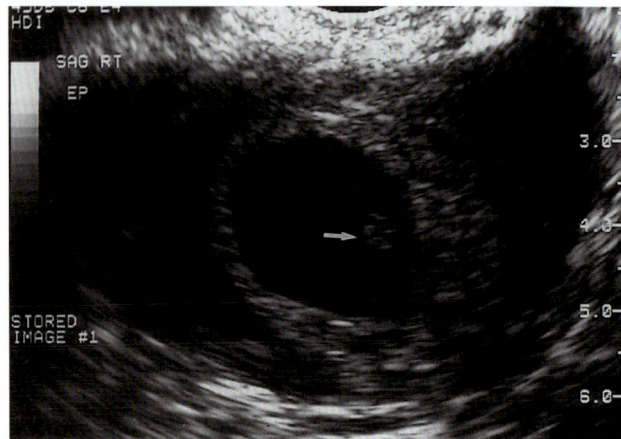

Figure 8–4 Ectopic embryo. An embryo (*arrow*) is identified within the ectopic gestational sac. Cardiac activity was noted.

abortion or very early intrauterine pregnancy (less than 5 weeks gestational age). Careful correlation with menstrual data and serum human chorionic gonadotropin (HCG) titers is helpful in distinguishing these entities. A subnormal rise or plateau of the serum HCG titers suggests a diagnosis of ectopic pregnancy.

An abnormal sac in the endometrial canal may represent an abnormal intrauterine pregnancy such as an incomplete abortion or a pseudogestational sac associated with an ectopic pregnancy. Duplex and color Doppler can distinguish these entities by demonstrating placental flow.[16] Endovaginal color flow imaging demonstrates placental flow as an area of increased vascularity around the periphery of the true gestational sac. Taylor et al described placental flow as a relatively high-velocity, low-impedance signal localized to the site of placentation during pulsed Doppler sampling.[17] He theorized that placental flow is related to the invasion of maternal tissues by trophoblastic villi. As the developing placenta invades the myometrium, maternal spiral arteries shunt blood into the intervillous space across a pressure gradient of ~60 mm Hg. This results in the low-resistance flow pattern observed during color and pulsed Doppler imaging.

Dillon et al showed that placental flow is noted in an intrauterine pregnancy ~36 days after the last menstrual period.[16] A velocity cut-off value of 21 cm/s was found to distinguish an intrauterine pregnancy from a pseudogestational sac. Pulsed Doppler sampling is performed with 0 degrees angle correction with manual manipulation of the transducer to obtain maximal Doppler velocity shifts.

The pseudogestational sac appears as an irregular saclike structure or thickening of the endometrial canal. This is related to a decidual reaction from an associated ectopic pregnancy. Unlike a normal gestational sac, the pseudogestational sac does not exhibit a double decidual lining, yolk sac, or fetal pole. Placental flow will not be identified around a pseudogestational sac.

The most specific sonographic appearance for ectopic pregnancy is an extrauterine sac or "tubal ring" (**Fig. 8–5**). The sac usually demonstrates a thick echogenic ring and may contain a yolk sac or fetal pole. The mass should be separate from the ovary to avoid confusion with a corpus luteum cyst. If the mass is not separate from the ovary, then follow-up endovaginal scans and serum HCG titers may be necessary for diagnosis.

Solid and complex adnexal masses may also represent an ectopic pregnancy in conjunction with an empty uterus and positive serum HCG titer. Placental flow may be demonstrated within these complex masses during endovaginal color flow imaging[7] (**Fig. 8–6**). These masses usually represent hemorrhage into the ectopic gestational sac or a ruptured ectopic pregnancy in the fallopian tube. They may also present as free intraperitoneal hematomas. Any extraovarian mass is suspicious for ectopic pregnancy in a pregnant patient without findings of intrauterine gestation.

In a recent study, placental flow was found in 55 (85%) of 65 ectopic pregnancies.[7] There was a sensitivity of 95% and specificity of 85% for the diagnosis of ectopic pregnancy with endovaginal color flow imaging. Detection of placental flow in an adnexal mass separate from the ovary is diagnostic of ectopic pregnancy. A velocity cutoff value is not required for the detection of placental flow in the adnexae. The detection of placental flow in adnexal lesions has been helpful in the diagnosis of ectopic pregnancy in the absence of an extrauterine sac or tubal ring.

Treatment of ectopic pregnancy includes surgical excision, preferably under laparoscopic guidance. Salpingectomy and salpingostomy are the most commonly performed procedures. There is a trend toward nonsurgical treatment utilizing methotrexate or expectant management. Methotrexate has been found to be efficacious in several series.[18,19] The risk of recurrent ectopic pregnancy is increased following tubal surgery, and close surveillance is recommended in subsequent pregnancies.

Ovarian Torsion

Ovarian torsion accounts for ~3% of gynecologic emergencies. Torsion usually occurs in premenopausal patients and is often associated with an ovarian mass. The mass serves as the focal point for the torsion, which involves both the ovary and the fallopian tube. Twenty percent of patients are pregnant at the time of diagnosis. Torsion can also occur in postmenopausal patients and may be associated with an ovarian neoplasm. Torsion of normal adnexa is uncommon but may be related to pregnancy or pelvic mass.

Patients with ovarian torsion present with acute, severe onset of unilateral pelvic pain. The right ovary is more commonly involved than the left.[20] Pain may be accompanied with nausea and vomiting, which mimics other conditions, including appendicitis or small bowel obstruction. Recurrent, intermittent bouts of pain may precede the current episode by days to weeks.

Sonography is the primary noninvasive examination for the diagnosis of ovarian torsion. Sonographic findings in ovarian torsion are variable. Most patients with torsion

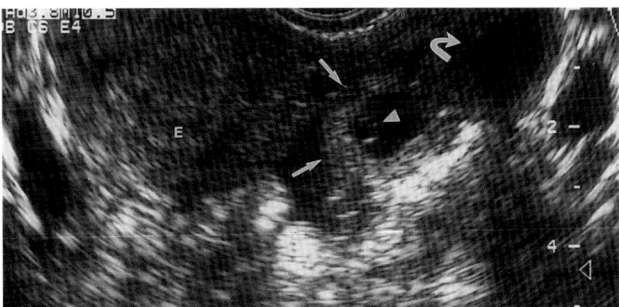

Figure 8–5 Ectopic gestational sac. An extrauterine gestational sac (*straight arrows*) with a yolk sac (*arrowhead*) is identified. Also note endometrial thickening (E) and left corpus luteal cyst (*curved arrow*).

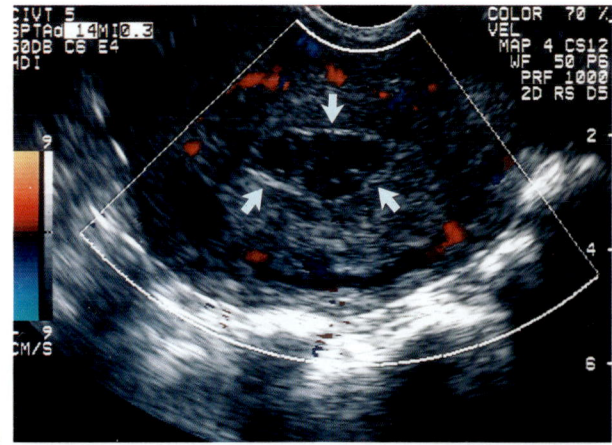

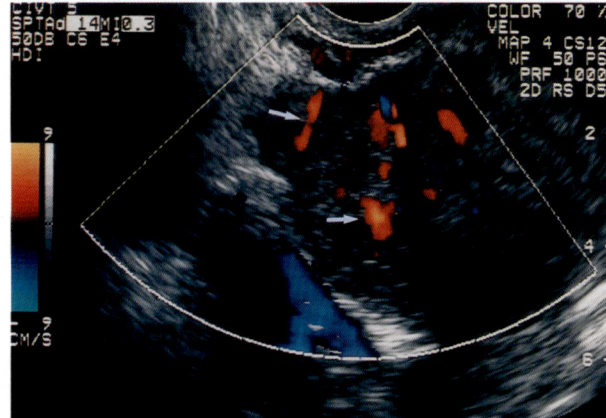
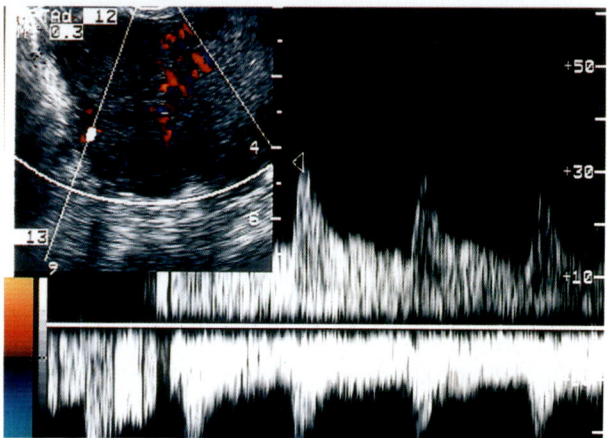

Figure 8–6 Solid ectopic with placental flow. **(A)** A pseudogestational sac (*arrows*) is seen in the uterus. Color flow imaging demonstrates no flow within the pseudogestational sac. **(B)** An ill-defined mass (arrows) is seen adjacent to the uterus (UT). The findings suggest small bowel, hematoma, or ectopic pregnancy. **(C)** Color flow imaging reveals flow (*arrows*) within the mass, confirming the location of the ectopic pregnancy. **(D)** Spectral analysis demonstrates low-impedance flow consistent with placental flow.

present with an enlarged ovary or mass. The sonographic appearance of the mass can vary from cystic to complex to completely solid.[20] The torsed ovary may contain hypoechoic areas representing hemorrhage or infarction. Venous and lymphatic obstruction produce edema and free intraperitoneal fluid. Clues to ovarian torsion include the presence of an enlarged ovary in an unusual location such as the cul-de-sac or above the uterus. The finding of a twisted or coiled vascular pedicle ("slinky sign") is also helpful. With partial torsion, the ovary can attain massive size due to edema from lymphatic obstruction. In pediatric patients, two sonographic patterns have emerged. In prepubertal girls, torsion tends to occur in enlarged, complex cystic masses, whereas in pubertal girls torsion occurs predominantly in solid, enlarged adnexal masses.[21]

The diagnosis of ovarian torsion is confirmed by the failure to detect arterial or venous flow from within ovarian parenchyma with color and pulsed Doppler (**Fig. 8–7**). The absence of flow within the torsed ovary during color flow, power, and pulsed Doppler is diagnostic. All color flow parameters must be optimized to ensure that the absence of flow is not related to technical factors such as high pulse repetition frequency (PRF), high wall filter, or low color gain settings. Arterial flow may be seen only around the periphery of the ovary with chronic torsion due to reactive inflammation. Decreased vascularity may be seen within the ovary with partial torsion. Several authors have described the presence of venous and arterial signals within surgically proven torsed ovaries.[21-23] This is likely related to the dual blood supply to the ovary from the ovarian artery and branches of the uterine artery. Thus, it is necessary to incorporate clinical and sonographic information to consider the diagnosis of ovarian torsion in difficult cases. The presence of an adnexal mass in a patient presenting with acute or recurrent pelvic pain should suggest the diagnosis of ovarian torsion.

Diagnostic laparoscopy is usually performed for ovarian torsion following sonographic evaluation. If the ovary appears viable, it is detorsed with removal of ovarian mass, if present. The ovary may be secured to prevent recurrent torsion. The ovary is removed if found to be nonviable or gangrenous.

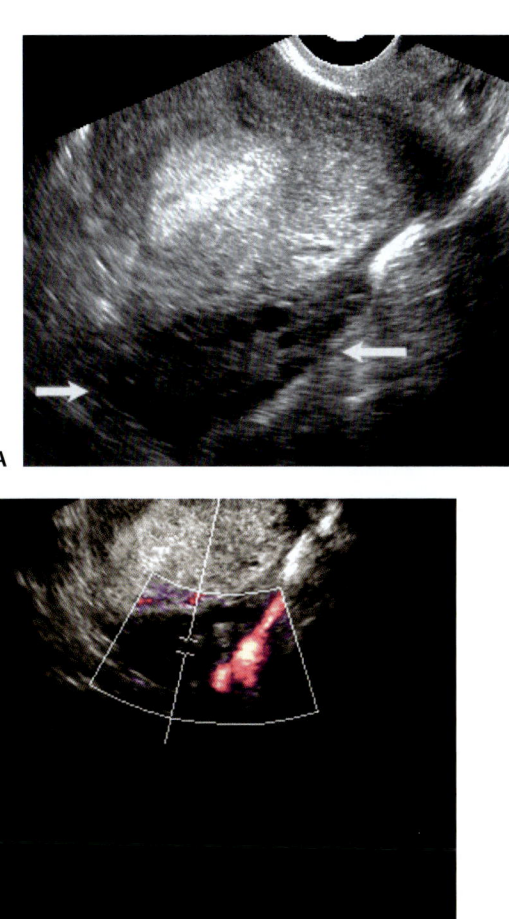
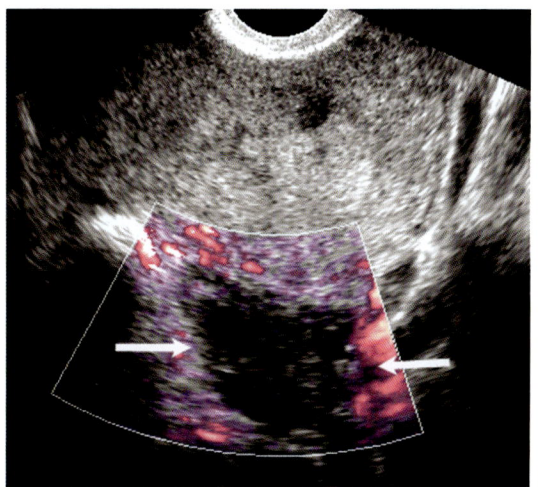

Figure 8–7 Ovarian torsion. **(A)** An enlarged ovary is seen behind the uterine fundus. Ovarian torsion. **(B)** No flow is identified within the mass during power Doppler imaging. **(C)** Pulsed Doppler evaluation fails to demonstrate arterial or venous flow within the mass consistent with ovarian torsion.

Pelvic Inflammatory Disease

Most cases of pelvic inflammatory disease (PID) are due to an ascending infection from the cervix to the endometrium. Continued spread to the fallopian tubes may occur due to reflux of menstrual blood with the eventual spill of exudate into the peritoneal cavity. Signs of a lower genital tract infection usually precede symptoms of PID. Most patients are premenopausal, with a typical history of multiple sexual partners and gonococcal or chlamydial infection.

TOA represents a severe complication of PID, occurring in ~15% of cases. This results from exudation of pus and microorganisms from the tube to the adjacent ovary or surrounding pelvic structures. This exudation leads to tissue destruction and the formation of loculations or abscess cavities affecting the tube, ovary, uterus, and bowel.

The most frequent symptom is bilateral lower abdominal or pelvic pain or tenderness. There may be associated nausea, vomiting, and fever, which reflect peritoneal inflammation. Physical examination may demonstrate cervical motion tenderness, palpable, tender adnexae, and leukorrhea. Laboratory data consistent with PID include leukocytosis, elevated erythrocyte sedimentation rate, and positive cultures for *Neisseria gonorrhoeae* or *Chlamydia trachomatis*.

Ultrasound is not reliable to detect subtle signs of salpingitis but can identify other signs of inflammation, including endometritis, pyosalpinx, TOA, and pelvic collections. The endovaginal examination is particularly uncomfortable and frequently results in the "chandelier sign." Sonographic signs of endometritis include fluid or gas within the endometrial cavity. Fluid or debris within the fallopian tube is suspicious for pyosalpinx. The tube typically tapers as it enters the uterus and distends distally. TOA appears as a cystic mass, which may demonstrate fluid levels or echogenic debris within the collection (**Fig. 8–8**). Occasionally, they may have a complex appearance with solid regions, nodularity, and septations. The ovary may not be identified separate from the mass. These masses may be hypervascular, a nonspecific finding.

Endometrial biopsy and laparoscopy are useful for confirming the diagnosis and obtaining cultures of the upper genital tract. These studies are particularly useful for patients failing antibiotic therapy due to severe disease or incorrect diagnosis.

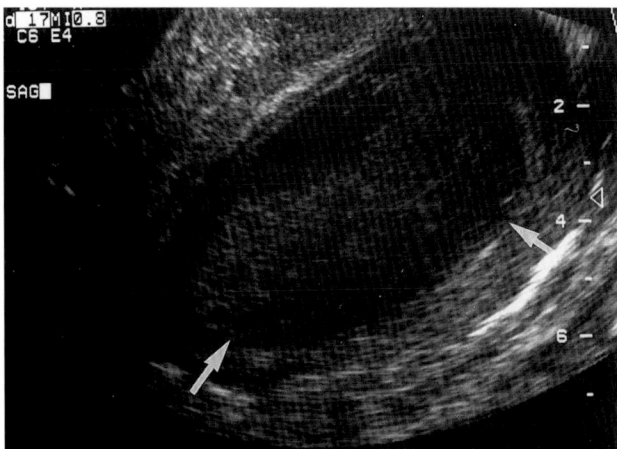

Figure 8–8 Tubo-ovarian abscess. A large complex mass (*arrows*) is filled with echogenic debris. The ovary was not identified separate from the mass.

Treatment for PID requires antibiotic therapy. Severe PID and TOA require hospitalization for intravenous administration of broad-spectrum antibiotics and percutaneous drainage. Surgical exploration is considered for patients who do not respond to medical therapy within 72 to 96 hours. Surgical drainage or total abdominal hysterectomy bilateral salpingo-oophorectomy (TAH-BSO) may be performed for impending abscess rupture or overwhelming sepsis.

Endometriosis

Endometriosis results from ectopic location of endometrial tissue outside the uterus within the peritoneal cavity and on the surfaces of pelvic organs and ligaments. Endometriosis less commonly presents with acute pelvic pain. The pain is described as aching and constant, beginning 2 to 7 days before the onset of menses and increasing in severity during menstruation. The patient may give a history of similar prior episodes of dysmenorrhea. Patients may also complain of infertility, dyspareunia, back pain, and uterine bleeding. Symptoms may relate to endometriosis at multiple sites, causing tenesmus, rectal bleeding, dysuria, flank pain, and urgency. Physical findings are variable and may include tenderness, nodularity, parametrial thickening, and adnexal masses.

Endometriosis is difficult to detect sonographically when the implants are small (< 5 mm). These implants may bleed and produce cystic or complex masses, which can be seen with ultrasound. These represent endometriomas and may contain low-level internal echoes consistent with hemorrhage (**Fig. 8–9**). The masses may contain nodules or septations that may simulate ovarian neoplasms. They may wax and wane in size and vascularity from cycle to cycle. These periodic changes are seen when comparing serial examinations and are diagnostic for this disease. Magnetic resonance imaging (MRI) confirms the presence of blood products within these adnexal masses and may find smaller implants in locations difficult to assess with ultrasound. Laparoscopy is considered the gold standard for this diagnosis because there is direct visualization and sampling of small implants.

The choice of treatment depends on the severity of symptoms and the extent of disease. Implants may be cauterized and adhesions lysed at laparoscopy. Hormonal suppression is reserved for invasive disease or cases resistant to laparoscopic treatment. Hysterectomy and oophorectomy are also options for severe cases.

Adnexal Tumors

Adnexal tumors are another uncommon cause of acute pelvic pain. Pain usually results from infection, torsion, or hemorrhage into the pelvic mass. Both benign and malignant ovarian tumors may torse. Acute pain and adnexal swelling with a decrease in the hematocrit are consistent with hemorrhage into a pelvic mass. Similarly, an elevated

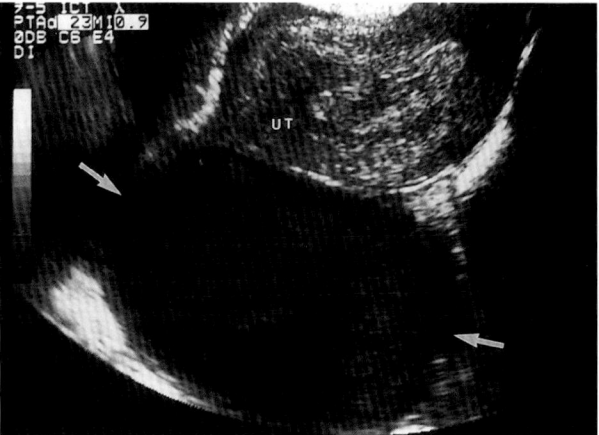
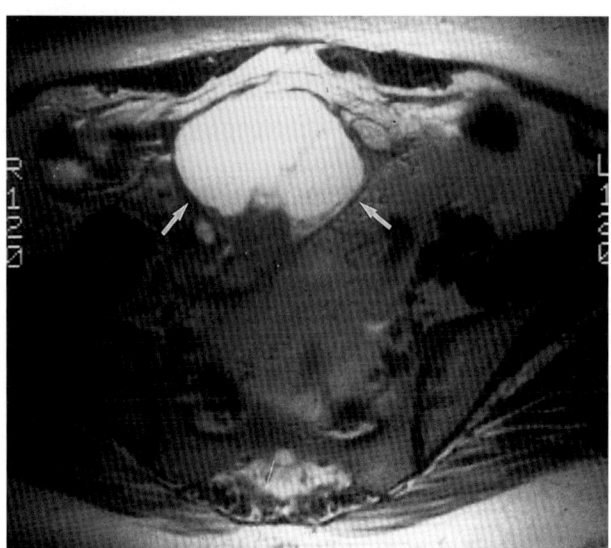

Figure 8–9 Endometrioma. **(A)** A complex cystic mass (*arrows*) is noted adjacent to the uterus (UT). **(B)** Magnetic resonance imaging demonstrates increased signal within the mass (*arrows*) consistent with hemorrhage.

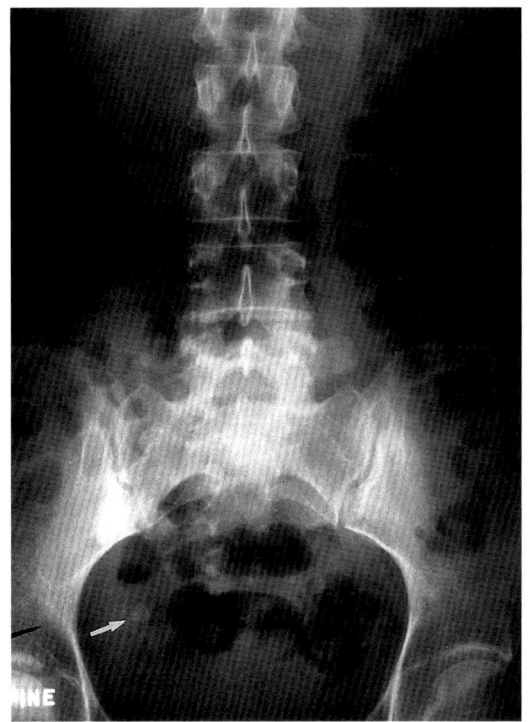 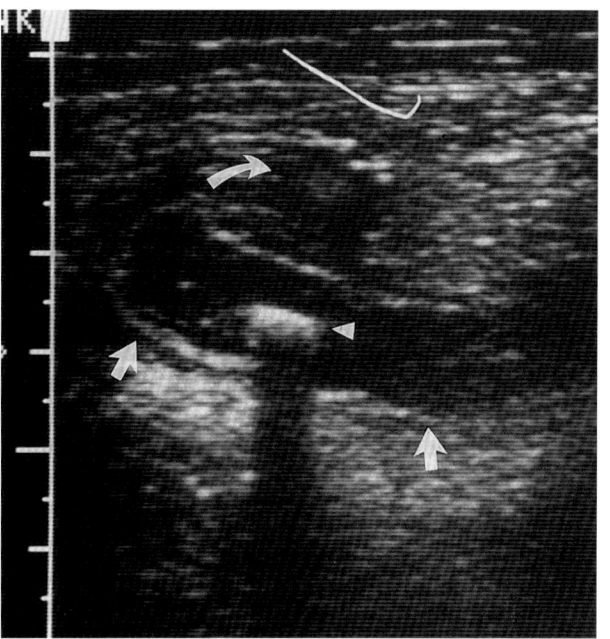

Figure 8–10 Appendicitis. **(A)** Abdominal radiograph demonstrates focal calcification (*arrow*) in the right lower quadrant consistent with an appendicolith. **(B)** A noncompressible, distended loop (*arrows*) is identified at the site of maximal tenderness. Note periappendiceal fluid (*curved arrow*) and fecalith (*arrowhead*).

white blood cell count, fever, and pelvic tenderness associated with an adnexal mass suggest superimposed infection.

Uterine fibroids can also undergo torsion, infection, or hemorrhage. MRI is helpful for identification of an adnexal mass as a fibroid. It is necessary to identify the uterine pedicle attachment of a pedunculated fibroid to distinguish a torsed fibroid from other adnexal masses. Color Doppler is particularly useful in demonstrating the vascular pedicle connection of the fibroid to the uterus.

Appendicitis

Appendicitis is one of the most common causes of acute abdominal/pelvic pain and is the most common indication for emergency laparotomy. Patients present with right lower-quadrant pain, which may be accompanied by fever, leukocytosis, and tenderness. Unfortunately, the clinical features are not specific. Thirty percent of patients will have an atypical presentation resulting in a high (20 to 46%) negative appendectomy rate.[24,25] The differential diagnosis includes all the gynecologic problems discussed earlier, as well as urolithiasis, diverticulitis, bowel obstruction, and other inflammatory conditions. A pregnancy test and endovaginal sonography are helpful to exclude other conditions.

Because appendicitis can mimic other clinical entities, the diagnostic evaluation should include the abdomen and pelvis. Radiography, ultrasound, and computed tomography (CT) are useful in the imaging workup. Plain-film radiographs may demonstrate right lower-quadrant calcification consistent with an appendicolith or findings suggestive of another process such as obstruction, ileus, or ureteral calculus.

Sonography is effective in the diagnosis of acute appendicitis with sensitivity of 80 to 89% and accuracy of 90 to 95%.[26–28] A graded compression technique is performed to demonstrate a distended, noncompressible appendix. A high-frequency (5 to 7 MHz) linear array transducer is used to gradually compress and disperse overlying bowel loops over the site of maximum tenderness. The inflamed appendix will appear as a noncompressible, aperistaltic blind loop on sagittal and transverse views (**Fig. 8–10**). The inflamed appendix demonstrates a "target" appearance on the transverse view with a diameter greater than 6 mm. An appendicolith is occasionally seen within the appendix. Sonography will also detect loculated periappendiceal fluid consistent with perforation and abscess formation. Gas can be seen within the appendix or adjacent abscess. Loss of the echogenic submucosal ring is associated with advanced infection and perforation.

CT is recommended for patients with suspected appendiceal perforation on clinical or sonographic grounds. CT can better define the extent of inflammation compared with ultrasound, and help guide percutaneous drainage procedures. Similarly, CT can better define abscesses or collections related to diverticulitis or Crohn's disease. CT should also be performed in patients with persistent symptoms without a diagnosis.

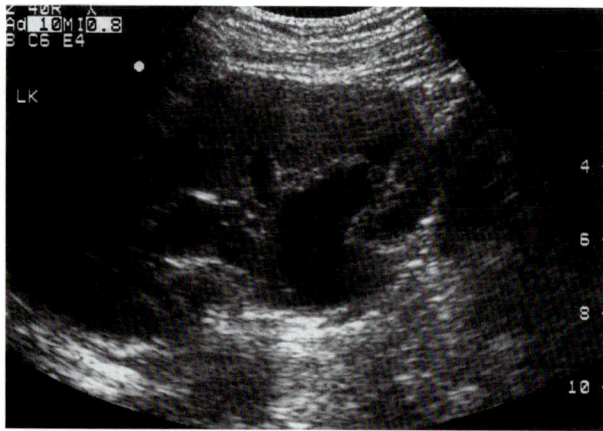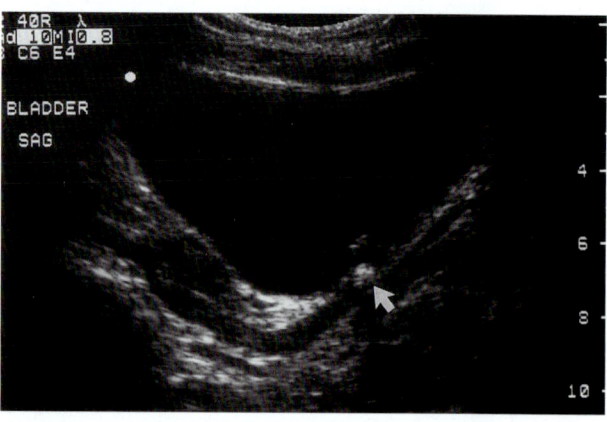

Figure 8–11 Ureteral calculus. **(A)** There is moderate left hydronephrosis. No obstructing calculus is seen. **(B)** Transvesical examination of the pelvis reveals a calculus (*arrow*) at the ureterovesical junction.

Ureteral Calculus

Patients with urinary obstruction related to ureteral calculus may also present with acute lower quadrant or pelvic pain. The pain is unilateral and may radiate to the back, flank, or pelvis. There may be associated hematuria, fever, and leukocytosis.

When the clinical presentation is nonspecific, the diagnostic evaluation should include the abdominal and pelvic organs. A KUB may demonstrate renal or ureteral calculi. Like appendicitis, sonography is employed to distinguish between gynecologic and nongynecologic processes. Although ultrasound may demonstrate dilatation of the renal collecting system, there may be minimal or no hydronephrosis with early obstruction.[29] Ultrasound is less sensitive than intravenous urography for the diagnosis of acute renal obstruction. Sonography and KUB may replace intravenous urography in patients with renal insufficiency or contrast allergy.[30] Unenhanced helical CT has proven accurate and reliable for the detection of ureteral calculi in patients with flank pain. A recent study demonstrated a 98% sensitivity and 100% specificity for the detection of ureteral calculi with noncontrast-enhanced spiral CT in patients referred with acute flank pain.[31]

When renal colic is suspected, a search for the level of obstruction should be performed. Careful sonographic examination of the pelvis, including the region of the ureterovesical junction (UVJ) may reveal the obstructing calculus (**Fig. 8–11**). Endovaginal sonography may be helpful in identification of the distal ureteral stone. The transducer is directed toward the posteroinferior aspect of the bladder at the level of the UVJ. A dilated distal ureter can be followed to the level of obstruction. An obstructing calculus appears as an echogenic structure with acoustic shadowing (**Fig. 8–12**). In patients without obstruction, an intermittent ureteral jet can be identified at the UVJ with color flow imaging. An absent or persistent ureteral jet suggests ureteral obstruction.

Summary

Acute pelvic pain is a common clinical problem with many possible etiologies. The clinical history, physical examination, and laboratory data are necessary to formulate the differential diagnosis. Ultrasound is the preferred first-line noninvasive imaging examination due to ready availability, low cost, and high diagnostic accuracy. Ultrasound can distinguish between gynecologic and nongynecologic causes of pelvic pain. Duplex and color Doppler may add important diagnostic information to improve diagnosis.

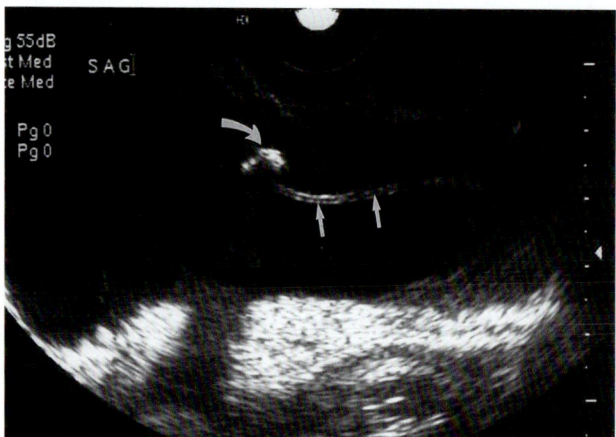

Figure 8–12 Ureteral calculus. Endovaginal sonogram reveals a calculus (*curved arrow*) in the distal ureter (*straight arrows*).

References

1. Ritchie WG. Sonographic evaluation of normal and induced ovulation. Radiology 1986;161:1–10
2. Hackeloer BJ, Fleming R, Robinson HP, et al. Correlation of ultrasonic and endocrinologic assessment of human follicular development. Am J Obstet Gynecol 1979;135:122–128
3. O'Herlihy C, Robinson HP, deCrispigny LJ. Mittelschmerz is a preovulatory symptom. BMJ 1980;280:986
4. Kerin JF, Edmonds DK, Warnes GM, et al. Morphological and functional relations of graafian follicle growth to ovulation in women

using ultrasonic, laparoscopic and biochemical measurements. Br J Obstet Gynaecol 1981;88:81-90
5. Queenan JT, O'Brien GD, Bains LM, et al. Ultrasound scanning of ovaries to detect ovulation in women. Fertil Steril 1980;34:99-105
6. Koninckx PR, Renaer M, Brosens IA. Origin of peritoneal fluid in women: an ovarian exudation product. Br J Obstet Gynaecol 1980;87:177-183
7. Pellerito JS, Taylor KJW, Quedens-Case C, et al. Ectopic pregnancy: evaluation with endovaginal color flow imaging. Radiology 1992;183:407-411
8. Taylor KJ, Burns P, Wells PNT. Ultrasound Doppler flow studies of the ovarian and uterine arteries. Br J Obstet Gynaecol 1985;92:240-246
9. Dillon EH, Quedens-Case C, Ramos IM, et al. Endovaginal pulsed and color flow Doppler in first trimester pregnancy. Ultrasound Med Biol 1993;19:517-525
10. Centers for Disease Control. Ectopic pregnancy: United States, 1986. MMWR Morb Mortal Wkly Rep 1989;38:481-484
11. Weckstein LN. Clinical diagnosis of ectopic pregnancy. Clin Obstet Gynecol 1987;30:236-244
12. Halpin TF. Ectopic pregnancy: the problem of diagnosis. Am J Obstet Gynecol 1970;106:227-236
13. Nyberg DA, Mack LA, Jeffrey RB, Laing FC. Endovaginal sonographic evaluation of ectopic pregnancy: a prospective study. AJR Am J Roentgenol 1987;149:1181-1186
14. Dashefsky SM, Lyons EA, Levi CS, et al. Suspected ectopic pregnancy: endovaginal and transvesical US. Radiology 1988;169:181-184
15. Cacciatore B, Stenman UH, Ylostalo P. Comparison of abdominal and vaginal sonography in suspected ectopic pregnancy. Obstet Gynecol 1989;73:770-774
16. Dillon EH, Feyock AL, Taylor KJW. Pseudogestational sacs: Doppler US differentiation from normal or abnormal intrauterine pregnancies. Radiology 1990;176:359-364
17. Taylor KJ, Ramos IM, Feyock AL, et al. Ectopic pregnancy: duplex Doppler evaluation. Radiology 1989;173:93-97
18. Stovall TG, Ling FW, Carson SA, Buster JE. Nonsurgical diagnosis and treatment of tubal pregnancy. Fertil Steril 1990;54:537-538
19. Kojima E, Abe Y, Morita M, et al. The treatment of unruptured tubal pregnancy with intratubal methotrexate injection under laparoscopic control. Obstet Gynecol 1990;75:723-725
20. Warner MA, Fleischer AC, Edell SL, et al. Uterine adnexal torsion: sonographic findings. Radiology 1985;154:773-775
21. Stark JE, Siegel MJ. Ovarian torsion in prepubertal and pubertal girls: sonographic findings. AJR Am J Roentgenol 1994;163:1479-1482
22. Rosado WM, Trambert MA, Gosink BB, Pretorius DH. Adnexal torsion: diagnosis by using Doppler sonography. AJR Am J Roentgenol 1992;159:1251-1253
23. Fleischer AC, Stein SM, Cullinan JA, Warner MA. Color Doppler sonography of adnexal torsion. J Ultrasound Med 1995;14:523-528
24. Abu-Yousef MM, Franken EA. An overview of graded compression sonography in the diagnosis of acute appendicitis. Semin Ultrasound CT MR 1989;10:352-363
25. Lewis FR, Holcroft JW, Boey J, et al. Appendicitis: a critical review of diagnosis and treatment in 1,000 cases. Arch Surg 1975;110:677-684
26. Abu-Yousef MM, Bleicher JJ, Maher JW, et al. High-resolution sonography of acute appendicitis. AJR Am J Roentgenol 1987;149:53-58
27. Puylaert JBCM. Acute appendicitis: US evaluation using graded compression. Radiology 1986;158:355-360
28. Jeffrey RB, Laing FC, Lewis FR. Acute appendicitis: high-resolution real-time US findings. Radiology 1987;163:11-14
29. Laing FC, Jeffrey RB, Wing VW. Ultrasound versus excretory urography in evaluating acute flank pain. Radiology 1985;154:613-616
30. Haddad MC, Sharif HS, Shahed MS, et al. Renal colic: diagnosis and outcome. Radiology 1992;184:83-88
31. Fielding JR, Steele G, Fox LA, et al. Spiral computerized tomography in the evaluation of acute flank pain: a replacement for excretory urography. J Urol 1997;157:2071-2073

9 Intraoperative Ultrasound
Robert A. Kane

Intraoperative ultrasound is a dynamic and highly interactive imaging study and is one of the most rapidly developing areas within ultrasonography. Unfortunately, many radiologists have been reluctant to spend a significant portion of time out of the department during the workday to perform and interpret intraoperative ultrasound studies, fearing that they will lose 1 or 2 hours of work time while waiting in the operating suite until the surgeon is ready for the scans to be performed. However, the information obtained during intraoperative ultrasound is often crucial for accurate diagnostic assessment and planning of surgical approaches to resection of the disease processes. Studies have shown that the impact of intraoperative ultrasound imaging on surgical decision making justifies the time and effort involved in terms of both efficacy and cost-benefit.[1] Our opinion, as well as that of many others with experience in the field, is that the benefits gained by intraoperative ultrasound imaging justify the time spent by the radiologists performing the procedure.

Technique for Efficient Performance of Intraoperative Ultrasound

We have evolved several means to improve the radiologists' efficiency when performing intraoperative ultrasound scans. These strategies typically allow a radiologist to perform the intraoperative ultrasound and return to the radiology department in ~30 minutes. The most effective strategies are as follows:

1. Intraoperative ultrasound studies are booked in advance with the ultrasound section whenever possible, which allows more planning and manipulation of the work schedule within the ultrasound section, and anticipation of the approximate time for performing the study.
2. Prepositioning of the intraoperative ultrasound scanner in the operating suite in advance of the examination may save a few minutes' waiting time for elevators.
3. The radiologist who will perform the examination may choose to work in surgical scrubs, thereby eliminating the need to change into scrubs when the call from the operating room arrives.
4. Mutual cooperation and respect between the surgeons and radiologists has resulted in an agreement that the surgeons will call for the intraoperative ultrasound scan 10 to 15 minutes before they are actually ready for scanning, and the radiologists and technologists guarantee their readiness to perform the scan within 10 to 15 minutes of the telephone call. This arrangement is usually successful in avoiding any unnecessary waiting by either the surgical team or the radiological team and thus maximizes efficiency.

In our institution, the radiologist scrubs in on the case and is gowned and gloved and performs the actual scanning. A typical intraoperative study can be completed within 5 to 10 minutes, assuming that the sonologist is experienced. Scanning performed by the surgeon with the radiologist observing at the bedside or by remote teleradiography is less optimal compared with the radiologist actually performing the scan. Scanning provides important hand-to-eye information, and the scanning technique of most surgeons cannot compare with that of a skilled and experienced sonologist. Even though intraoperative ultrasound scanning has removed many of the noise-generated barriers to excellent image quality, proper scanning technique, understanding of image artifacts, and recognition of subtle findings such as isoechoic tumor nodules are best achieved by someone with extensive experience in ultrasonography. In a busy hospital setting, with frequent utilization of intraoperative ultrasonography, a remote teleradiography linkage to the intraoperative ultrasound images may be an acceptable alternative, providing that the surgeon performing the intraoperative scans has sufficient experience at intraoperative scanning.

If possible, it is optimal to sterilize the intraoperative ultrasound probes before the operation. We have had excellent success using gas sterilization with ethylene oxide for many of our intraoperative probes. However, many manufacturers are reluctant to allow gas sterilization, fearing that the transducers will be damaged by the high temperatures of aeration that are required by ethylene oxide gas sterilization, although we have not experienced any problems. Some operating suites will allow prolonged immersion in Cidex (glutaraldehyde; Johnson & Johnson, Arlington, Texas) as an adequate method of probe sterilization, but other institutions do not consider this sufficiently sterile for open intraoperative use, and there have been some adverse patient contrast reactions to the glutaraldehyde if it has not been sufficiently rinsed prior to patient exposure. In our institution, direct patient contact with glutaraldehyde-soaked equipment is not allowed, and therefore sterile probe covers are utilized. The application of probe covers may add 1 or 2 minutes to the time of the procedure as the cover is being applied, and there is some risk of compromise of sterile technique should the probe cover rip, which can occur occasionally. Therefore, when using equipment with sterile probe covers, we soak the probes in glutaraldehyde for 30 minutes before the procedure in case there is a break in sterile technique. The probes are thoroughly rinsed and, as an additional precaution, sterile gel is used inside the probe cover. It is preferable to use specifically designed transducer sheaths that fit snugly over the transducer head because loose-fitting covers may cause imaging artifacts due to trapped gas or folds in the sheath. Standard endoscopic sheathes can be used to cover the entire transducer cord.

Our preferred method of sterilization currently utilizes the Sterrad system (Advanced Sterilization Products, Irvine, California), which is gas-plasma technology using low-temperature sterilization, thereby avoiding some of the problems with the high-temperature ethylene oxide systems. Sterilization is adequate to allow direct patient contact with the probes, thereby avoiding the necessity for probe covers. There are no hazardous emissions and, hence, sterilization time is shorter because prolonged aeration and ventilation are not required.

Application of Intraoperative Ultrasound

Intraoperative ultrasound has many uses, and the applications are extensive and growing. In neurosurgery, intraoperative ultrasound is used effectively in surgery on the brain and spinal cord, and, in intraabdominal surgery, the uses are principally in the liver, biliary tract, and pancreas. Intraoperative assessment of vascular surgical disease and intraoperative ultrasound imaging post endarterectomy or reconstructive procedures is now on the increase. Other newly developing areas of use include intraoperative localization of breast tumors; applications in the genitourinary systems, such as evaluation of small renal cell carcinomas; as well as in gynecologic surgery; and, finally, to provide guidance for interventional procedures, such as prostate cryosurgery and tumor ablations in the liver. One of the most exciting and rapidly developing new areas is that of laparoscopic ultrasound (LUS) imaging, which is being applied to assessment of diseases of the liver, pancreas, and biliary tract within the abdomen and has also been used to help detect lung tumors during thoracoscopic resections. Another new and exciting application is the use of catheter-mounted, high-frequency ultrasound transducers for endoluminal intraoperative use in the bile ducts and ureters, for gynecologic procedures, and for vascular intraluminal assessment. Given the limitations of space, this discussion focuses on selected neurosurgical and intraabdominal applications.

Neurosurgical Applications

Brain

Intraoperative ultrasound scans of the brain can be obtained through a burr hole, using specially designed small burr hole probes or endoluminal probes, such as are used for prostate or transvaginal scanning. More commonly, intraoperative ultrasound scans are obtained through an open craniotomy flap. Excellent images can be obtained transdurally as well as directly on the brain surface after incision of the dura. The optimal frequency for brain imaging ranges from 5 to 7.5 MHz in frequency, and the best probe configuration is found in the endfire sector type probes, either mechanical or electronic convex array or phased array probes. The dura or brain surface is moistened with a small amount of sterile saline solution, which provides acoustic coupling for the transducer. Meticulous scanning technique is essential, with particular care to avoid applying significant pressure on the brain. A very light contact with the moistened dura or brain surface is sufficient for adequate acoustic coupling.

The principal use of intraoperative ultrasound is to accurately locate and localize masses within the brain substance that cannot be visualized directly by the neurosurgeon, and of course the brain cannot be palpated. Even masses a few millimeters deep to the cortical surface are difficult or impossible to detect visually. The vast majority of primary and metastatic brain tumors are markedly hyperecholc in comparison with the surrounding normal brain structures.[2] The sulcal convolutions on the brain surface are somewhat echogenic, but most of the brain substance is of relatively low and homogeneous echogenicity. Consequently, most tumors

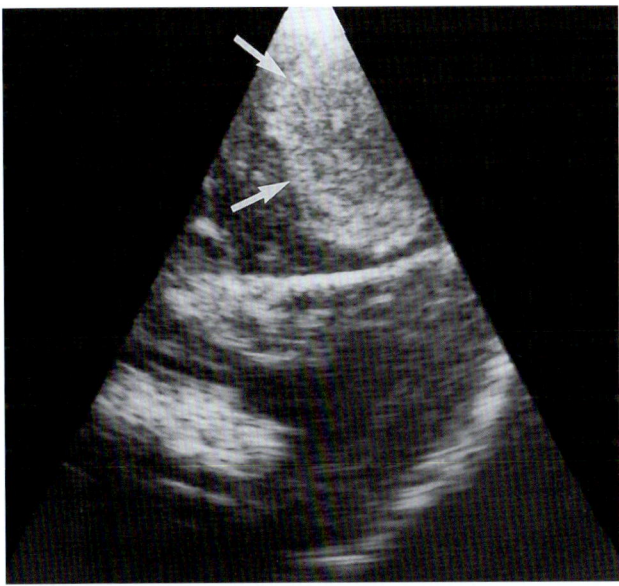

Figure 9–1 Hyperechoic glioma. Ultrasound scan shows a glioma (arrows) in the occipital lobe.

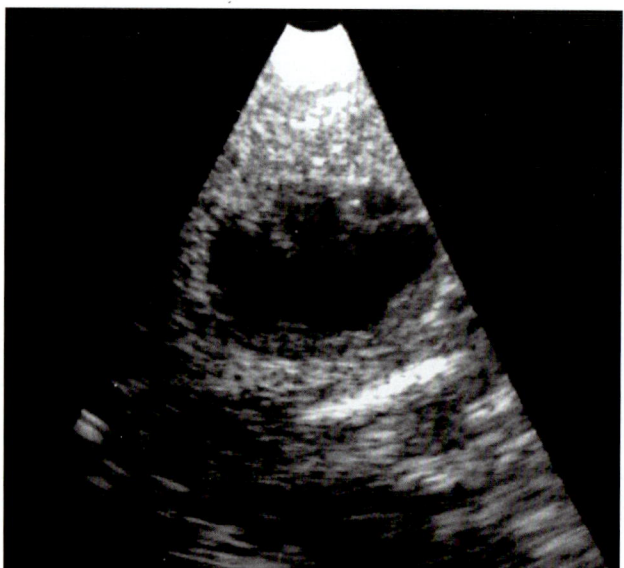

Figure 9–2 Predominantly cystic astrocytoma. Ultrasound scan clearly shows mural nodularity and septation.

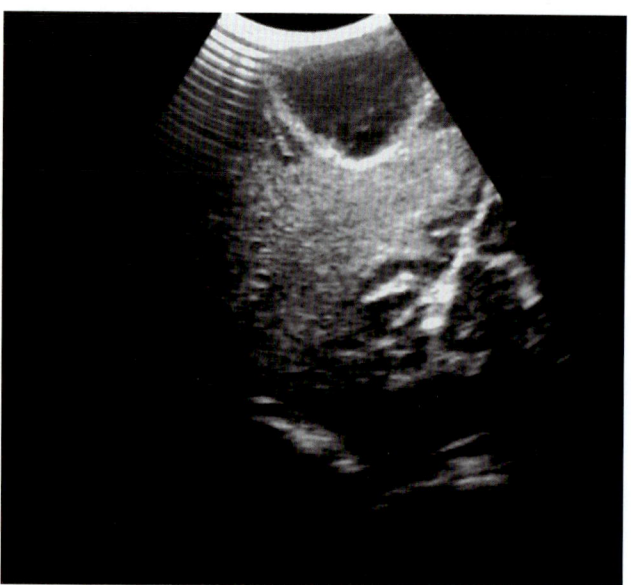

Figure 9–3 Poorly differentiated brain metastasis from primary lung carcinoma. Ultrasound scan shows an echogenic rim, but the central portion is hypoechoic due to liquefaction necrosis. Note the gyral and sulcal detail, which is obliterated by brain edema surrounding the tumor nodule.

stand out dramatically as hyperechoic lesions against a relatively hypoechoic background (**Fig. 9–1**). The reactive edema associated with brain tumors can decrease even further the echogenicity of brain substance and increase the conspicuity of focal masses.[3] Meningiomas are the most highly echogenic primary brain tumors, and usually have a relatively smooth contour and sharp margination. Calcifications within meningiomas occur frequently and result in a further increase in echogenicity. Glioblastomas are also markedly hyperechoic and are often well marginated, but may have less well-defined margins when they are aggressive and invasive.[4] Cystic degeneration may occur in glioblastomas as well as in cystic astrocytomas (**Fig. 9–2**), and the septations, cyst cavities, and areas of solid tumor and mural nodularity are well depicted by intraoperative ultrasound.[5,6] The complex nature of these cystic neoplasms is more completely portrayed with intraoperative ultrasound than with other imaging modalities, including computed tomography (CT) and even magnetic resonance imaging (MRI). Complete definition of the various spaces and cystic compartments may be important to guide surgical decompression of cystic tumors by aspiration. Most brain metastases are also hyperechoic and well circumscribed (**Fig. 9–3**), with an appearance similar to meningiomas and gliomas.[7] Liquefaction necrosis, which may occur spontaneously or as the result of therapy, may diminish the echogenicity of tumors centrally (**Fig. 9–3**). Low-grade astrocytomas can present a much more difficult imaging problem because they tend to be less echogenic and also to have very poorly defined infiltrative margins, insinuating into the adjacent brain substance in a very ill-defined manner.[8,9] In addition, chronic edema associated with low-grade astrocytomas may actually increase brain echogenicity adjacent to the tumor, thus making tumor margins even more poorly defined.[10]

In addition to defining the tumor site and assessing margins, intraoperative ultrasound is helpful to the neurosurgeon in selecting an approach to resection of the tumor that will hopefully minimize damage to surrounding functional brain tissue. Following resection, intraoperative ultrasound can be utilized to evaluate completeness of surgical resection by rescanning after filling the surgical cavity with sterile saline and seeking any residual tumor nodules.

Intraoperative ultrasound imaging is also very helpful in guiding biopsy procedures, again with the goal of minimizing trauma to adjacent brain tissues.[11] Specially designed probes can be used through a modified burr hole to allow precise needle placement with minimal patient trauma.[12] Biopsies can be performed with electronic real-time biopsy guides, or freehand under direct real-time visualization.[13] High-resolution endfire endoluminal probes have been quite useful to perform accurate real-time biopsies through small craniotomy sites utilizing electronic biopsy guidance (**Fig. 9–4**). Utilization of color flow imaging may help to choose a path for the biopsy needle that will minimize disruption of major blood vessels between the cortical surface and the tumor site.

Real-time guidance can also be successfully used for tumor ablative techniques, placement of ventricular shunt catheters, and drainage of intracranial fluid collections and

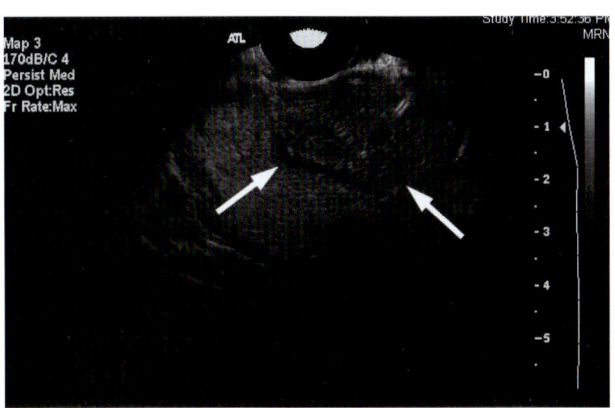 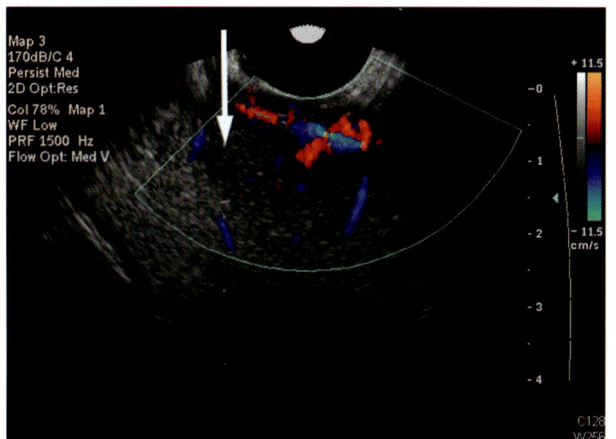

Figure 9–4 **(A)** Left temporal glioblastoma (arrows). **(B)** Color flow imaging helps target a safe, less vascular path for biopsy. The linear cursor (arrow) demarks the planned position of the biopsy needle.

abscesses (**Fig. 9–5**).[14] Following ultrasound-guided needle biopsies, we routinely rescan the patient for several minutes after the biopsy to assess for any bleeding within the lesion. Acute bleeding may appear as a small, highly echogenic focus within the mass or in the surrounding brain parenchyma. Occasionally, fluid/fluid levels may be seen, particularly when there is bleeding into a mass with cystic degeneration (**Fig. 9–6**). Scanning for several minutes is usually sufficient to ensure that any bleeding has stabilized.

Gray-scale, Doppler, and color flow imaging have been used in neurosurgical approaches to aneurysms and arteriovenous malformations (AVMs).[15] Assessment of blood flow is important during clipping or resection of aneurysms. Many AVMs are poorly visualized on gray-scale intraoperative ultrasound imaging, but the use of color flow imaging has been very helpful in defining their location and boundaries.

Many neurosurgical procedures now utilize frame-based or nonframe-based image guidance systems utilizing preoperative image information derived from MRI or CT scans, as a guide to surgical exploration and resection. However, brain tissue movement during surgery can be a significant source of error during image-guided surgical interventions. To compensate for this tissue motion, intraoperative ultrasound has been utilized to detect brain deformation during neurosurgery. Interactive image overlay systems allow projection of the region of interest on

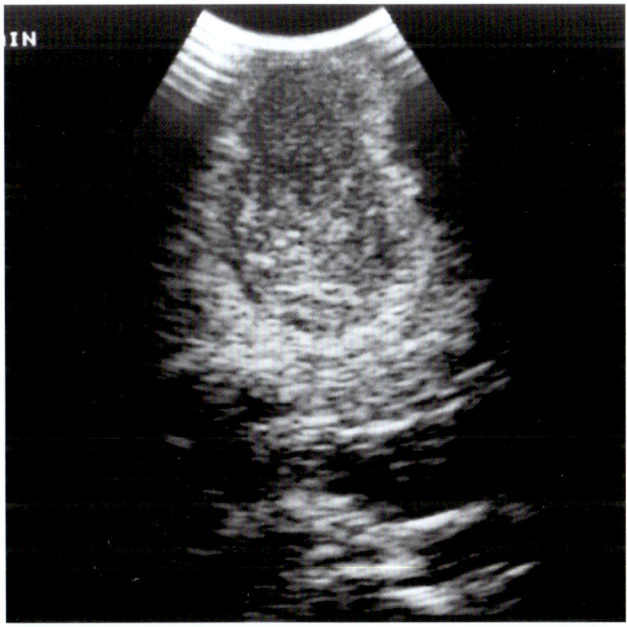

Figure 9–5 Frontal lobe abscess. Ultrasound scan shows an echogenic rim and centrally located, moderately echogenic purulent material. Ultrasound-guided aspiration and evacuation of the abscess was performed.

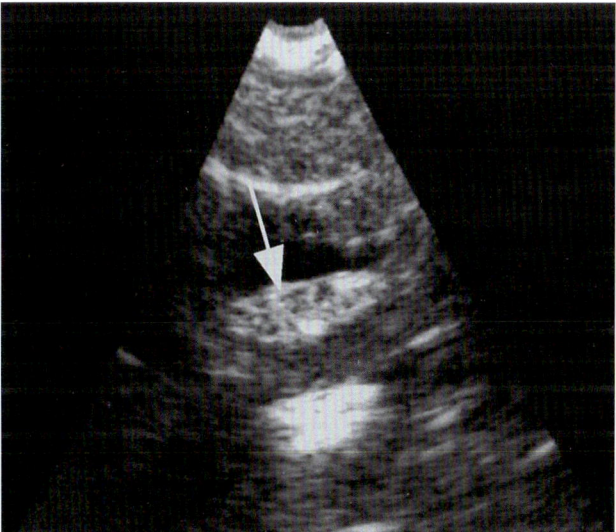

Figure 9–6 Astrocytoma. Ultrasound scan shows fluid-blood level (arrow) within the cystic cavity of an astrocytoma after needle biopsy.

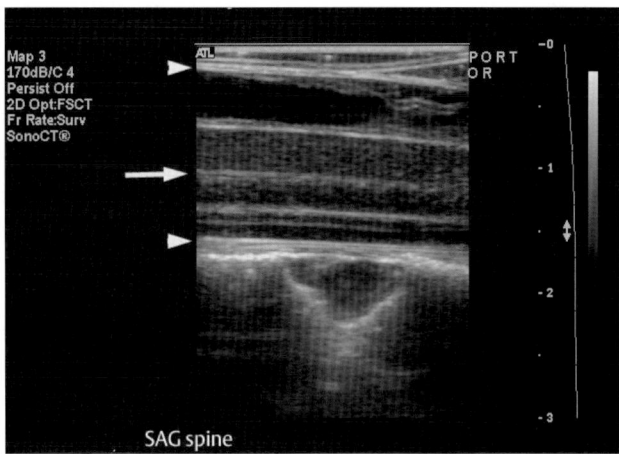
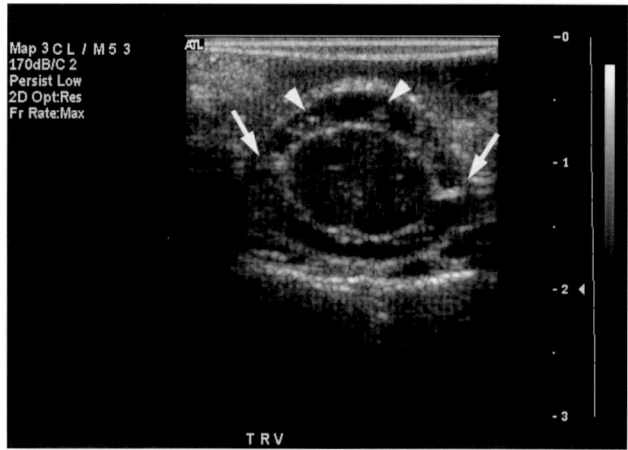

Figure 9–7 Thoracic cord. Sagittal ultrasound scans show the central spinal canal (arrow) as a paired linear echogenic structure. The dura (arrowheads) is well seen posteriorly and anteriorly.

Figure 9–8 Transverse ultrasound scan of the cervical cord demonstrates dentate ligaments (arrows) and several nerve roots cut in cross section (arrowheads) within the posterior dural sac.

intraoperative ultrasound to overlay an associated MR image, helping the surgeon correlate the ultrasound anatomy to the more familiar MR images. The small discrepancies between the ultrasound and preoperative MR images can thus be utilized to assess tissue motion during neurosurgery.[16] Indeed, even today, there are advocates for intraoperative ultrasound as a much simpler, less expensive, and equally efficacious technique for guiding intraoperative procedures in comparison with the elegant, but highly complex and exceedingly expensive intraoperative MRI systems.[17]

Spine

The uses of intraoperative ultrasound imaging in the evaluation of spinal cord abnormalities are similar to those for brain imaging. Endfire probes are essential and the optimal frequency would be in the 7 to 10 MHz range, although 5 MHz probes can be successfully utilized. Electronic curved array or linear array probes are preferable because they allow concomitant utilization of color flow imaging, but mechanical endfire probes can also be utilized. The surgical laminectomy site is filled with sterile degassed saline to provide an acoustic coupling medium. The probe is then placed onto the pool of degassed saline solution. Images are usually obtained through the dura without direct contact with the spinal cord.

Both axial and sagittal planes are utilized. The spinal cord itself has a relatively low to moderate echogenicity and is quite homogeneous in texture.[18] The central spinal canal or indentation of the cord at the site of the central canal can be visualized as an echogenic single or paired set of lines relatively central within the spinal cord, which is otherwise featureless (**Fig. 9–7**). The central spinal canal is an important normal landmark that is frequently disrupted by pathological conditions within the cord. The arachnoid membrane is difficult to visualize, but the dura is well seen both dorsally and ventrally, and a small amount of fluid is usually present between the dura and the arachnoid. The dentate ligaments are well visualized in axial views (**Fig. 9–8**). They arise from the dorsal and lateral margins of the sac and extend laterally to the adjacent spinal canal. Nerve roots are inconsistently imaged in the cervical and thoracic spine, but are well seen at the conus medullaris and distally in the region of the cauda equina. Nerve roots appear to be hypoechoic or anechoic, but are readily visualized within the spinal fluid by highly reflective dorsal and ventral margins, appearing as two parallel echogenic lines. Pulsations can be imaged in real time from the anterior spinal artery, which is deep to the cord. Color flow imaging and power Doppler imaging will show the vascularity in a more complete fashion.

Assessment of the location and extent of masses is one of the principal uses of spinal intraoperative ultrasound. Lesion location can be assessed as intramedullary or extramedullary, and intradural and extradural components can be evaluated.[19] This capability can be particularly useful in depicting tumors such as neurofibromas, which may have both intradural and extradural components. The spinal cord cannot be retracted extensively, and intraoperative ultrasound imaging can provide important information as to the full extent of such tumors.[20] Many intramedullary tumors of the cord, including ependymomas, dermoids, and many metastases, are hyperechoic. Astrocytomas, however, are frequently isoechoic with extremely ill-defined margins, and consequently are very poorly visualized. These lesions may be recognized by effacement of the landmark echoes from the central spinal canal, as well as by fusiform swelling of the cord. Other nonneoplastic inflammatory and posttraumatic conditions can also cause swelling of the cord and may not be readily distinguishable from astrocytomas.[21] Astrocytomas may show cystic degeneration, which can also be seen in ependymomas and hemangioblastomas

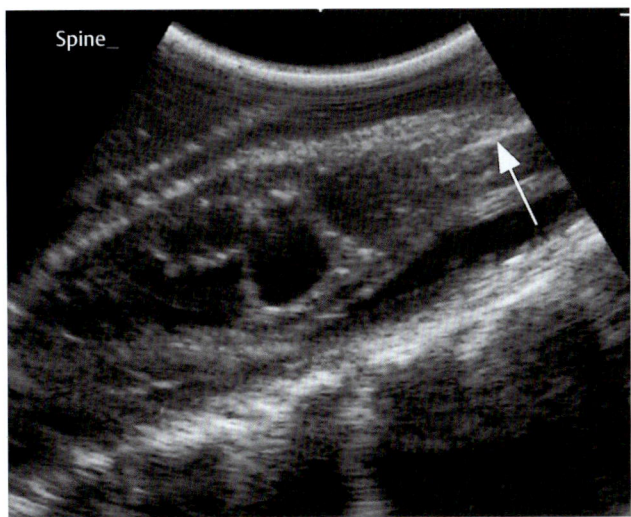

Figure 9–9 Hemangioblastoma of the cervical cord. Ultrasound scan shows multiple cystic components and interruption of the central spinal canal (arrow), which indicates the presence of an intramedullary mass.

(**Fig. 9–9**). These tumors can form fairly large cystic cavities and simulate syringomyelia. However, the presence of solid masses, mural nodules, or irregularly thickened septations will help to distinguish cystic tumors from a benign syrinx.[22,23]

Extramedullary tumors include meningiomas (**Fig. 9–10**), neurofibromas, lipomas, and dermoids, as well as malignant tumors, which are most often metastatic. Other conditions can also produce an extramedullary mass effect, including protruding discs, bony lesions (spurs and fracture fragments), hematomas, abscesses, and arachnoid cyst. Most of the neoplastic lesions appear as moderately echogenic masses with displacement or compression of the adjacent spinal cord and displacement of other structures, including nerve roots. Bony spurs and fragments are highly echogenic and may be associated with acoustic shadow. Herniated disc fragments are moderately echogenic, but substantially less so than bony spurs.[24] Hematomas appear hyperechoic acutely,[25] but may have a variable appearance, depending on their age and degree of liquefaction, whereas most abscesses and cysts have predominantly fluid components and increased transmission of sound through the fluid.

Intraoperative ultrasound is very useful in evaluating the extent of surgical resections,[26,27] as well as in guiding biopsies, particularly biopsies of tumors with extensive cystic or necrotic components. Intraoperative ultrasound and color flow imaging can be useful in identifying the more viable solid components of the tumor, thereby avoiding the necrotic components and diminishing the number of biopsies required to establish a diagnosis. Drainage of epidural abscesses and hematomas can also be aided by ultrasound guidance, as well as the drainage of cystic tumor cavities and the cavities of syringomyelia, both by real-time guidance of needle placement into the various component cavities and assessment of completeness of evacuation of cyst fluid. Finally, placement of intracystic shunt catheters within a syrinx can also be facilitated by intraoperative ultrasound guidance, and intraoperative ultrasound can demonstrate the adequacy of neural tissue decompression when spinal fractures are treated with Harrington rod fixation.[28]

Abdominal Applications

Gallbladder and Bile Ducts

Intraoperative imaging of the gallbladder and extrahepatic bile ducts is best performed using an endfire probe with a center frequency of 7 or 7.5 MHz. Either linear array or

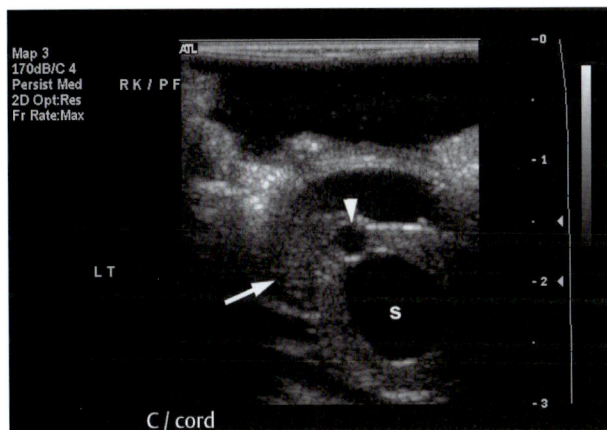
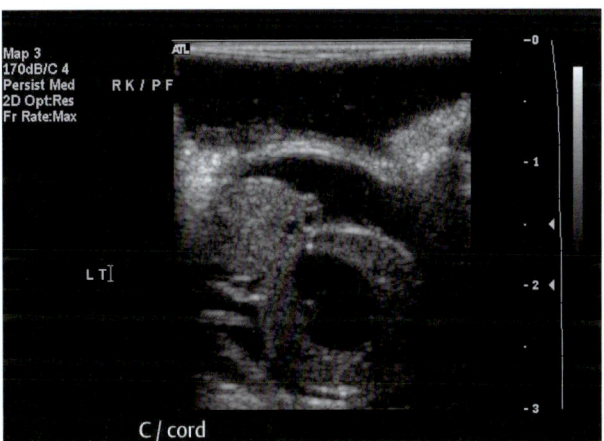

Figure 9–10 Cervical hemangioblastoma. **(A)** Transverse scan demonstrating the intramedullary portion of this tumor (arrow), including a small cystic component (arrowhead). A secondary syrinx (S) is noted centrally in the cord. **(B)** A scan at a slightly different level reveals the large extramedullary intradural component of this mass.

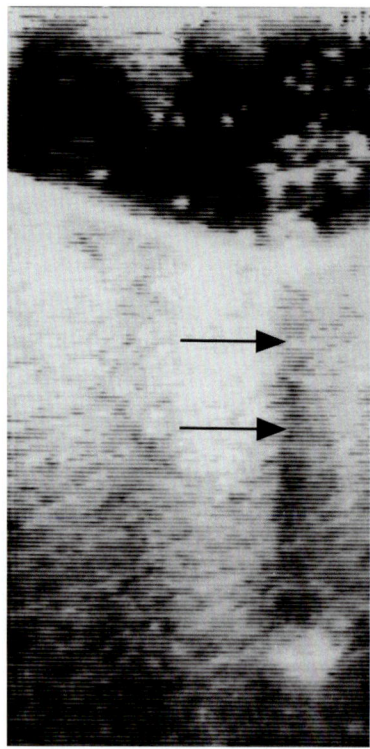

Figure 9–11 Gallbladder stones. Intraoperative ultrasound scan of the gallbladder shows numerous tiny, submillimeter stones not seen on preoperative studies. Arrows indicate acoustic shadowing from the conglomeration of these tiny stones.

sector formats are acceptable. Imaging at 5 MHz is probably also acceptable, but may require a standoff mechanism, such as filling the abdominal cavity with sterile saline or using a water-filled glove, to avoid near-field artifacts which may detract from imaging these structures. Scanning is performed directly in contact with the common bile duct or gallbladder, and scanning can be performed in any anatomical plane desired. If a complete study requires imaging of the intrahepatic bile ducts, then the endfire probe may be satisfactory for the central ducts, but a complete evaluation of the peripheral ducts may require a sidefire liver-type probe. Intraoperative ultrasound of the gallbladder is not frequently required because preoperative ultrasound studies are usually more than adequate. Routine screening for gallstones is performed on patients with morbid obesity who are undergoing gastric bypass or stapling procedures because these patients frequently develop acute cholecystitis after substantial weight loss. Therefore, if stones are present, then the gallbladder is usually removed at the time of gastric surgery. These patients may be difficult, if not impossible, to image adequately because of their body habitus and, therefore, if the preoperative study is unsatisfactory, intraoperative ultrasound imaging of the gallbladder can be rapidly performed and may be capable of demonstrating stones that were not visualized preoperatively (**Fig. 9–11**).[29]

Intraoperative ultrasound may be useful in assessing gallbladder masses discovered incidentally at surgery or to assess the extent of a known gallbladder carcinoma (**Fig. 9–12**), particularly regarding potential invasion into the adjacent liver bed, which would require a more aggressive surgical resection.[30] Intraoperative ultrasound is nearly as accurate as frozen section to determine the depth of invasion.[31] If the tumor is resectable but also invading the liver, most surgeons would advocate a wedge resection of liver parenchyma to obtain a tumor-free margin at the time of intraoperative ultrasound. A careful search for more distant hepatic metastases or lymph node metastases should be performed to avoid unnecessary radical surgery in patients with advanced metastatic disease.

Intraoperative ultrasound of the bile ducts has been regarded by several surgical groups as a competitive or possibly superior modality to radiographic intraoperative cholangiography.[32,33] There is also a substantial amount of interest in the use of laparoscopic ultrasound

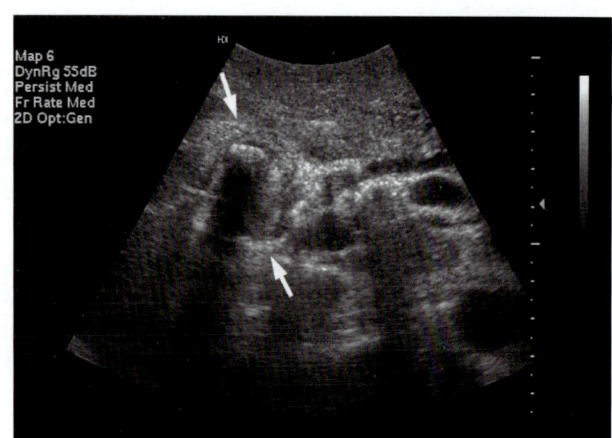

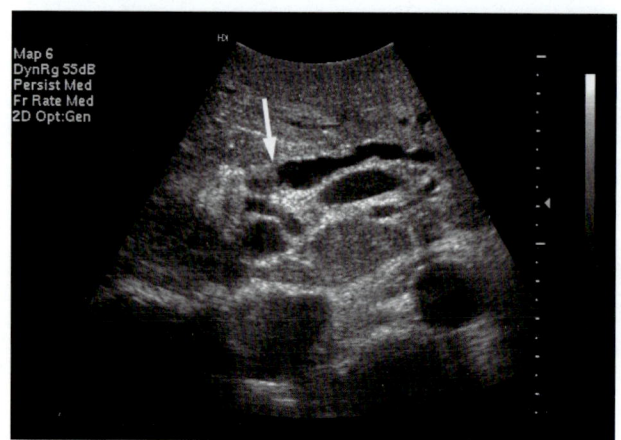

Figure 9–12 Gallbladder carcinoma. **(A)** Large solid mass in the gallbladder fossa (arrows), engulfing a gallstone that exhibits posterior acoustic shadowing. **(B)** Small isoechoic metastasis (arrow) causing obstruction and dilatation of the left hepatic bile duct.

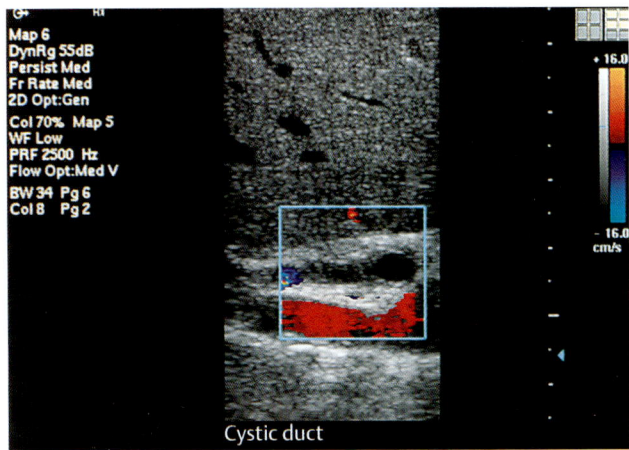

Figure 9–13 Transverse view of the common duct. Color flow Doppler image allows distinction of the biliary ducts from the adjacent portal vein (red) and hepatic artery (blue). This image shows the entry of the cystic duct into the common duct.

imaging for bile duct assessment in patients with potential choledocholithiasis undergoing laparoscopic cholecystectomy. The common bile duct, common hepatic duct, and intrahepatic bile ducts can be well visualized with both open and laparoscopic intraoperative ultrasound (**Fig. 9–13**).[34,35] Therefore, intraoperative ultrasound or LUS can be quite effective in demonstrating bile duct stones, and because laparoscopic cholangiography is somewhat arduous and difficult to perform, LUS may provide a superior alternative,[36] although no directly comparative studies have been performed. Routine use of LUS for every laparoscopic cholecystectomy is unwarranted due to the low yield of unsuspected pathology.[37] In our own institution, however, when choledocholithiasis is suspected clinically, endoscopic retrograde cholangiopancreatography is performed preoperatively both for diagnosis and, when positive, for therapeutic intervention via endoscopic sphincterotomy and stone extraction. If this approach is undertaken, the need for any form of intraoperative bile duct evaluation is substantially diminished.

Benign strictures and malignant obstructions in the biliary tract can be well evaluated by intraoperative ultrasound or LUS imaging to define the precise site and extent of the obstruction and help plan the type of biliary bypass procedure to be performed.[38] The sclerosing form of cholangiocarcinoma can be difficult to fully assess even with intraoperative ultrasound imaging because the tumor is an infiltrative and intensely sclerosing type lesion with poorly identified margins. Other forms of cholangiocarcinoma, particularly the papillary types, can be well defined by intraoperative ultrasound imaging (**Fig. 9–14**). In patients with central Klatskin type cholangiocarcinomas, we have occasionally been asked to scan the liver to identify large dilated intrahepatic ducts that might prove suitable for a peripheral hepaticojejunostomy, when a central decompression is mechanically impossible. This has been successfully accomplished in particular in the left lobe along the ligamentum teres, where large ducts draining segments 2 and 3 can, at times, be identified. More frequently now, however, patients with this large central type tumor are drained externally by percutaneous or endoscopic techniques.

Liver

Intraoperative ultrasound of the liver is most frequently performed on patients who are undergoing possible surgical resection of liver cancer, either primary or metastatic.

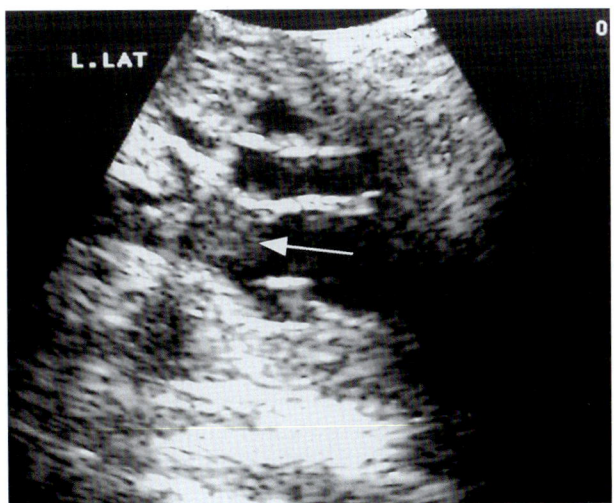
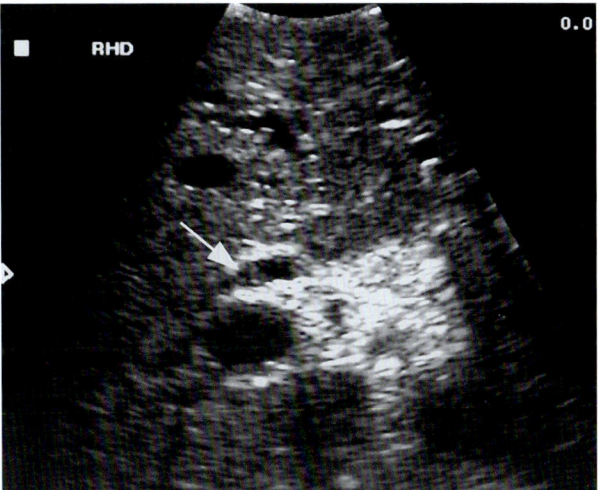

Figure 9–14 Klatzkin-type cholangiocarcinoma. **(A)** Ultrasound scan shows dilatation of the left hepatic duct, with tumor invasion (arrow). **(B)** Ultrasound scan shows dilatation of the peripheral ducts in the left medial segment, but the right hepatic duct (arrow) has a normal caliber and is free of tumor. This finding allowed a left hepatectomy and right hepaticojejunostomy to be performed.

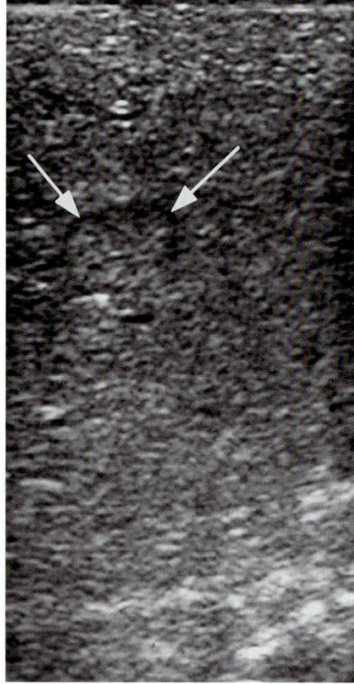
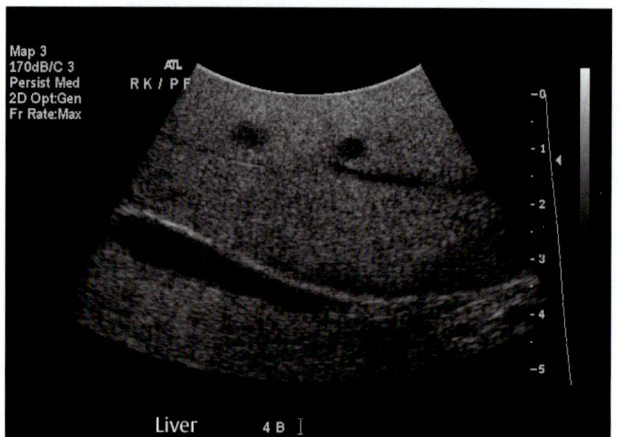

Figure 9–15 Occult liver metastases seen only with intraoperative ultrasound imaging. **(A)** A 1.2 cm isoechoic colon metastasis visible only because of the hypoechoic rim (arrows). **(B)** Two out of seven additional occult breast metastases identified at intraoperative ultrasound, each measuring 4 mm in diameter.

This examination is best performed using a side-fire probe with center frequency of 5 MHz, which allows full penetration of the liver from front to back, even in the right lobe where 12 cm of tissue can be adequately imaged. Although higher center frequencies of 7 or 7.5 MHz are excellent for biliary pancreatic imaging, only ~6 cm of liver can be effectively imaged at this higher frequency, and therefore a complete examination of the liver would be significantly lengthened in time and made more difficult because scans along the undersurface of the liver are less satisfactory due to the irregular contours and possible adhesions. A sidefire linear array or convex array configuration is also important to fit the probe between the liver and the diaphragm or the liver and the lateral rib cage, where there is very little space. By cradling the sidefire probe in the fingers, all portions of the liver can be adequately reached and scanned even without full mobilization of the liver. Scanning is optimal in the transverse plane beginning at the dome of the left edge of the liver and proceeding from cephalad to caudad. The next field should slightly overlap the original field while moving from left to right across the liver. With this overlapping field of view, the entire liver can be adequately assessed in 5 to 10 minutes.[39] The principal advantages of intraoperative ultrasound imaging of the liver are as follows:

1. The most complete detection of primary and metastatic tumors in the liver
2. Real-time definition of lobar and segmental liver anatomy as well as normal and aberrant vascular supply and drainage
3. Assessment of the feasibility of resection, planning of the most appropriate type of resection, and identification of deep tumor margins in patients undergoing nonsegmental wedge-type resections
4. Real-time guidance for tumor biopsy procedures and aspiration of fluid collections
5. Real-time guidance for ablative techniques such as cryosurgery, radiofrequency ablation, or alcohol ablation

The spatial resolution of intraoperative ultrasound imaging in the liver is unsurpassed, allowing for imaging of cysts as small as 1 to 3 mm and solid lesions as small as 3 to 5 mm (**Fig. 9–15**). Until the advent of multidetector CT and faster MRI allowing multiple-phase contrast imaging, intraoperative ultrasound would routinely detect 25 to 30% more lesions.[40] The vast majority of lesions detected by intraoperative ultrasound, but not by preoperative imaging studies or palpation are 1 cm or less in diameter, which in part, reflects the spatial resolution limits of preoperative studies.[41] CT arterial portography can definitely increase the sensitivity for detection of liver lesions to the range of 85 to 90%,[42] but this results in somewhat less specificity, particularly in attempts to detect lesions well under 1 cm in size. False-positive results for CT arterial portography

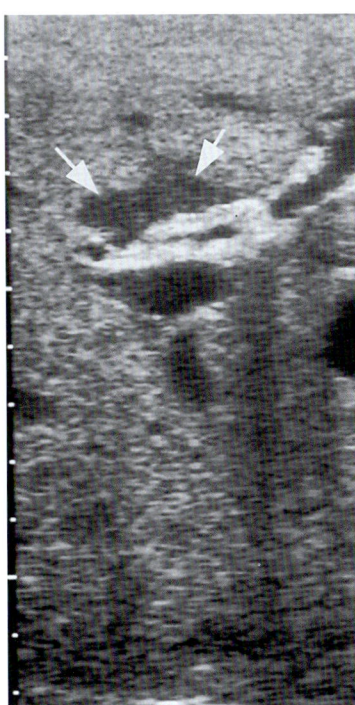

Figure 9–16 Diffuse fatty infiltration of the liver. Ultrasound scan shows diffuse fatty infiltration with sparing (arrows) at the porta hepatis. This sparing caused false-positive results on computed tomographic arterial portography.

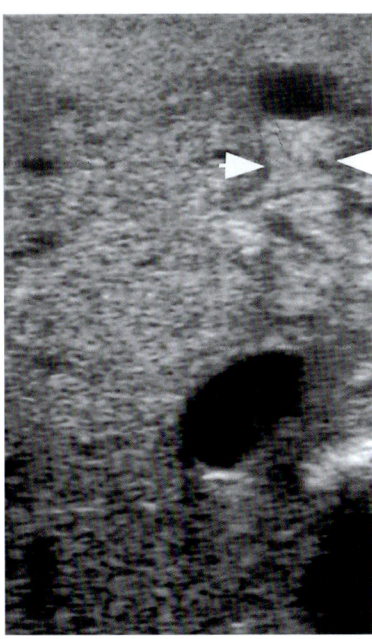

Figure 9–17 Hepatic cyst. Ultrasound scan shows an enhanced 5 mm cyst (arrowheads), which caused a false-positive computed tomographic reading.

are encountered with some frequency due to perfusion abnormalities (**Fig. 9–16**) and small hepatic cysts (**Fig. 9–17**).[43,44] Recent advances in MRI, multidetector CT, and positron emission tomographic (PET) scanning have reduced the additional intraoperative ultrasound lesion detection rate to 5 to 10%.[45-47]

In our institution and others, patients who may be candidates for resection of liver tumors initially undergo laparoscopy to attempt to identify patients with diffusely metastatic disease outside the liver, which would render the patient inoperable. Laparoscopic ultrasound of the liver can be combined with this approach to identify the maximum number of detectable liver lesions because additional tumors detected by LUS, but not on preoperative imaging, may also render a patient inoperable due to multiplicity of lesions or involvement of multiple lobes of the liver. LUS has the same capacity for detecting small liver lesions as open intraoperative ultrasound and is even more important in this situation because the surgeon is unable to palpate the liver, and only a minority of small liver tumors can be directly visualized with the laparoscope.[48,49] LUS is technically more challenging and much more time consuming than open intraoperative ultrasound imaging of the liver and may have slightly less sensitivity for lesion detection, as has been suggested in preliminary studies.

However, with further evolution of the technique and improvement in the equipment for laparoscopic ultrasound imaging, the small differences in sensitivity may diminish. State-of-the-art intraoperative ultrasound equipment allows the use of color flow or power Doppler imaging to assess the vascularity of liver tumors (**Fig. 9–18**). In addition, careful assessment of the vascular supply of the liver can have a major impact on surgical approach (**Fig. 9–19**). The presence of an accessory inferior right hepatic vein, which drains into the inferior vena cava distal to the hepatic confluence, may allow performance of a more extensive left trisegmentectomy. Similarly, an accessory or replaced left hepatic artery arising from the left gastric artery (**Fig. 9–20**), or a right hepatic artery arising from the superior mesenteric artery may influence the type of resection

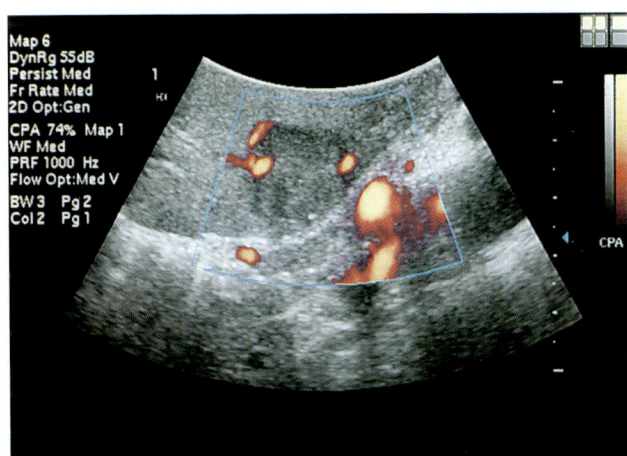

Figure 9–18 Colorectal metastasis. Power Doppler image demonstrates a hypovascular tumor with vessels being displaced around the periphery of the tumor nodule.

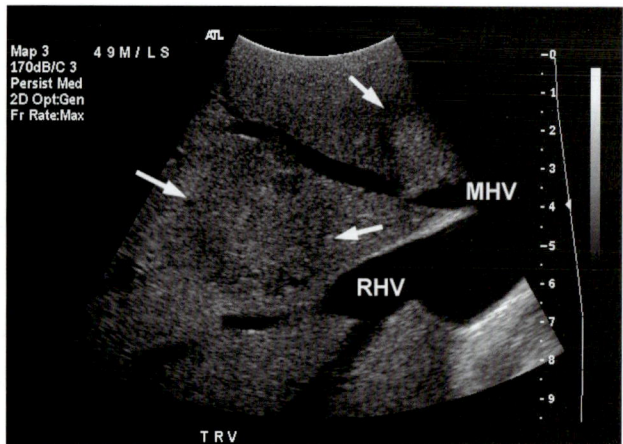

Figure 9–19 Two large isoechoic colorectal metastases (arrows) with deformity of the middle hepatic vein (MHV) and immediate contiguity to the right hepatic vein (RHV). The involvement or immediate proximity to the hepatic veins made resection technically impossible.

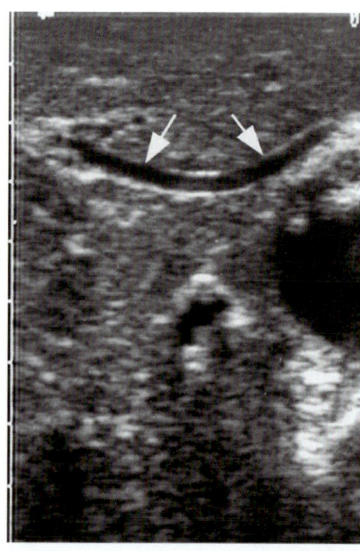

Figure 9–20 Replaced left hepatic artery. Ultrasound scan shows the point at which the left hepatic artery (arrows) enters the liver, along the ligamentum venosum.

performed.[50] The demonstration of major vessels surrounding masses or cystic lesions may influence the direct surgical approach to excision, drainage, or unroofing of a cyst (**Fig. 9–21**).

Lymphadenopathy can be readily assessed both in the porta hepatis as well as in the peripancreatic and celiac nodal groups. Demonstration of enlarged nodes in these areas may be important (**Fig. 9–22**) in determining resectability of a liver lesion because metastatic lymphadenopathy would generally render the patient inoperable for cure. Confirmation of lymph node metastases can be obtained directly by ultrasound-guided lymph node biopsies. Intraoperative ultrasound is not effective in demonstrating serosal implants or seeding of the mesentery by tumor, but this type of metastatic disease is often well detected by palpation or direct visual inspection or inspection via the laparoscope.

In patients with primary hepatocellular carcinoma, venous invasion is a frequent occurrence and is well detected both in the portal venous system as well as in the hepatic venous system.[51] Hepatic venous invasion can be life threatening at the time of surgery if the clot extends into the inferior vena cava or into the right atrium. Careful assessment of the full extent of venous invasion is therefore essential. Occasionally, during assessment of a patient with liver tumor of unknown origin, the site of the primary tumor may be visualized. In particular, the pancreas

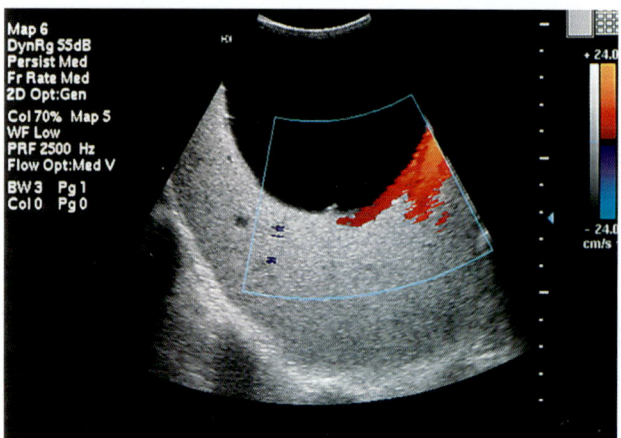

Figure 9–21 Hepatic cyst. Color flow imaging demonstrates displacement of the hepatic vasculature deep to the large hepatic cyst, distant from the area of planned surgical unroofing.

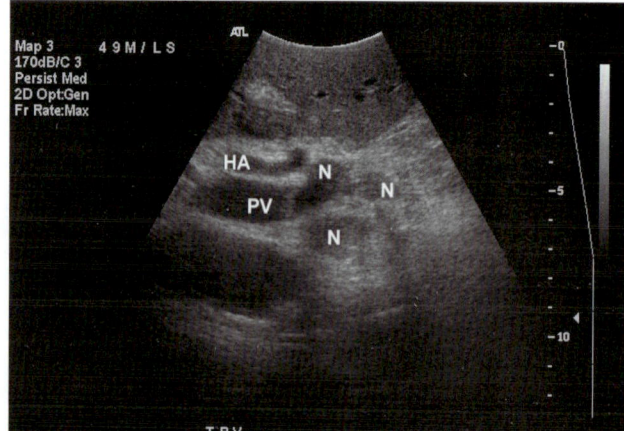

Figure 9–22 Metastatic lymphadenopathy. Multiple enlarged lymph nodes (N) were identified at intraoperative ultrasound and confirmed by biopsy to represent metastatic colorectal cancer. Planned hepatic metastasectomy was thereby canceled. HA, hepatic artery; PV, portal vein.

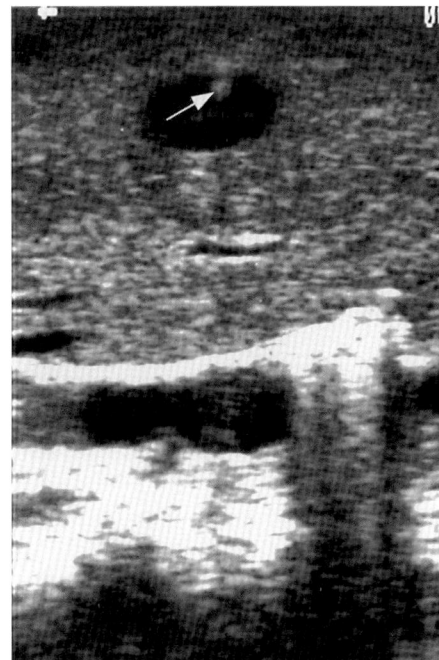 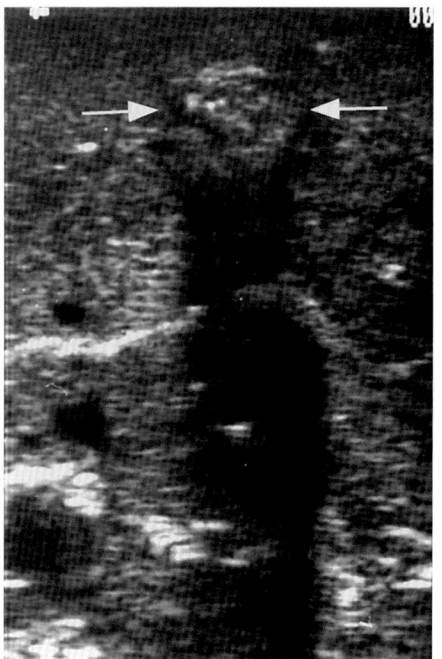

Figure 9–23 Hepatocellular carcinoma. **(A)** Ultrasound scan shows needle tip (arrow) penetrating a small tumor nodule. **(B)** On ultrasound scan, the nodule (arrows) is echogenic, with acoustic shadowing, after ethanol injection for tumor ablation.

should be closely assessed as a possible source of an unknown primary adenocarcinoma.

Most interventional intraoperative ultrasound-guided procedures, including biopsies, aspirations, and drainages, can be successfully performed with freehand real-time ultrasound guidance. Tumor ablation techniques, such as cryosurgery, radiofrequency, and ethanol injection (**Fig. 9–23**) are successfully performed and monitored under real-time intraoperative ultrasound guidance. At present however, guidance for procedures under laparoscopic ultrasound control is much more difficult. There are no commercially available systems equipped with electronic biopsy guidance systems similar to those used extensively and successfully in the diagnostic ultrasound laboratory. Consequently, LUS-guided interventional procedures are much more difficult, whether they involve biopsies, drainages, or tumor ablations. Freehand biopsies can be performed with LUS guidance (**Fig. 9–24**) by using specially designed long needles that puncture through the abdominal wall and enter the liver adjacent to the LUS probe, with the angle and depth of penetration controlled with real-time guidance. The degree of difficulty in performing these procedures is substantially greater than with open intraoperative ultrasound imaging, however, particularly for small, deep-seated lesions. It is hoped that eventually electronic biopsy guidance systems or interactive, stereotactic fusion imaging with preoperative CT or MRI will be developed by the manufacturers for use with LUS probes.

Pancreas

Intraoperative ultrasound imaging of the pancreas requires an endfire probe, either linear or sector format, with a center frequency ranging from 5 to 7.5 MHz. The sidefire configuration, which serves well for liver imaging, is unsuited for imaging the pancreas because this configuration will not allow satisfactory contact with the pancreas, particularly in large, deep abdominal cavities. The sector

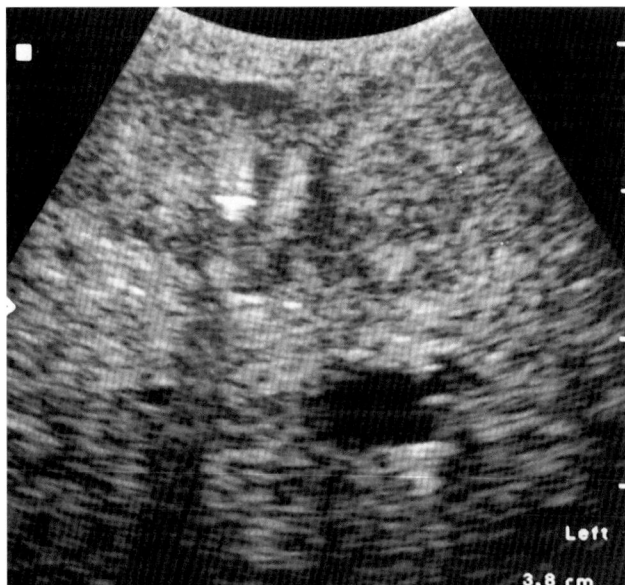

Figure 9–24 Hepatocellular carcinoma. During freehand laparoscopic ultrasound-guided biopsy, ultrasound scan shows the needle tip as an echogenic line within the tumor nodule.

format is favored because it shows a wider area of anatomy in each image section. When intraoperative ultrasound is used to evaluate neoplastic lesions in the pancreas, the liver should also be scanned for evidence of metastatic disease, which is commonly seen in ductal adenocarcinoma as well as in islet cell tumors of the pancreas.

Virtually all islet cell tumors of the pancreas produce hormones that can be detected by pathological studies using special stains or electron microscopy, but only a subset of these tumors produce clinical symptomatology. Patients with symptomatic islet cell tumors often have extremely small-sized tumors that are difficult to image by preoperative techniques. Many competitive and complementary strategies have evolved, including the use of multidetector CT, MRI with gadolinium, octreotide nuclear scans, superselective angiographic techniques, and portal venous sampling as well as endoscopic ultrasound imaging. Although each technique has its advocates, none is wholly satisfactory, with sensitivities ranging from 70 to 85%. Intraoperative ultrasound imaging is the single most effective technique for detection of functioning islet cell tumors[52,53] and, at times, can detect even nonpalpable lesions as small as 3 to 5 mm. Most islet cell tumors are homogeneous and therefore hypoechoic; they are thus well detected against the background of hyperechoic pancreatic parenchyma. Most islet cell tumors have smooth well-marginated borders, whether benign or malignant, because these tumors are seldom locally aggressive, even when malignant.

The pancreas can be scanned from the head and uncinate process to the tail in a matter of minutes, either before or after mobilization techniques have been performed. It may be useful to fill the abdominal cavity with degassed saline solution to serve as an acoustic window, although excellent images can often be obtained with direct contact imaging or even by scanning through compressed bowel and mesentery. Occasionally, the lateral segment of the liver may provide an acoustic window to the pancreatic body and tail. As with the liver and biliary tract, a systematic imaging study with overlapping fields is essential to evaluate the entire pancreas.

Insulinomas are usually solitary (**Fig. 9–25**) and benign,[54] but all islet cell tumors have malignant potential. Gastrinomas are also frequently extrapancreatic in location,[55] lying in the so-called gastrinoma triangle between the common duct, head of the pancreas, and second and third portions of the duodenum. In patients with the multiple endocrine neoplasia syndrome (MEN-1), the insulinomas may also be multiple.[56] In fact, these tumors often arise in the wall of the duodenum or in extrapancreatic tissues and adjacent lymph nodes (**Fig. 9–26**). Malignant islet cell tumors frequently involve local lymph nodes in the pancreatic, portal, and celiac beds. Liver metastases are also frequent and may be widespread and very small, exhibiting either a decreased or increased echogenicity. Glucagonomas and somatostatinomas are often somewhat larger than the other functional islet cell tumors and are

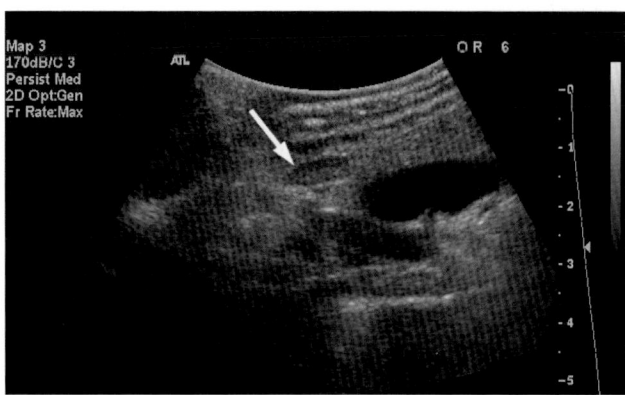

Figure 9–25 Insulinoma. This nonpalpable 3 × 7 mm insulinoma (arrow) in the head of the pancreas is well demonstrated at intraoperative ultrasound.

frequently located more distally in the pancreas, are usually solitary, and are also most often malignant. The so-called nonfunctional islet cell tumors (those that do not produce clinical symptomatology) often present as very large pancreatic masses, which usually exhibit locally benign behavior even when malignant and metastatic. Therefore, these tumors are usually well marginated, with passive displacement of surrounding vessels and infrequent vascular or neural invasion (**Fig. 9–27**).

Laparoscopic ultrasound of the pancreas has also been described as a sensitive and successful method in localizing insulinomas.[57] This method may be particularly important for small lesions localized to the body or tail of the pancreas because laparoscopic partial pancreatic resections

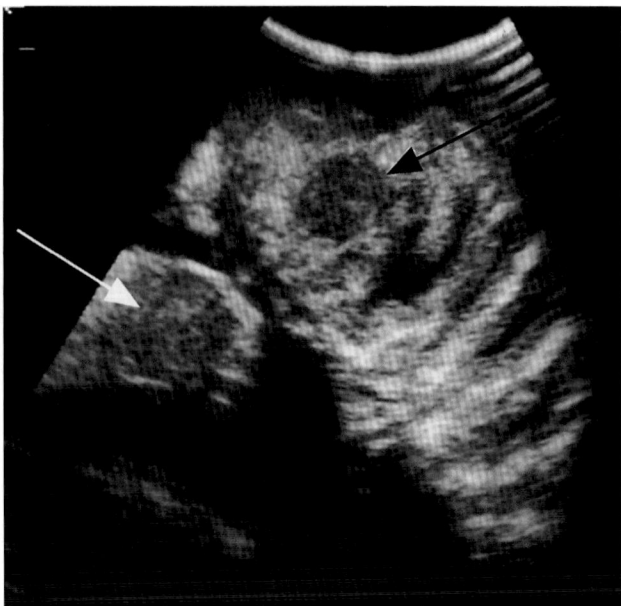

Figure 9–26 Gastrinoma. Ultrasound scan shows 0.7 cm gastrinoma arising in the wall of the duodenum (black arrow), with adjacent 1.2 cm metastasis (white arrow) in the lymph node.

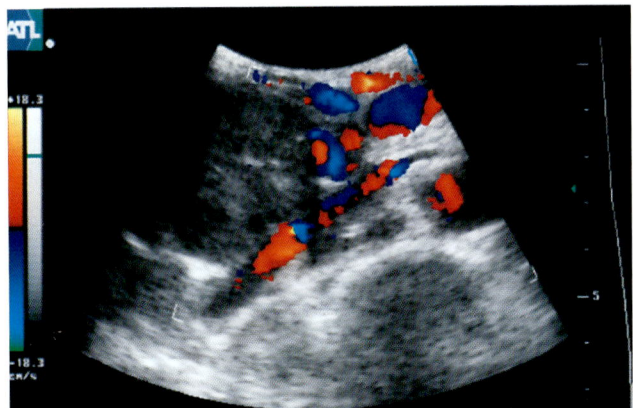

Figure 9–27 Nonfunctioning pancreatic islet cell tumor. Color flow Doppler imaging demonstrates passive displacement of the pancreatic vasculature around the large 5 cm hypoechoic mass, without evidence of vascular invasion. These tumors tend to be locally nonaggressive, even when malignant.

can be performed, thus avoiding a more prolonged hospitalization and recovery time from an open surgical resection. The LUS approach to the pancreas is best performed by utilizing a right upper or left upper quadrant port, allowing the probe to be oriented along the long axis of the pancreas in a relatively transverse plane. This allows for better orientation than attempting to image in the sagittal oblique plane across the short axis of the pancreas. At times, however, the head/neck and uncinate processes of the pancreas are better imaged in a more sagittal approach from a periumbilical port, which may also be more useful in allowing concurrent imaging of the liver for potential metastatic disease.

Intraoperative ultrasound imaging is seldom required for detection of ductal adenocarcinoma of the pancreas because this lesion is usually readily palpable, although identification of tumor by palpation can be difficult when there is extensive surrounding pancreatitis and, in this setting, intraoperative ultrasound imaging may be of help. Intraoperative and especially laparoscopic ultrasound imaging can be useful to assess for signs of unresectability in small pancreatic adenocarcinomas.[58] Preoperative imaging studies, especially high-quality multidetector CT arteriography, can be very accurate in predicting unresectability, but these techniques are still evolving and are not yet widely available. In many settings, laparoscopy is performed before open laparotomy and resection[59] to visually assess for metastatic disease in the mesentery and peritoneal surfaces, as well as on the surface of the liver. LUS can be utilized in conjunction with this approach to assess local resectability of pancreatic tumors (**Fig. 9–28**) by assessing the integrity of the pancreatic vasculature, particularly the superior mesenteric vein (SMV), splenic vein, as well as the superior mesenteric artery (SMA) and celiac artery. Direct vascular invasion of the SMV/portal vein confluence or the celiac artery or SMA would render the patient inopera-

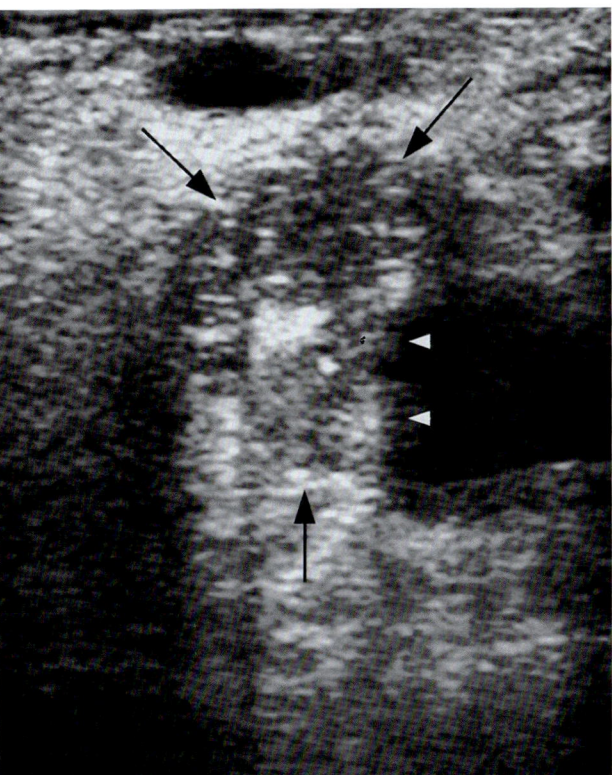

Figure 9–28 Pancreatic ductal adenocarcinoma. Ultrasound scan shows a mass (black arrows), which has invaded the lateral wall of the superior mesenteric vein (arrowheads). This invasion makes the tumor unresectable.

ble. As with other types of tumors, assessment of metastatic disease to local lymph nodes and to the liver can also be performed. A combination of the visual laparoscopic and LUS techniques can help to minimize the number of patients subjected to open laparotomy, only to prove ultimately unresectable.[60,61]

Intraoperative ultrasound can also be used in assessing cystic neoplasms of the pancreas.[62] Serous microcystic adenomas of the pancreas, which are almost always benign, can be well assessed by intraoperative ultrasound imaging (**Fig. 9–29**). The cyst cavities should be thin walled, as well as the septations, and most of the cysts are under 1 to 2 cm in size, many as small as a few millimeters in diameter. Conversely, the presence of thick, irregular septa, mural nodules, or solid components is most consistent with a mucinous cystadenoma or cystadenocarcinoma (**Fig. 9–30**), both of which require surgical resection because malignancy cannot be excluded by imaging criteria, and even the benign cystadenoma is considered premalignant. Intraductal papillary mucinous neoplasms (IPNM) of the pancreas often present difficulties in surgical judgment as to the exact extent of the neoplasm and, therefore, the extent of required pancreatic resection. Intraoperative ultrasound provides an excellent means of assessing patients with IPNM, particularly in defining small hyperechoic masses within the main pancreatic duct or branch ducts,

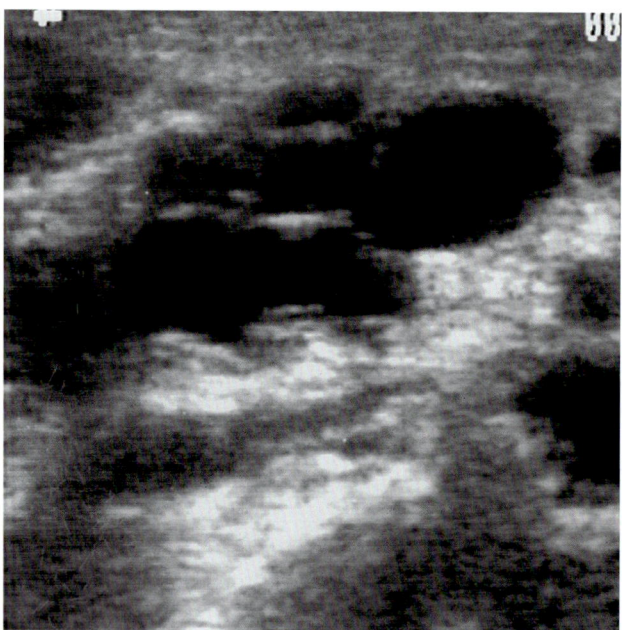

Figure 9–29 Microcystic pancreatic adenoma. Ultrasound scan shows multiple thin-walled cysts, all well under 2 cm in size, with no septal thickening or nodularity.

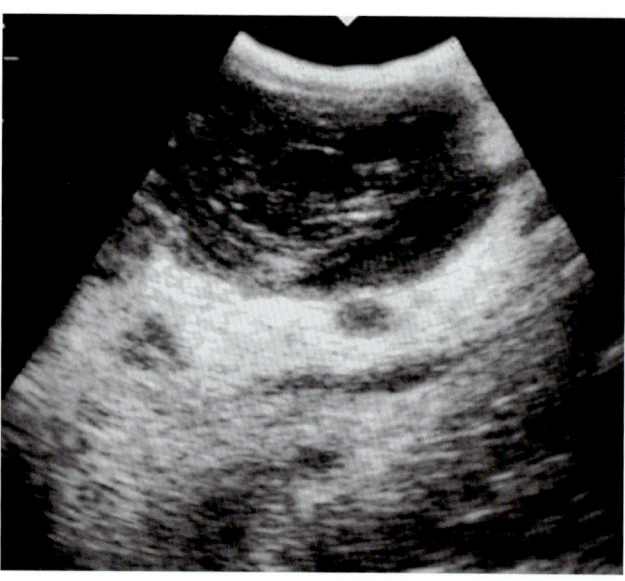

Figure 9–30 Mucinous cystadenocarcinoma of the pancreas. Ultrasound scan shows a large 3 cm cystic mass with thickened irregular septations and an adjacent small solid nodule.

as well as more accurately defining the extent of multifocal lesions, proving more sensitive than endoscopic retrograde cholangiopancreatography (ERCP) and endoscopic ultrasonography and thereby proving valuable for planning surgical strategy.[63]

Intraoperative ultrasound imaging can be useful in patients with pancreatitis who are undergoing surgery for biliary bypass or pancreatic drainage procedures (**Fig. 9–31**). The extent of pseudocysts and pancreatic ductal abnormalities can be well demonstrated as well as the potential communications between the pancreatic duct and the pseudocyst cavities.[64,65] If the pancreatic duct is obstructed, drainage of the pseudocysts may prove inadequate and drainage of the pancreatic duct itself may be required for adequate therapy. The pancreatic duct may be difficult to localize by palpation in an enlarged, fibrotic, and rock-hard pancreas, whereas identification of the dilated pancreatic duct is simple and highly accurate with

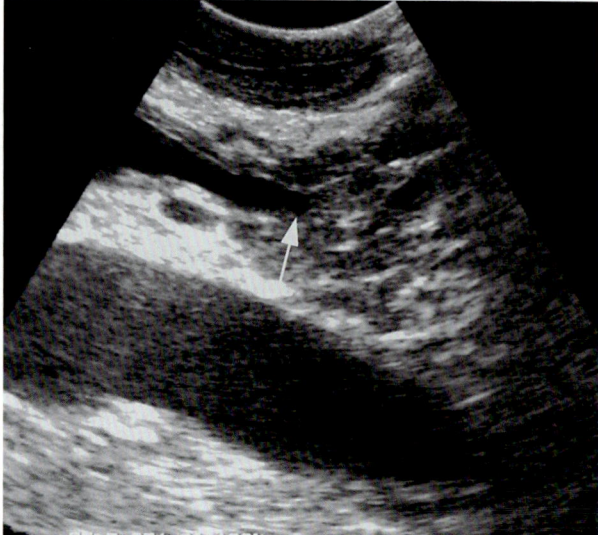

A

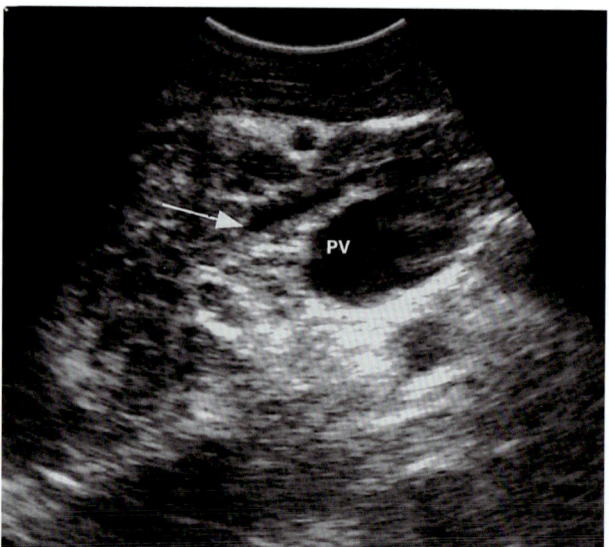

B

Figure 9–31 Calcific pancreatitis. **(A)** Sagittal ultrasound scan demonstrates a stricture of the common bile duct (arrow) at the entrance of an enlarged head of the pancreas. **(B)** Transverse ultrasound scan shows an obstruction of the pancreatic duct (arrow). Pancreatitis rather than neoplasm was suggested by the lack of a hypoechoic mass and by diffuse enlargement with calcification. This diagnosis was confirmed by multiple biopsies. A biliary bypass was performed, and pancreatic resection was avoided. PV, portal vein.

intraoperative ultrasound, thereby identifying the optimal site for incision and drainage via a Puestow procedure. The use of color flow imaging and power Doppler can be important in evaluating focal peripancreatic fluid collections to assess for possible pseudoaneurysms. Intraoperative ultrasound guidance can also be employed for biopsy of pancreatic masses, drainage of fluid collections, and diagnostic punctures of the pancreatic duct.

Conclusion

Intraoperative ultrasound is an important and rapidly expanding field. The demand from surgeons for access to this highly effective modality is growing continuously. The rapidly developing capacity of laparoscopic surgery is adding further to increased demand for ultrasound imaging via laparoscopic approaches.

The techniques and applications presented in this chapter will hopefully increase the interest of radiologists in performing and interpreting intraoperative ultrasound and LUS studies, as well as to assist them in a more efficient use of their time when performing these studies. Intraoperative ultrasound studies have a profound impact on patient care and strongly influence surgical decision making. The necessity for high-quality intraoperative ultrasound scans is unquestionable and, in this author's opinion, the best-quality scans will be obtained when the radiologist scrubs in and both performs and interprets the study using the scanning skills and observational ability that can only be acquired by years of experience with ultrasound imaging studies.

References

1. Kane RA, Hughes LA, Cua EJ, et al. The impact of intraoperative ultrasonography on surgery for liver neoplasms. J Ultrasound Med 1994;13:1–6
2. Knake JE, Chandler WF, McGillicuddy JE, et al. Intraoperative sonography for brain tumor localization and ventricular shunt placement. AJR Am J Roentgenol 1982;139:733–738
3. Enzmann DR, Wheat R, Marshall WH, et al. Tumors of the central nervous system studied by computed tomography and ultrasound. Radiology 1985;154:393–399
4. Rubin JM, Dohrmann GJ. Intraoperative neurosurgical ultrasound in the localization and characterization of intracranial masses. Radiology 1983;148:519–524
5. Latchaw RE, Gold LHA, Moore JS Jr, et al. The nonspecificity of absorption coefficients in the differentiation of solid tumors and cystic lesions. Radiology 1977;125:141–144
6. Kjos BO, Brant-Zawadzki M, Kucharczyk W, et al. Cystic intracranial lesions: magnetic resonance imaging. Radiology 1985;155: 363–369
7. Lange SC, Howe JF, Shuman WP, et al. Intraoperative ultrasound detection of metastatic tumors in the central cortex. Neurosurgery 1982;11:219–222
8. Knake JE, Chandler WJ, Gabrielson TO, et al. Intraoperative sonographic delineation of low-grade brain neoplasms defined poorly by computed tomography. Radiology 1984;151:735–739
9. Hatfield MK, Rubin JM, Gebarski SS, et al. Intraoperative sonography in low-grade gliomas. J Ultrasound Med 1989;8:131–134
10. Smith SJ, Vogelzang RL, Marzano MI, et al. Brain edema: ultrasound examination. Radiology 1985;155:379–382
11. Tsutsumi Y, Andoh Y, Inoue N. Ultrasound-guided biopsy for deep-seated brain tumors. J Neurosurg 1982;57:164–167
12. Berger MS. Ultrasound-guided stereotactic biopsy using a new apparatus. J Neurosurg 1986;65:550–554
13. Sutcliffe JC, Battersby RD. Intraoperative ultrasound-guided biopsy of intracranial lesions: comparison with freehand biopsy. Br J Neurosurg 1991;5:163–168
14. Shanley DJ, Eline MJ. Intracerebral hematoma localization and removal using intraoperative ultrasound. Milit Med 1992;157:622–624
15. Black KL, Rubin JM, Chandler WF, et al. Intraoperative color flow Doppler imaging of AVMs and aneurysm. J Neurosurg 1988;68: 635–639
16. Comeau RM, Fenster A, Peters TM. Intraoperative US in interactive image-guided neurosurgery. Radiographics 1998;18:1019–1027
17. Rubin JM, Quint DJ. Intraoperative US versus intraoperative MR imaging for guidance during intracranial neurosurgery. Radiology 2000;215:917–918
18. Rubin JM, Dohrmann GJ. Intraoperative ultrasonography of the spine. Radiology 1983;146:173–175
19. Platt JF, Rubin JM, Chandler WF, et al. Intraoperative spinal sonography in the evaluation of intramedullary tumors. J Ultrasound Med 1988;7:317–325
20. Quencer RM, Montalvo BM, Green BA, et al. Intraoperative spinal sonography of soft-tissue masses of the spinal cord and spinal canal. AJR 1984;143:1307–1315
21. Post MJD, Quencer RM, Montalvo MB, et al. Spinal infection: evaluation with magnetic resonance imaging and intraoperative ultrasound. Radiology 1988;169:765–771
22. Hutchins WW, Vogelzang RL, Neiman HL, et al. Differentiation of tumor from syringohydromyelia: intraoperative neurosonography of the spinal cord. Radiology 1984;151:171–174
23. Quencer RM, Montalvo BM, Naidich TP, et al. Intraoperative sonography and spinal dysraphism and syringohydromyelia. AJR Am J Roentgenol 1987;148:1005–1013
24. Montalvo BM, Quencer RM, Brown MD, et al. Lumbar disk herniation and canal stenosis: value of intraoperative sonography in diagnosis and surgical management. AJR Am J Roentgenol 1990;154: 821–830
25. Mirvis SE, Geisler FH. Intraoperative sonography of cervical spinal cord injury: results in 30 patients. AJR Am J Roentgenol 1990;155: 603–609
26. Lunardi P, Acqui M, Ferrante L, Fortuna A. The role of intraoperative ultrasound imaging in the surgical removal of intramedullary cavernous angiomas. Neurosurgery 1994;34:520–523
27. Dempsey RJ, Moftakhar R, Pozniak M. Intraoperative Doppler to measure cerebrovascular resistance as a guide to complete resection of arteriovenous malformations. Neurosurgery 2004;55:155–161
28. Quencer RM, Montalvo BM, Eismont FJ, Green BA. Intraoperative spinal sonography in thoracic and lumbar fractures: evaluation of Harrington rod instrumentation. AJR Am J Roentgenol 1985;145: 343–349
29. Herbst CA, Mittlestaedt CA, Staab EV, et al. Intraoperative ultrasonography evaluation of the gallbladder in morbidly obese patients. Ann Surg 1984;200:691–692
30. Machi J, Sigel B, Zaren HA, Kurohiji T, Yamashita Y. Operative ultrasonography during hepatobiliary and pancreatic surgery. World J Surg 1993;17:640–645

31. Azuma T, Yoshikawa T, Araida T, et al. Intraoperative evaluation of the depth of invasion of gallbladder cancer. Am J Surg 1999;178: 381–384
32. Sigel B, Coelho JCU, Nyhus LM, et al. Comparison of cholangiography and ultrasonography in the operative screening of the common bile duct. World J Surg 1982;6:440–444
33. Sigel B, Machi J, Beitler JG, et al. Comparative accuracy of operative ultrasonography and cholangiography in detecting common duct calculi. Surgery 1983;94:715–720
34. Yamashita Y, Kurohiji T, Hayashi J, et al. Intraoperative ultrasonography during laparoscopic cholecystectomy. Surg Laparosc Endosc 1993;3:167–171
35. Stiegmann GV, McIntyre R, Yamamoto M, et al. Laparoscopy-guided intracorporeal ultrasound accurately delineates hepatobiliary anatomy. Surg Endosc 1993;7:325–330
36. Jakimowicz J. Laparoscopic intraoperative ultrasonography, equipment, and technique. Semin Laparosc Surg 1994;(1):52–61
37. Rothlin MA, Schlumpf R, Largiader F. Laparoscopic sonography. Arch Surg 1994;129:694–700
38. vanDelden OM, deWit LT, vanDijkum EJMN, et al. Value of laparoscopic ultrasonography in staging of proximal bile duct tumors. J Ultrasound Med 1997;16:7–12
39. Kane RA. Intraoperative ultrasound. In: Wilson SR, Charboneau JW, Leopold GR, eds. Ultrasound: A Categorical Course Syllabus. San Francisco, CA: American Roentgen Ray Society; 1993:341–350
40. Clarke MP, Kane RA, Steele DG, et al. Prospective comparison of preoperative imaging and intraoperative ultrasonography in the detection of liver tumors. Surgery 1989;106:849–855
41. Kane RA, Longmaid HE, Costello P, Finn JP, Roizental M. Noninvasive imaging in patients with hepatic masses: a prospective comparison of ultrasound, CT and MR imaging [abstract]. Am J Roentgenol 1993;160(Suppl):133
42. Soyer P, Levesque M, Elias D, Zeitoun G, Roche A. Detection of liver metastases from colorectal cancer: comparison of intraoperative US and CT during arterial portography. Radiology 1992;183: 541–544
43. Matsui O, Takahashi S, Kadoya M, et al. Pseudolesion in segment IV of the liver at CT during arterial portography: correlation with aberrant gastric venous drainage. Radiology 1994;193:31–35
44. Nelson RC, Thompson GH, Chezmar JL, Harned RK, Fernandez MP. CT during arterial portography: diagnostic pitfalls. Radiographics 1992;12:705–718
45. Sahani DV, Kalva SP, Tanabe KK, et al. Intraoperative US in patients undergoing surgery for liver neoplasms: comparison with MR imaging. Radiology 2004;232:810–814
46. Milson JW, Jerby BL, Kessler H, et al. Prospective, blinded comparison of laparoscopic ultrasonography vs. contrast-enhanced computerized tomography for liver assessment in patients undergoing colorectal carcinoma surgery. Dis Colon Rectum 2000;43:41–49
47. Rydzewski B, Dehdashti F, Gordon BA, et al. Usefulness of intraoperative sonography for revealing hepatic metastases from colorectal cancer in patients selected for surgery after undergoing FDG PET. AJR Am J Roentgenol 2002;178:353–358
48. Kane RA, Roizental M, Kruskal JB, et al. Preliminary investigation of liver and biliary imaging with a dedicated laparoscopic US system [abstract]. Radiology 1994;193(P):287
49. John TG, Greig JD, Crosbie JL, Miles WF, Garden OJ. Superior staging of liver tumors with laparoscopy and laparoscopic ultrasound [comments]. Ann Surg 1994;220:711–719
50. Kruskal JB, Kane RA. Intraoperative ultrasonography of the liver. Crit Rev Diagn Imaging 1995;36:175–226
51. Kruskal JB, Kane RA. Correlative imaging of malignant liver tumors. Semin Ultrasound CT MR 1992;13:336–354
52. Gorman B, Charboneau JW, James EM, et al. Benign pancreatic insulinoma: preoperative sonographic localization. AJR Am J Roentgenol 1986;147:929–934
53. Zeiger MA, Shawker TH, Norton JA. Use of intraoperative ultrasonography to localize islet cell tumors. World J Surg 1993;17:448–454
54. Charboneau JW, Gorman B, Reading CC, et al. Intraoperative ultrasonography of pancreatic endocrine tumors. In: Rifkin MD, ed. Intraoperative and Endoscopic Ultrasonography. New York, NY: Churchill Livingstone; 1987:123–134
55. Sugg SL, Norton JA, Fraker DL, et al. A prospective study of intraoperative methods to diagnose and resect duodenal gastrinomas. Ann Surg 1993;218:138–144
56. Akerstrom G, Johansson H, Grama D. Surgical treatment of endocrine pancreatic lesions in MEN-1 (review). Acta Oncol 1991;30: 541–545
57. Lo CY, Lo CM, Fan ST. Role of laparoscopic ultrasonography in intraoperative localization of pancreatic insulinoma. Surg Endosc 2000;14:1131–1135
58. Alberti A, Dattola P, Littori F, et al. [Intraoperative ultrasonography in the staging of pancreatic head neoplasms] L'ecografia intraoperatoria nella stadiazione delle neoplasie cefalopancreatiche. Chir Ital 2002;54:59–64
59. John TG, Greig JD, Carter DC, Garden OJ. Carcinoma of the pancreatic head and periampullary region: tumor staging with laparoscopy and laparoscopic ultrasonography. Ann Surg 1995;221:156–164
60. Hann LE, Conlon KC, Bach AM, Dougherty EC, et al. Laparoscopic sonography of peripancreatic tumors: preliminary experience. Am Roentgenol 1997;169:1257–1262
61. vanDelden OM, Smits NJ, Bemelman WA, et al. Comparison of laparoscopic and transabdominal ultrasonography in staging of cancer of the pancreatic head region. J Ultrasound Med 1996;15:207–212
62. Kubota K, Noie T, Sano K, et al. Impact of intraoperative ultrasonography on surgery for cystic lesions of the pancreas. World J Surg 1997;21:72–76
63. Kaneko T, Nakao A, Inoue S, et al. Intraoperative ultrasonography by high-resolution annular array transducer for intraductal papillary mucinous tumors of the pancreas. Surgery 2001;129: 55–65
64. Sigel B, Machi J, Ramos JR, et al. The role of ultrasound imaging during pancreatic surgery. Ann Surg 1984;200:486–493
65. Printz H, Klotter HJ, Nies C, et al. Intraoperative ultrasonography in surgery for chronic pancreatitis. Int J Pancreatol 1992;12:233–237

Index

Note: Page numbers followed by *f* and *t* represent figures and tables respectively.

A
Abdominal bruit
  celiac axis stenosis and, 76, 76*f*
  midaortic syndrome and, 76–77
  renal arteriovenous fistulas and, 76, 77*f*
  renovascular hypertension and, 67, 68*t*, 70–71, 71*f*
Abscess
  epididymal tail, 91, 91*f*
  frontal lobe, intraoperative ultrasound and, 114–115, 115*f*
  testicular, 92, 92*f*
  tubo-ovarian, 102, 107–108, 107*f*
ACAS. *See* Carotid Atherosclerosis Study
Accessory vessels, in renovascular hypertension evaluation, 74
Acquired immunodeficiency syndrome, deep vein thrombosis differential diagnosis in, 2, 3*f*
ACR (American College of Radiology), deep vein thrombosis imaging methods and, 3
Acute pelvic pain
  appendicitis and, 109, 109*f*
  diagnostic evaluation in
    nonimaging tests, 102
    sonographic, 102–110, 103*f*–110*f*
  differential diagnosis of, 102
  ectopic pregnancy and, 104–105, 104*f*–105*f*
  endometrioma and, 108, 108*f*
  endometriosis and, 108, 108*f*
  inflammatory disease and, 107–108, 107*f*
  ovarian cysts and, 102–104, 103*f*–104*f*
  ovarian torsion and, 102, 105–106, 107*f*
  ureteral calculus and, 109–110, 110*f*
Acute scrotal pain
  diagnostic evaluation in, 81–82
  diagnostic imaging in. *See* Color duplex sonography
  differential diagnosis of, 81, 81*t*
Adenocarcinoma, pancreatic ductal, intraoperative ultrasound of, 125, 125*f*
Adenoma, pancreatic microcystic, 125, 125*f*
Adnexal tumors, 108–109
AIDS (acquired immunodeficiency syndrome), deep vein thrombosis differential diagnosis in, 2, 3*f*
American College of Radiology, deep vein thrombosis imaging methods and, 3, 4*t*
Aneurysm, popliteal venous, in deep venous thrombosis differential diagnosis, 2, 2*f*
Angioneurotic edema, upper extremity swelling and, 54
Angioplasty, superficial femoral and popliteal artery, 25
Appendicitis, acute pelvic pain and, 109, 109*f*
Appendix testis torsion
  Doppler findings in, 96, 96*f*
  imaging findings in, 95–96, 95*f*–96*f*
Arm swelling
  diagnostic evaluation of, 54–55
    ultrasound role in, 64
  differential diagnosis in, 53–54, 53*f*
  ultrasound imaging of, 55–57, 55*f*–60*f*, 62
    accuracy, 62–63
    limitations, 61*f*–64*f*, 63–64
Arterial insufficiency, lower extremity, 17
  duplex ultrasound imaging in, 19–25, 21*f*–23*f*, 25*f*
  history and physical examination in, 17
  imaging tests in (other than ultrasound), 19
  nonimaging diagnostic tests, 18–19, 18*f*
Arterial occlusion
  in carotid artery disease, total *vs.* subtotal, 47, 47*f*
  lower extremity, duplex Doppler diagnosis of, 23
Arterial stent stenosis, lower extremity, duplex Doppler examination of, 25, 25*f*
Arteriovenous fistulas
  as pulsatile groin mass, 36–37, 36*f*–39*f*
  with pseudoaneurysm, 31, 32*f*
  renal, 76, 77*f*
Arteriovenous malformations, intraoperative ultrasound and, 115
Astrocytoma, intraoperative ultrasound and, 115, 115*f*
Atheroembolism
  and carotid artery disease, 42
  risk estimation in, 50
AVMs (arteriovenous malformations), intraoperative ultrasound and, 115
Axillary artery, in arm swelling evaluation, 55, 55*f*

B
Baker's cyst, in deep venous thrombosis differential diagnosis, 1*f*, 2
"Bell-clapper sign," scrotal pain and, 81–82
Bile duct disorders, intraoperative ultrasound in, 117–119, 118*f*–119*f*
Brain, intraoperative ultrasound of, 113–116, 113*f*–116*f*
  metastases, 114, 114*f*
Breast cancer, axillary dissection and radiation therapy for, arm swelling after, 53
Bruit
  abdominal. *See* Abdominal bruit
  carotid, ultrasound evaluation in, 49–50
Bursitis, in lower extremity joints. *See* Baker's cyst
Bypass grafts, lower extremity, duplex Doppler examination of, 24–25

C
Calcifications, pancreatic, intraoperative ultrasound of, 126, 126*f*
Calculus disease, ureteral, 109–110, 110*f*
Calf, intermittent claudication in, 17
Calf veins, in deep vein thrombosis imaging, 6–7, 7*f*
  limitations, 11–13, 12*f*–13*f*
  scanning technique, 8
Carcinoma
  cholangiocarcinoma, Klatskin-type, 119, 119*f*
  gallbladder, 118, 118*f*
  hepatocellular, 122–123, 123*f*
Cardiac pacing wire, in subclavian vein, arm swelling and, 58, 61*f*
Cardiac pulsatility, in upper extremity swelling evaluation, 58, 60*f*–61*f*

Carotid artery disease
    differential diagnosis of, 42–43
    stroke and transient ischemic events linked to, 42
    ultrasound imaging in
        accuracy, 43–45, 44f–45f
        carotid plaque, 43, 44f
        contralateral stenosis, 47–48
        efficacy, 42–43
        indications for, 49
        stenosis grading, 45–46, 46f, 46t
        total vs. subtotal occlusions, 47, 47f
Carotid artery stenosis
    color Doppler evaluation of, 44–45, 44f
    contralateral, 47–48
    grading of, 45–46, 46f, 46t
Carotid Atherosclerosis Study, 43
    carotid stenosis grading and, 43, 46, 46t
Carotid bruits, carotid sonography in, 49–50
Carotid endarterectomy, clinical trial findings in, 42, 43
Carotid plaque
    characterization of, 43, 48–49, 48f
    echolucent, 43, 48
    and stroke association, 43, 44f
    ulcerated, 43, 48–49, 49f
Carotid sonography
    and atheroembolism risk estimation, 50
    in carotid bruits, 49–50
    indications for
        in stroke, 49
        in transient ischemic attack, 49
Catheterization
    in groin interventional procedures, 28
        complications. See Pulsatile groin mass, in postcatheterization patient
    upper extremity swelling and, 54
DS. See Color Doppler sonography
Celiac axis stenosis, abdominal bruit and, 76, 76f
Cellulitis
    scrotal, 92–93, 93f
    upper extremity swelling and, 53, 53f
Central catheter, upper extremity swelling and, 54
Cervical hemangioblastoma, intraoperative ultrasound and, 116–117, 117f
Cervical spinal cord, intraoperative ultrasound and, 116, 117f
CFDI. See Color flow Doppler imaging
Chlamydia trachomatis, pelvic inflammatory disease and, 107
Cholangiocarcinoma, Klatskin-type, 119, 119f
Chronic venous insufficiency syndrome
    diagnosis of, 14, 14f
    ultrasound-guided treatment for, 14
Chronic venous thrombosis, diagnosis of, 13, 13f–14f
Cidex, for probe sterilization, 112–113
Claudication, defined, 17
Color Doppler sonography. See also Color duplex sonography
    of carotid artery stenoses, 44–45, 44f
    in carotid plaque evaluation, 43, 44f
    in deep vein thrombosis evaluation, 2
    in intrarenal artery evaluation, 73–74f, 73–74f
    of pseudoaneurysm in groin, 30–31, 30f
    in renovascular hypertension, 70–72, 70f–71f
    in upper extremity evaluation, 57–58, 58f–61f
Color duplex sonography
    advantages of, 19

    in appendix testis torsion, 96, 96f
    clinical utility of, 19
    in epididymitis, 93–95, 94f–95f
    in epididymo-orchitis, 93–95, 94f–95f
    of extremity arteries, 20
    investigative purpose of, 19–20
    in lower extremity arterial occlusion, 23
    in lower extremity arterial stenosis, 20–21, 21f–23f
        accuracy, 21–23, 24t
        grading criteria, 20–21, 21t, 22t
    in lower extremity bypass graft examination, 24–25
    in orchitis, 93–95, 94f–95f
    postangioplasty examination with, 25, 25f
    in scrotal pain evaluation, 82
        equipment and machine setup, 82–83
        rationale for using, 83
        technique, 83–85, 83f–84f
    technical limitations of, 19
    in testicular evaluation
        torsion, 89–90, 89f–90f
        trauma, 98
        tumors, 97, 97f
Color flow Doppler imaging
    in chronic venous thrombosis, 13, 13f–14f
    in deep vein thrombosis evaluation, 2, 2f, 3
        accuracy, 9f, 10–11
        classic findings in, 9–10, 9f–11f
        examination protocol, 7
        limitations, 11–13, 12f–13f
        normal findings, 4–5, 5f
    of pancreatic islet cell tumor, 125f
Colorectal metastases, intraoperative ultrasound and, 121, 121f–122f
Common femoral vein
    in chronic venous thrombosis evaluation, 13, 14f
    in deep vein thrombosis evaluation, 5, 6f
        classic findings, 9f, 10
        limited compression examination, 7–8
Compression
    thoracic outlet, 62
    ultrasound-guided. See Ultrasound-guided compression
Computed tomography
    in arm swelling evaluation, 54
    in deep vein thrombosis evaluation, 3
    multidetector. See Multidetector row computed tomography
Computed tomography angiography
    in deep vein thrombosis evaluation, 4
    in lower extremity arterial insufficiency, 19
    in renovascular hypertension evaluation, 69–70, 70f
Computed tomography arterial portography, liver lesion detection by, 120–121, 121f
Contrast venography
    in arm swelling evaluation, 54
    in deep vein thrombosis evaluation, 3
Corpus luteal cysts, 103–104, 103f
    hemorrhagic, 104, 104f
CT. See Computed tomography
CTA. See Computed tomography angiography
Cystadenocarcinoma, pancreatic mucinous, intraoperative ultrasound of, 125–126, 126f
Cyst(s)
    Baker's, 1f, 2
    corpus luteum. See Corpus luteal cysts
    hepatic, 121, 121f–122f
    ovarian, 102–104, 103f–104f

D

D-dimer test, in deep vein thrombosis diagnosis, 2
Deep vein thrombosis
  chronic venous thrombosis and, 13, 13f–14f
  diagnosis of
    accuracy of presentation in, 1–2
    D-dimer test in, 2
    imaging evaluation in, 3–4, 4t
    implications for, 1
  differential diagnosis of, 1f, 2, 2f–3f
  ultrasound imaging in, 4
    accuracy, 9f, 10–11
    classic findings, 9–10, 9f–11f
    complications, 11
    examination protocol, 7
    limitations, 11–13, 12f–13f
    limited compression examination and, 7–8
    normal findings, 4–5, 5f–6f
    technique, 5–9, 6f–7f
    unilateral vs. bilateral scanning, 8–9
Doppler flow imaging. *See also* Color flow Doppler imaging
  in deep vein thrombosis evaluation, 2, 11f
  in extremity arterial evaluation, 18, 18f
  intrarenal, 75–76
  renal response to revascularization and, 75
Doppler spectral analysis, in deep vein thrombosis evaluation, 3
  limitations of, 11–13, 12f–13f
  normal findings, 4–5, 5f–6f
DRASTIC (Dutch Renal Stenosis Intervention Cooperative) study, 68
Duplex ultrasound. *See* Color duplex sonography
Duplication, of calf veins, in deep vein thrombosis evaluation, 7, 13
Dutch Renal Stenosis Intervention Cooperative study, 68
DVT. *See* Deep vein thrombosis

E

Early systolic compliance peak, 73, 73f, 74
Echogenicity
  of carotid plaque, 43, 48–49, 49f
  of chronic thrombus, 13, 13f
Echolucent plaque, 43, 48
ECST. *See* European Carotid Surgery Trial
Ectopic pregnancy, 104–105, 104f–106f
Edema
  angioneurotic, in upper extremity, 54
  with pain, in lower extremity. *See* Deep vein thrombosis
Embolic phenomena, and carotid artery disease, 42
Endometrioma, acute pelvic pain and, 108, 108f
Endometriosis, 108, 108f
Endovaginal sonography, 102, 110, 110f
Epididymis
  scrotal pain and. *See* Acute scrotal pain; Epididymitis
  sonographic evaluation of, 83–85, 83f, 84f
    Doppler findings, 87f, 88
    normal findings, 85
    in testicular torsion, 88–90, 88f–90f
Epididymitis, imaging findings in, 90–92, 91f
  Doppler findings, 93–95, 94f–95f
Epididymo-orchitis, imaging findings in, 92, 92f
  Doppler findings in, 93–95, 94f–95f
ESP (early systolic compliance peak), 73, 73f, 74
Essential hypertension, clinical characteristics of, 68t

European Carotid Surgery Trial, 43
  carotid stenosis grading and, 45
EVS. *See* Endovaginal sonography
Extrauterine pregnancy, 104–105, 104f–106f
Extremities
  lower. *See* Lower extremities
  upper, swelling in. *See* Arm swelling

F

False-negatives
  in arm swelling evaluation, 55
  in deep vein thrombosis imaging, 12
False-positives
  in arm swelling evaluation, 55
  in liver lesion detection, 120–121, 121f
Female pelvis, acute pain in, 102–110
Femoral veins, in deep vein thrombosis imaging, 7
Fistula, arteriovenous. *See* Arteriovenous fistulas
Follicular cysts, ovarian, 103–104, 103f
Fournier's gangrene, scrotal cellulitis and, 93, 93f
Frontal lobe abscess, intraoperative ultrasound and, 114–115, 115f

G

Gallbladder, intraoperative ultrasound of, 117–119, 118f–119f
  in gallbladder cancer, 118, 118f
  gallstones, 118, 118f
Gastrinoma, intraoperative ultrasound of, 124, 124f
Genital system, male, acute scrotal pain and, 81–101
Glioblastoma, intraoperative ultrasound and, 114, 115f
Glioma, hyperechoic, intraoperative ultrasound and, 113, 114f
Glucagonomas, intraoperative ultrasound of, 124
Granuloma, sperm, postvasectomy pain and, 99–100, 99f–100f
Greater saphenous vein, ultrasound guided ablation of, 14
Groin mass, pulsatile. *See* Pulsatile groin mass, in postcatheterization patient
GSV (greater saphenous vein), ultrasound guided ablation of, 14

H

Hemangioblastoma of cervical cord, intraoperative ultrasound and, 116–117, 117f
Hematoma
  in deep venous thrombosis differential diagnosis, 2
  as pulsatile groin mass, 28, 29f, 30
Hepatic artery, accessory or replaced, intraoperative ultrasound and, 120–121, 121f
Hepatic cysts, intraoperative ultrasound and, 121, 121f–122f
Hepatic metastases, intraoperative ultrasound and, 120, 120f
Hepatocellular carcinoma, intraoperative ultrasound and, 122–123, 123f
Hernia, inguinal, with scrotal extension, 100, 100f
Hypertension
  essential, characteristics of, 68t
  renovascular. *See* Renovascular hypertension

I

Iliac veins, in deep venous thrombosis evaluation, 10, 11f
  imaging limitations, 11f, 12

Impedance plethysmography, in deep vein thrombosis evaluation, 3
Infection
  epididymal. See Epididymitis; Epididymo-orchitis
  pelvic inflammatory disease and, 107
  testicular torsion vs., in acute scrotal pain differentiation, 81–82
Inguinal hernia, with scrotal extension, 100, 100f
Innominate vein
  color duplex ultrasound of, 58, 60f
  stenosis of, 58, 60f
Insulinoma, intraoperative ultrasound of, 124, 124f
Intermittent claudication
  defined, 17
  in lower extremity arterial insufficiency, 17
Internal jugular vein, in arm swelling evaluation, 54–55
Intraoperative ultrasound
  abdominal applications of, 117–127
    gallbladder and bile ducts, 117–119, 118f–119f
    liver, 119–123, 120f–123f
    pancreas, 123–127, 124f–126f
  background in, 112
  efficient, technique for, 112–113
  neurosurgical application of, 113–117
    brain, 113–116, 113f–116f
    spine, 116–117, 116f–117f
  probe sterilization for, 112–113
Intrarenal artery evaluation, in renovascular hypertension diagnosis, 72–75, 73f–74f
Intratesticular vessels, sonographic evaluation of, 85
  Doppler findings, 86–88, 86f–87f
Ischemic stroke. See Stroke
Islet cell tumors, intraoperative ultrasound of, 124, 125f

K
Kidneys. See Renal entries
Klatskin-type cholangiocarcinoma, 119, 119f

L
Lactic acid, in ischemic muscles, 17
Laparoscopic surgery, for ectopic pregnancy, 105
Laparoscopic ultrasound, 113
  of pancreas, 124–125
Laser ablation, for chronic venous insufficiency, 14
Legs. See Lower extremities
Liquefactive necrosis, epididymal tail, 91, 91f
Liver. See also Hepatic and Hepato- entries
  intraoperative ultrasound of, 119–123, 120f–123f
Lower extremities
  in deep vein thrombosis evaluation, 4–5, 5f–6f
  vessels commonly visualized, 6, 6f
  painful, after walking. See Arterial insufficiency, lower extremity
  swelling with pain or edema in. See Deep vein thrombosis
LUS. See Laparoscopic ultrasound
Lymph nodes
  hyperemic, simulating pseudoaneurysm, 37, 40f
  metastases to, intraoperative ultrasound and, 122, 122f
Lymphoma, non-Hodgkin's, in differential diagnosis of deep vein thrombosis, 2

M
Magnetic resonance angiography
  in arm swelling evaluation, 55
  in lower extremity arterial insufficiency, 19
  in renovascular hypertension evaluation, 69, 69f
Magnetic resonance venography, in deep vein thrombosis evaluation, 4
Male genital system, acute scrotal pain and, 81–101
MDC. See Multidetector row computed tomography
Metastases, intraoperative ultrasound and
  brain, 114, 114f
  colorectal, 121, 121f–122f
  hepatic, 120, 120f
  lymph node, 122, 122f
Microbubble ultrasound contrast agents, in calf vein scanning, 8–9
Midaortic syndrome, abdominal bruit and, 76–77
Mittelschmerz, 102–103
MRA. See Magnetic resonance angiography
Mucinous tumors, pancreatic, intraoperative ultrasound of, 125–126, 126f
Multidetector row computed tomography
  in deep vein thrombosis evaluation, 3–4
  in liver lesion detection, 120–121

N
NASCET. See North American Symptomatic Carotid Endarterectomy Trial
Neisseria gonorrhoeae, pelvic inflammatory disease and, 107
Non-Hodgkin's lymphoma, in differential diagnosis of deep vein thrombosis, 2, 3f
North American Symptomatic Carotid Endarterectomy Trial, 42
  carotid stenosis grading and, 45–46, 46f, 46t

O
Orchitis, imaging findings in, 92, 92f
  Doppler findings, 93–95, 94f–95f
Ovarian cysts, 102–104, 103f–104f
Ovarian torsion, 102, 105–106, 107f

P
Paget-Schroetter syndrome, 54, 62
Pain
  pelvic, acute. See Acute pelvic pain
  postvasectomy, 99–100, 99f–100f
  right lower quadrant, appendicitis and, 109, 109f
Pancreas
  adenocarcinoma of, intraoperative ultrasound of, 125, 125f
  intraoperative ultrasound of, 123–127, 124f–126f
Pancreatitis, calcific, intraoperative ultrasound in, 126, 126f
Peak systolic velocity
  in lower extremity arterial insufficiency evaluation, 20–21, 21t
  in renovascular hypertension diagnosis, 72
Pelvic inflammatory disease, 107–108, 107f
Pelvic pain, acute. See Acute pelvic pain
Peroneal veins, in deep vein thrombosis imaging, 6, 7f
  classic findings in, 10f
Physical examination, in scrotal pain evaluation, 82
Physiological testing, in extremity arterial evaluation, 18–19, 18f
PI (pulsatility index), in renovascular hypertension evaluation, 74–75
Popliteal vein, in deep vein thrombosis evaluation, 12, 12f
  aneurysm diagnosis and, 2, 2f
  classic findings in, 9f, 10
Postangioplasty examination, lower extremity duplex Doppler for, 25, 25f

Power Doppler imaging. *See* Color duplex sonography
Pregnancy, extrauterine, 104–105, 104*f*–106*f*
Pseudoaneurysm
  in deep venous thrombosis differential diagnosis, 2, 3*f*
  hyperemic lymph nodes simulating, 37, 40*f*
  as pulsatile groin mass, 30–31, 30*f*–32*f*
    complications, 31
    ultrasound-guided compression, 31–35, 33*f*–35*f*
  right common femoral artery, in differential diagnosis of deep vein thrombosis, 2, 3*f*
  traumatic, of lower extremity, 35, 35*f*
PSV. *See* Peak systolic velocity
Pulsatile groin mass, in postcatheterization patient, 28
  ultrasound evaluation of, 28, 29*f*
    arteriovenous fistulas, 36–37, 36*f*–39*f*
    hematomas, 28, 29*f*, 30
    pitfalls, 37, 39, 40*f*, 41
    pseudoaneurysm, 30–35, 30*f*–35*f*
Pulsatility index, in renovascular hypertension evaluation, 74–75
Pulsus tardus, intrarenal artery and, 73, 73*f*–74*f*

R
Radiofrequency ablation, for chronic venous insufficiency, 14
Radionuclide venography
  in arm swelling evaluation, 54
  in deep vein thrombosis evaluation, 3
RAR (renal:aortic ratio), in renovascular hypertension diagnosis, 72
Renal arteries
  color Doppler imaging of, 70–72, 70*f*–71*f*
  Doppler analysis and, 75–76
Renal arteriovenous fistula, abdominal bruit and, 76, 77*f*
Renal:aortic ratio, in renovascular hypertension diagnosis, 72
Renovascular hypertension
  cause of, 67
  clinical characteristics of, 68*t*
  differential diagnosis of, 67–68
  imaging evaluation in, 69–70, 69*f*–70*f*
    sonographic, 70–76, 70*f*–71*f*, 73*f*–74*f*
  nonimaging evaluation in, 68–69
  prevalence of, 67
  workup for at-risk patients, 67–68
Resistive index, in renovascular hypertension evaluation, 74–75
Respiratory phasicity, in deep vein thrombosis evaluation, 4–5, 5*f*–6*f*, 12, 12*f*
Revascularization, for renovascular hypertension, 75
RI (resistive index), in renovascular hypertension evaluation, 74–75
"Ring of fire" appearance, ovarian follicular cyst and, 103–104, 103*f*
RLQ (right lower quadrant pain), appendicitis and, 109, 109*f*
RVH. *See* Renovascular hypertension

S
Salpingectomy/Salpingostomy, 105
Scintigraphy, in renovascular hypertension evaluation, 69
Scrotal cellulitis, 92–93, 93*f*
Scrotal pain, acute. *See* Acute scrotal pain
Scrotum
  acute pain in. *See* Acute scrotal pain
  Doppler evaluation of, 83. *See also* Color duplex sonography
  inguinal hernia and, 100, 100*f*
SFVs (superficial femoral veins), in deep vein thrombosis imaging, 6, 7
Somatostatinomas, intraoperative ultrasound of, 124
Sperm granuloma, postvasectomy pain and, 99–100, 99*f*–100*f*
Spermatic cord thrombosis, imaging findings in, 98–99, 98*f*
  Doppler findings, 99
Spermatic cords
  scrotal pain and. *See* Acute scrotal pain
  sonographic evaluation of, 83–85, 84*f*
    Doppler findings, 87–88, 87*f*
    normal, 85
    in testicular torsion, 88–90, 88*f*–90*f*
Spinal cord, intraoperative ultrasound of, 116–117, 116*f*–117*f*
Spinal dysraphism, intraoperative ultrasound of, 116–117, 116*f*–117*f*
Stenosis(es)
  arterial, duplex Doppler grading of
    accuracy, 21–23, 24*t*
    criteria, 20–21, 21*f*–23*f*, 21*t*, 22*t*
    mild form, 21, 21*f*
    moderate form, 21, 22*f*
    severe form, 21, 23*f*
  carotid artery, color Doppler evaluation of, 44–45, 44*f*
  celiac axis, abdominal bruit and, 76, 76*f*
  Doppler assessment of, 20
  innominate vein, 58, 60*f*
  lower extremity arterial stent, duplex Doppler examination of, 25, 25*f*
Stenting, of superficial femoral and popliteal artery, 25, 25*f*
Sterilization, of intraoperative ultrasound probes, 112–113
Sterrad sterilization system, 113
"String-of-beads" appearance, in trilobed pseudoaneurysm in groin, 31, 31*f*
Stroke
  and carotid plaque association, 43, 44*f*
  carotid sonography in, indications for, 49
Subclavian vein, in arm swelling evaluation, 54–55
Superficial femoral veins, in deep vein thrombosis imaging, 6, 7
Superior mesenteric artery and vein, intraoperative ultrasound of, 125, 125*f*
Superior vena cava, in arm swelling evaluation, 54
  cephalid portion, 55, 56*f*
  ultrasound technique in, 56–57, 56*f*–57*f*
SVC. *See* Superior vena cava
Swelling
  in lower extremity, with pain or edema. *See* Deep vein thrombosis
  in upper extremity. *See* Arm swelling

T
TAH-BSO (total abdominal hysterectomy-bilateral salpingo-oophorectomy), 108
Testes, scrotal pain and, sonographic evaluation of, 83–85, 84*f*. *See also* Color duplex sonography
  acute pain, 81–82, 81*t*
  in appendix testis torsion. *See* Appendix testis torsion
  Doppler findings in, 86–87, 86*f*–88*f*
  in infection. *See* Epididymitis; Epididymo-orchitis
  normal findings in, 85
  in testicular torsion, 88–90, 88*f*–90*f*

Testes, scrotal pain and, sonographic evaluation of (*continued*)
    trauma and. *See* Testicular trauma
    tumors and. *See* Testicular tumors
Testicular torsion
    imaging findings in, 88–89, 88*f*–89*f*
        Doppler findings, 89–90, 89*f*–90*f*
    infection *vs.*, in acute scrotal pain differentiation, 81–82
Testicular trauma, imaging findings in, 97, 97*f*–98*f*
    Doppler findings, 98
Testicular tumors, imaging findings in, 96–97, 97*f*
    Doppler findings, 97, 97*f*
Thoracic inlet veins, upper extremity anatomy and, 55, 55*f*
Thoracic outlet compression, 62
Thoracic outlet syndrome, 62
Thoracic spinal cord, intraoperative ultrasound and, 116, 116*f*
Thrombosis
    deep vein. *See* Deep vein thrombosis
    spermatic cord, 98–99, 98*f*
    upper extremity swelling and, 53–54, 53*f*
    of variocele, 100, 100*f*
TIA. *See* Transient ischemic attack
Tibial veins, in deep vein thrombosis imaging, 6, 7*f*
    classic findings, 10*f*
TOA (tubo-ovarian abscess), 102, 107–108, 107*f*
Torsion
    appendix testis. *See* Appendix testis torsion
    ovarian, 102, 105–106, 107*f*
    testicular. *See* Testicular torsion
Total abdominal hysterectomy-bilateral salpingo-oophorectomy, 108
Transient ischemic attack
    and carotid artery disease, 42
    carotid sonography in, indications for, 49
Trauma, to testes. *See* Testicular trauma
Tubo-ovarian abscess, 102, 107–108, 107*f*
Tumors. *See also individually named tumors*
    adrenal, 108–109
    islet cell, intraoperative ultrasound of, 124, 125*f*
    mucinous pancreatic, 125–126, 126*f*
    testicular, 96–97, 97*f*

U

Ulcerated plaque, 43, 48–49, 49*f*
Ultrasound-guided compression
    of common femoral artery, deep vein thrombosis and, 7–8
    of pseudoaneurysm in groin, 31–35, 33*f*–35*f*
Upper extremity swelling. *See* Arm swelling
Ureteral calculus, acute pelvic pain and, 109–110, 110*f*

V

Valsalva maneuver
    in deep vein thrombosis evaluation, 4, 5*f*
    in upper extremity swelling evaluation, 58–59
Variocele, thrombosis of, 100, 100*f*
Vas deferens, postvasectomy pain and, 99, 99*f*
Vasectomy, pain following, 99–100, 99*f*–100*f*
Venous enhanced subtracted peak arterial technique, in MR venography, 4, 13
Venous outflow obstruction, upper extremity swelling and, 54
Venous stasis, upper extremity swelling and, 54
Venous thrombosis, upper extremity swelling and, 53–54, 53*f*
VESPA (venous enhanced subtracted peak arterial) technique, in MR venography, 4, 13

W

Walking, painful legs after. *See* Arterial insufficiency, lower extremity
Women, acute pelvic pain in, 102–110. *See also* Acute pelvic pain

Y

"Yin-yang" color Doppler pattern, in groin pseudoaneurysm, 30–31, 30*f*
    ultrasound-guided compression and, 33, 34*f*